INTRODUCTION TO EPIDEMIOLOGY

Distribution and Determinants of Disease in Humans

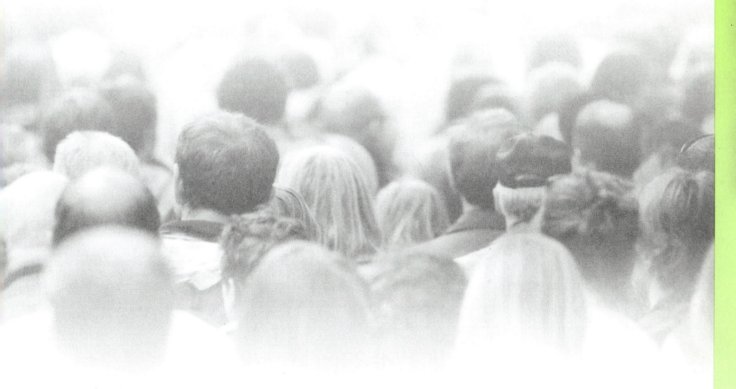

PUBLIC HEALTH BASICS

PUBLIC HEALTH BASICS

INTRODUCTION TO EPIDEMIOLOGY

Distribution and Determinants of Disease in Humans

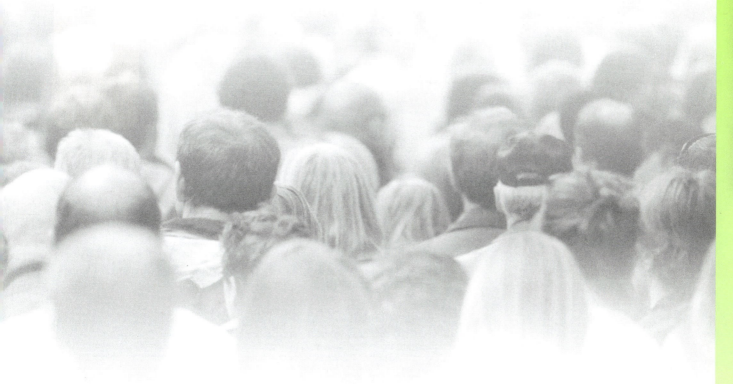

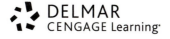

Caroline A. Macera ▪ Richard A. Shaffer ▪ Peggy M. Shaffer

Series Editor: Carleen H. Stoskopf

DELMAR
CENGAGE Learning

Australia • Brazil • Japan • Korea • Mexico • Singapore • Spain • United Kingdom • United States

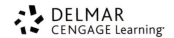

Introduction to Epidemiology: Distribution and Determinants of Disease in Humans, First Edition
Caroline A. Macera
Richard A. Shaffer
Peggy M. Shaffer

Vice President, Careers & Computing: Dave Garza

Director of Learning Solutions: Matthew Kane

Senior Acquisitions Editor: Tari Broderick

Managing Editor: Marah Bellegarde

Associate Product Manager: Meghan E. Orvis

Editorial Assistant: Nicole Manikas

Vice President, Marketing: Jennifer Baker

Marketing Director: Kristin McNary

Associate Marketing Manager: Scott Chrysler

Senior Director, Production: Wendy Troeger

Production Manager: Andrew Crouth

Content Project Manager: Brooke Greenhouse

Senior Art Director: Jack Pendleton

Media Editor: Bill Overocker

Cover Image: © iStock.com

Library of Congress Control Number: 2012940912

ISBN-13: 978-1-111-54030-2

ISBN-10: 1-111-54030-6

Delmar
5 Maxwell Drive
Clifton Park, NY 12065-2919
USA

Cengage Learning is a leading provider of customized learning solutions with office locations around the globe, including Singapore, the United Kingdom, Australia, Mexico, Brazil, and Japan. Locate your local office at: **international.cengage.com/region**

Cengage Learning products are represented in Canada by Nelson Education, Ltd.

To learn more about Delmar, visit **www.cengage.com/delmar**

Purchase any of our products at your local college store or at our preferred online store **www.cengagebrain.com**

Notice to the Reader

Publisher does not warrant or guarantee any of the products described herein or perform any independent analysis in connection with any of the product information contained herein. Publisher does not assume, and expressly disclaims, any obligation to obtain and include information other than that provided to it by the manufacturer. The reader is expressly warned to consider and adopt all safety precautions that might be indicated by the activities described herein and to avoid all potential hazards. By following the instructions contained herein, the reader willingly assumes all risks in connection with such instructions. The publisher makes no representations or warranties of any kind, including but not limited to, the warranties of fitness for particular purpose or merchantability, nor are any such representations implied with respect to the material set forth herein, and the publisher takes no responsibility with respect to such material. The publisher shall not be liable for any special, consequential, or exemplary damages resulting, in whole or part, from the readers' use of, or reliance upon, this material.

Printed in the United States of America
1 2 3 4 5 6 7 16 15 14 13 12

Contents

CHAPTER 3   MEASURING DISEASE OCCURRENCE AND EXPOSURE   39

CHAPTER 4   DATA SOURCES   59

CHAPTER 5 STUDY DESIGN 81

PART II   Applications in Epidemiology   175

CHAPTER 8   INFECTIOUS DISEASES   176

CHAPTER 13   DIABETES MELLITUS   365

Preface

INTRODUCTION

Introduction to Epidemiology: Distribution and Determinants of Disease in Humans, First Edition, is a text developed to introduce undergraduates to the field of epidemiology. This is a relatively new area to undergraduate education, although it has been a staple of public health graduate programs for many years. Although many texts designed for undergraduates have been written using the same format as graduate student text, this text differs because it takes advantage of younger students' facility with electronic media and is organized with more introductory material initially (such as basic biostatistical concepts, as well as disease concepts) so that the remaining material will have context. Anyone teaching introductory epidemiology at the undergraduate level will find this text right on target for the level of their students. The text and examples come from a basic presentation of the concepts, but they do not overwhelm students who are just hearing these concepts for the first time. Students will get a basic understanding of the major diseases in humans and be able to see how the concepts of epidemiology are applied to study the impact of these diseases. This book text assist with gradually "immersing" the students into the subject as they begin their learning process about the fundamental science of public health: epidemiology.

WHY WE WROTE THIS TEXT

After 30 years of teaching epidemiology to graduate students, we have recently had the opportunity to teach epidemiology to undergraduate students. Even more noteworthy is the recent opportunities we have had to work with high school students interested in epidemiology. None of us had even heard of epidemiology when we were undergraduates, let alone in high school. Like so many students back then, if asked about a career in epidemiology, they would have asked, "Isn't that a skin doctor?"

When we first started teaching epidemiology to undergraduates, as expected, it was a very different experience than teaching our graduate classes. We started out using textbooks that we had used for years at the graduate level, but *very* quickly found them to be difficult for undergraduate students. In so many sections of the classic epidemiology textbooks, we had to backtrack during our lectures to explain the foundations and basics of the concepts explained in the texts because the students had not been exposed to very basic concepts that we take for granted at the graduate level. We do not think this is because the undergraduates are unable to excel in epidemiology; in fact, we are convinced that it is the best time to be teaching the basics of the distribution and determinants of disease. But by definition, undergraduates have not had as much time in their education careers to be exposed to many health and public health concepts, so epidemiology is daunting at that stage. So we have found that successfully teaching epidemiology to undergraduates is based on an understanding of where they are in their lifelong education of health and public health.

ORGANIZATION OF THE TEXT

The text is presented in two parts. Part I consists of Chapters 1 through 7 and focuses on basic concepts of epidemiology including the history of epidemiology, integration of epidemiology into public health, disease occurrence, data sources, accuracy, and study design. These topics are presented without any expectations that students have a background in epidemiology. The second part of the textbook contains Chapters 8 through 15 and provides a unique presentation of the high-impact diseases and conditions in epidemiology. The goal of these chapters is not just to acquaint students with the diseases, but also help students to learn about the distribution and determinants of the diseases as well. Disease areas include cardiovascular disease, cancer, diabetes, and infectious disease. Because most undergraduates are expected to have a global perspective, the final chapter is focused on the practice of epidemiology in developing countries.

ANCILLARY PACKAGE

The complete supplement package for *Introduction to Epidemiology: Distribution and Determinants of Disease in Humans* was developed to achieve two goals:

1. To assist students in learning and applying the information presented in the text, and

2. To assist instructors in planning and implementing their courses in the most efficient manner and provide exceptional resources to enhance their students' experience.

Instructor Companion Website to Accompany Introduction to Epidemiology

ISBN 13: 978-1-111-54031-9

Spend less time planning and more time teaching with Delmar Cengage Learning's Instructor Resources to Accompany *Introduction to Epidemiology: Distribution and Determinants of Disease in Humans*. The Instructor Companion Website can be accessed by going to http://www.cengage.com/login to create a unique user log-in. The password-protected Instructor Resources include the following:

Instructor's Manual

An electronic Instructor's Manual provides instructors with invaluable tools for preparing class lectures and examinations. Following the text chapter-by-chapter, the Instructor's Manual reiterates objectives, provides a synthesized recap of each chapter's main points and goals, and houses the answers to each chapter's review questions.

Computerized Test Bank in Exam View™

An electronic test bank makes and generates tests and quizzes in an instant. With a variety of question types, including short answer, multiple-choice, true or false, and matching exercises, creating challenging exams will be no barrier in your classroom. This test bank includes a rich bank of 450 questions that test students on retention and application of what they have learned in the course. Answers are provided for all questions so instructors can focus on teaching, not grading.

Instructor PowerPoint Slides

A comprehensive offering of more than 500 instructor support slides created in Microsoft® PowerPoint outlines concepts and objectives to assist instructors with lectures.

CourseMate to Accompany Introduction to Epidemiology

Visit http://www.cengagebrain.com to access the following resources:

- Printed Access Code ISBN 13: 978-1-111-54037-1
- Instant Access Code ISBN 13: 978-1-111-54034-0

CourseMate complements your textbook with several robust and noteworthy components:

- An interactive eBook, with highlighting, note taking, and search capabilities.
- Interactive and engaging learning tools, including flashcards, quizzes, videos, games, PowerPoint presentations, and much more!
- Engagement Tracker, a first-of- its-kind tool that monitors student participation and retention in the course.

About the Authors

Caroline A. Macera, Ph.D. is a Professor of Epidemiology at the Graduate School of Public Health at San Diego State University. Dr. Macera has more than 30 years' experience teaching epidemiology and has published extensively in the field of epidemiology and public health.

Richard A. Shaffer, Ph.D. is a Professor of Epidemiology at the Graduate School of Public Health at San Diego State University. Dr. Shaffer has taught epidemiology to undergraduate, graduate, and doctoral students for 13 years.

Peggy M. Shaffer, M.D. is a general pediatrician who has been practicing medicine for over 20 years. More recently, Dr. Shaffer has joined her husband in teaching public health to undergraduate students.

About the Public Health Basics Series

Lead by series editor, Dr. Carleen Stoskopf, PUBLIC HEALTH BASICS is a series that brings to life the interdisciplinary nature of public health and the integration of multiple scientific approaches to public health problem solving through surveillance, critical data analysis, planning and implementation of interventions and programs, evaluation, and management of constrained resources. Through this book series students will grapple with the major public health issues we are facing locally and globally, while learning and putting to practice the principles of public health.

Acknowledgments

We would like to give a special thanks to all our colleagues, friends, and family members who supported us throughout this project. A thank you also goes to the many reviewers of our first draft who provided important insights, as well as to our publishers for their help and enduring support.

We also would like to thank the professionals whose feedback was vital to the development of this first edition.

Larissa R. Bunner Huber, Ph.D.
Associate Professor of Epidemiology
University of North Carolina
Charlotte, North Carolina

Leslie Elliott, Ph.D., MPH
Assistant Professor of Epidemiology
University of Nebraska Medical Center
College of Public Health
Omaha, Nebraska

John J. Hsieh, Ph.D.
Professor of Biostatistics & Epidemiology
School of Community Health Sciences
University of Nevada
Reno, Nevada

Arlene Keddie, Ph.D.
Assistant Professor
Health Promotion and Health Education Programs
Northern Illinois University
DeKalb, Illinois

Melissa D. Zullo, Ph.D., MPH
Assistant Professor of Epidemiology
College of Public Health
Kent State University
Kent, Ohio

How to Use This Text

A GUIDED WALK THROUGH

Learning Objectives

Upon completion of this chapter, you should be able to:

1. Describe the concept of natural history of disease.
2. Explain the model of disease known as the epidemiology triangle.
3. Describe disease occurrence in terms of person, place, and time.
4. List the guidelines used to assess causality in epidemiological stu infectious and noninfectious diseases.
5. Explain the difference between primary, secondary, and tertiary prev

LEARNING OBJECTIVES: Learning Objectives are presented at the beginning of each chapter and introduce the core concepts you should be able to master after reading and studying each chapters. These can be a great review tool as well.

Key Terms

causality	indirect cause	preclinical
cause	Koch's postulates	primary prevention
clinical	latency period	screening test
dependent variable	levels of prevention	secondary prevention
descriptive epidemiology	morbidity	sensitivity
direct cause	mortality	specificity
epidemiologic triangle	nonclinical	study population
exposure	outcome	subclinical
incubation period	positive predictive value	tertiary prevention
independent variables		

KEY TERMS: The Key Terms listing introduces important terminology covered in the chapter. Definitions of these terms appear in the margin closest to where they are first presented in the chapter. This provides a quick and easy way to familiarize yourself with important terms and concepts.

Chapter Outline

Introduction
Natural History of Disease
Epidemiology Triangle
Disease Occurrence
    Person
    Place
    Time
Causality
    Causality of Infectious Diseases: Koch's Postulates
    Causality of Noninfectious Diseases: Bradford Hill
Levels of Prevention
Screening Tests
    Sensitivity and Specificity

CHAPTER OUTLINE: Use this Chapter Outline as an excellent reference guide to direct your learning and to ensure that you are competent and knowledgeable about each section of the chapter.

HISTORICAL NOTES: Historical Notes present unique and significant people and events in history that have shaped the study of disease and its determinants throughout the world. These tidbits give you an interesting glimpse into epidemiology's past and its significance to the modern study of disease.

Historical Note 2-1

Robert Koch, 1843–1910, was one of the most important and influential bacteriologists in history. He is credited with developing many innovative and fundamental laboratory techniques—some of which are still used today—and proving that microorganisms caused anthrax, cholera, and tuberculosis. His work was essential in proving the germ theory of disease and in establishing that such diseases were contagious. Koch was also instrumental in applying the germ theory to public health and hygiene practices in order to prevent disease in his native Germany and elsewhere. He won the Nobel Prize for Physiology or Medicine in 1905 and received many other medals and honors during his lifetime and after his death.

Images from the History of Medicine (NIH): www.fm nlm.gov

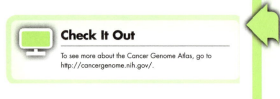

Check It Out

To see more about the Cancer Genome Atlas, go to http://cancergenome.nih.gov/.

CHECK IT OUT: Use the Internet and its various tools to educate yourself on a variety of topics and assessment tools about individual health or a worldwide disease. These boxes direct you to certain websites and organizations that can help enhance the impact of the chapter content.

GLOBAL PERSPECTIVE: Taking a different glance at disease and its impact not only at a national level, but also with a global perspective will introduce you to statistics and important public health problems across the globe for a more well-rounded view of a particular issue.

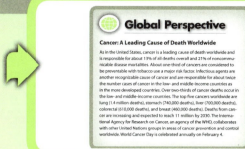

SUMMARY: The chapter Summary is a great place to ensure that you completely understand the information in the chapter and are able to apply it. Look back to the Learning Objectives and make sure that you have met those goals by the end of the Summary.

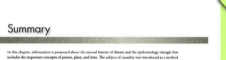

A CLOSER LOOK: A Closer Look is a creative and in-depth look at the heart of the chapter content. In one chapter, it may concern data quality, whereas in another chapter, the feature box may focus on the spread of a deadly disease at a certain point in history. These are incredibly rich sources of insight and real-world applications of essential chapter concepts and discussions.

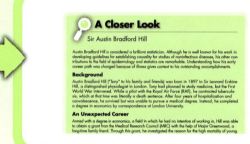

REVIEW QUESTIONS: Test your understanding of the information presented in the chapter with a variety of review style questions, including critical thinking. Use this practice to identify areas in the chapter that you may need to go back and reread until you are confident in answering those questions.

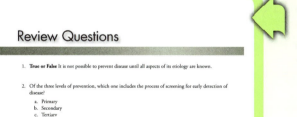

WEBSITE RESOURCES: Connect with public health organizations and learn about different government initiatives by utilizing the website resources section at the end of the chapter for further learning and networking opportunities.

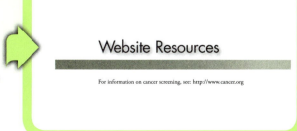

PART I

METHODS OF EPIDEMIOLOGY

Often called the "cornerstone of public health," epidemiological methods are used to understand the distribution, determinants, and control of diseases in human populations. The goals of Part I chapters are to introduce advanced undergraduate students to basic epidemiologic concepts and to apply these methods in identifying the distribution of disease in a population according to time, place, and person.

Using this text, you will be able to describe the basic study designs used in epidemiological research, including experimental, observational, cross-sectional, case control, prospective, ecological, and cohort, as well as the analytic techniques applicable to each design. You will also be able to explain the fundamental epidemiology concepts of natural history of disease, prevalence, incidence, rates, relative risk, attributable risk, precision, bias, validity, accuracy, and confounding.

The skills and tools found in Part I will allow you to be able to evaluate the evidence in favor of and against the likelihood that associations between diseases and potential risk factors that are observed in epidemiologic studies are causal. Understanding these methods will be important when learning about the applications of epidemiology in Part II of this text.

Chapter 1

INTRODUCTION TO EPIDEMIOLOGY

Learning Objectives

Upon completion of this chapter, you should be able to:

1. Describe three basic uses of epidemiology.
2. Explain how a scientific hypothesis is developed.
3. Name the key elements of the scientific method.
4. List four basic ethical elements present when conducting research among human populations.
5. Describe three major issues relating to research misconduct.

Key Terms

agent

chronic disease

determinants

distribution

endemic

epidemic

epidemic threshold

epidemiology

etiology

health-related states or conditions

human subject

hypothesis

infectious disease

informed consent

modifiable risk factors

natural history

nonmodifiable risk factors

null hypothesis

pandemic

plagiarism

risk factors

Chapter Outline

INTRODUCTION

epidemiology: the study of the distribution (who has the problem) and determinants (things that influence the problem) of health-related conditions in human populations and the application of this method to the control of health problems

infectious disease: refers to a contagious or transmissible disease

chronic disease: refers to a disease that is long-lasting

health-related states or conditions: diseases or events that cause illness, death, or disability. Examples are heart attacks or car accidents that can cause death, illness, or disability. Conditions that may not cause death but are very important because they cause disability include autism or arthritis.

distribution: refers to time, place, and types of persons affected by a particular disease or condition (demographics)

Epidemiology is the study of a scientific method of problem solving that helps "disease detectives" understand how people get sick and die, who gets sick and dies, and how to avoid getting sick. This technique has been around for centuries and is still valid today. Like all scientific disciplines, the field of epidemiology has its own language. The terms that researchers use to talk to each other are common words but may have unique meanings in epidemiology. These general definitions occur at the beginning of each chapter and are used within that chapter.

The word "epidemiology" literally means: *epi* = among, *demos* = people, *logos* = study or studies conducted among human populations. Although the field of epidemiology was originally focused on the study of **infectious disease** (contagious or transmittable diseases), the scope has expanded to include **chronic disease** (long-lasting diseases) and **health-related conditions** (diseases or events that cause illness, death, or disability). The current definition of epidemiology is the study of the **distribution** (who has the problem) and **determinants** (things that influence the problem) of health-related conditions in human populations and the application of this method to the control of health problems.

The strength of epidemiology lies in its problem-solving methods. Depending on the question to be investigated, several research techniques are available, including surveillance, observation, and experiments. Before learning more details about these

determinants: physical, biological, social, cultural, and behaviors that influence health

techniques in subsequent sections, this chapter will provide important information on basic scientific processes and on the ethical aspects of conducting research among human populations.

USES OF EPIDEMIOLOGY

The science of epidemiology is used to answer a number of questions related to health problems in human populations and will be introduced here and discussed in more detail in subsequent chapters. Overall, epidemiology is important to describe disease occurrence, to identify the causes of disease, and to find factors that increase a person's risk of disease. Epidemiology is also used to describe the extent of disease in a population and the **natural history** (the course of a disease if left untreated) and characteristics of a disease, as well as to evaluate preventive measures and guide policy decisions.

Initially, epidemiology can be used to describe both healthy and unhealthy populations. The first step in any investigation is to describe the population demographically by age, race, sex, education, and other relevant indicators. In addition, the tools of epidemiology can be used to track trends (how many people have a particular disease over time) and determine if particular diseases are increasing or decreasing in the population. To do this, surveys are used to measure the status of the population at a given point in time and to compare the results of the survey to the same population at another point in time. For example, surveys could be used to compare the percentage of children who are overweight now to the percentage who were overweight in 1960 to help understand trends in disease or health-related states (in this case, overweight status or obesity).

Epidemiologic methods can also establish **risk factors** (characteristics associated with disease development). Some risk factors are **nonmodifiable** (such as age or sex), whereas others are **modifiable** (such as quitting to smoke). Identifying modifiable risk factors that can be changed can lead to prevention programs designed to control the disease. For example, epidemiologic research can help answer questions such as "Are people who smoke because they are stressed less likely to be able to quit than people who smoke for other reasons?" Results of these types of inquiries may suggest that smoking cessation programs may want to include ways to manage stress as an integral part of their program.

In using epidemiology, we can determine the health of a community by counting the number of people with specific diseases or poor health habits who live in that area. In the era of tight budgets and limited money to prevent diseases (as opposed to treating diseases), public health agencies need to know where to best use their limited resources. The study of epidemiology can help in making these decisions. For example, if the number of people who smoke in a particular local area is very low, limited resources might be more effective in dealing with another unhealthy behavior that may be more common, such as low levels of physical activity. And finally, epidemiology can be used very effectively in understanding the causes of disease. Using sound scientific methods, epidemiology has helped us understand the adverse effects smoking has on several diseases, including lung cancer and heart disease, among others.

natural history: the course of a disease if left untreated

risk factors: characteristics associated with disease development

nonmodifiable risk factors: those risk factors that cannot be changed or eradicated

modifiable risk factors: those risk factors that can be changed or eradicated with lifestyle changes

Specialties in Epidemiology

All epidemiologists have an understanding of methods and study design, and many have a strong background in medicine and biology. However, the individual area of expertise may vary considerably among epidemiologists, and it is important to recognize the diversity that exists within the field. Similar to what is found in medicine, there are many specialties. Table 1-1 shows a sample of specialties in epidemiology as defined by their content areas. Although one person cannot be expected to be an expert in all of the content areas, a good epidemiologist will have a strong grounding in methodology with a specialization in one or more content area. Epidemiologists often work with teams of scientists, each one contributing unique expertise to solve a problem.

TABLE 1-1 Epidemiology Specialties

Specialization	Description
Chronic disease	Studies the occurrence and risk factors for disease such as cancer, heart disease, and diabetes that are slow to develop but span many years
Behavioral	Studies lifestyle factors that may be associated with disease status; examples include smoking, lack of physical activity, poor diet
Environmental	Studies the effect of the environment on human health; can subspecialize in water quality, air pollution, chemical exposures, radiation, and others
Forensic	Studies the joint integration of law enforcement functions and public health in criminal contexts (e.g., bioterrorism)
Genetic	Studies the role of genetics in disease development; can include infectious or chronic diseases
Infectious disease	Studies diseases that are acute and contagious; can include long-lasting diseases that are transmissible
Injury	Studies the distribution and risk factors for injuries, either accidental or intentional
Perinatal	Studies health problems of newborns
Reproductive health	Studies normal reproductive processes and problems that can occur, including infertility, birth defects, and low birth weight
Social epidemiology	Studies the effect of community socioeconomic factors on health
Violence	Studies the effect of violence on health

EPIDEMIOLOGY AND RESEARCH

> **hypothesis:** a tentative explanation for a scientific problem that can be tested by further investigation

Most improvement of the health of populations is to the result of an understanding of basic epidemiologic methods. An important role of epidemiology is to monitor the health status of a population and search for risk factors that can be modified to improve the health status of a population. Once a general **hypothesis**, or tentative explanation, is developed, there are several steps that are typically completed to conduct the study. First, there is a descriptive analysis of the problem (who has it; where they are living; when did they get it; how old they are; how many men,

Historical Note 1-1

John Snow

John Snow (1813-1858) was one of the most important contributors to the field of epidemiology. Using scientific methods, he developed testable ideas (hypotheses) about disease and its spread, transmission, and control. Most notably, he conducted an investigation of outbreak of the London cholera epidemic of 1853. At the time, many held the belief that a cloud of disease hung close to earth and infected everyone, but lower altitudes were more susceptible than higher ones.

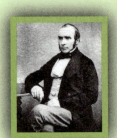

Courtesy of Wikipedia Commons: http://en.wikipedia.org/wiki/File:John_Snow.jpg

Snow disagreed because he thought cholera was transmitted through contaminated water, so he conducted a house-to-house survey to learn where people who died of cholera had obtained their water. He compared the location of deaths to the water supply, thus providing conclusive evidence as to the source of the contamination. There were two water companies in London; one pulled water downstream from sewage, and one pulled clean water from upstream. The majority of the deaths occurred around water pumps from the downstream company. He was able to identify and turn off the suspicious pump, thus controlling the spread of disease. From this event, it is clear that, although it is important to know the etiology of a disease, it is also important to observe characteristics of those who become ill. John Snow's historic experiment tested the hypothesis that cholera was transmitted by contaminated water, even though the bacterium that caused cholera, *Vibrio cholerae*, was unknown at that time.

women, and children have it; and other general characteristics of the population with the problem). Then a study is conducted using an appropriate study design (see Chapter 5, Study Design) to test the hypothesis. The approach may vary depending on whether the health problem under study is an acute problem (such as influenza) or a problem that has developed over time (such as heart disease). The science of epidemiology is designed to describe the health status of a population, to help explain **etiology** (the biological cause of a disease), and to serve as a basis for developing prevention and control programs. To do this requires the use of a rigorous set of rules often referred to as the *scientific method.*

> **etiology:** the biological cause of a problem or disease

Scientific Method

> **agent:** capable of causing an illness

The steps used to conduct epidemiologic research and specific examples are shown in Table 1-2. In this table, the examples are based on the cholera epidemic in London in 1853, although not all of the information regarding the **agent** or the cause of cholera was known at the time of the study. These steps can be applied to other diseases.

Hypothesis

> **null hypothesis:** a hypothesis that is stated as if there is no relationship between the study factors and the disease

Good science and epidemiology begin with a well-thought-out tentative explanation or hypothesis. For example, if water pump "A" was suspected as the source of an outbreak, the hypothesis can be stated as: Individuals obtaining water from pump "A" are more likely to develop the disease than individuals obtaining water from another pump. The purpose of a hypothesis is to develop a statement based on sound biological theories that can be tested. Once the hypothesis is developed, the work begins to test it. It is standard to state the research hypothesis as if there is no relationship, and this is known as the **null hypothesis**. The null hypothesis is stated as if the investigator believes that there will be no relationship between the study factors and the outcome, even though the investigator really believes (and expects) that there will be a relationship. Then the investigator will test the null hypothesis. For the cholera and pump "A" example, a null hypothesis is: Individuals obtaining water from pump "A" are ***not*** more likely to develop the disease than individuals obtaining water from another pump.

EPIDEMICS

There have been many important breakthroughs that have contributed to building the field of epidemiology. In ancient Greece, Hippocrates (460-377 BC) used epidemiology principles to understand disease occurrence; he is often called the Father of Medicine and the First Epidemiologist. The prevailing notion of the time was that disease was caused by gods and superstition; he was the first to recognize and document that different diseases occurred in different places under different conditions. Hippocrates contributed the idea of observation and the terms "epidemic" and "endemic."

TABLE 1-2 Steps Used to Conduct Epidemiologic Research

Steps	Examples as Applied to Cholera
Determine primary agent.	In this case, the cause of illness was a bacterium, *Vibrio cholerae*, which was not known in 1853.
Understand causation.	Exposure to *Vibrio cholerae* resulted in symptoms recognized in 1853 as cholera.
Determine characteristics of agent.	*Vibrio cholerae* can survive for up to 12 days in water, although this was not known in 1853.
Determine mode of transmission.	In 1853, the spread of cholera was correctly suspected to occur through drinking contaminated water.
Determine contributing factors.	The general health and immune status of the affected individuals were established.
Assess geographic patterns.	Cholera was found to be more common in warm areas or in areas with crowded population centers.
Define natural history.	The time from exposure to symptoms is 1-5 days for *Vibrio cholerae*, but this was not known in 1853.
Determine control measures.	Once symptoms appear, rapid treatment is required to prevent complications. For cholera, that includes rehydration to account for the excessive loss of body fluid.
Determine prevention measures.	To establish prevention measures, it was necessary to identify the source of exposure to *Vibrio cholerae*.
Plan health services.	To control the spread of disease, it is necessary to have strategies in place to address early response to symptoms.
Determine hypothesis (or tentative explanation).	A specific water pump was suspected to be the source of the illness known as cholera in 1853.

© Cengage Learning 2013

epidemic: refers to a disease or condition that affects a greater than expected (normal) number of individuals within a population, community, or region at the same time

endemic: the normal occurrence of a disease or condition common to persons within a localized area

The term **epidemic** refers to a disease or condition that affects a greater than expected (normal) number of individuals within a population, community, or region at the same time. Commonly used by people outside of epidemiology, the term is likely to be misused. Many people will use the term "epidemic" whenever there appears to be a large number of one specific event or occurrence. But in an epidemic, the number of events is far less important than the change from the normal occurrence in the past. The normal occurrence of disease in a population is known as the **endemic** level.

Diseases that occur in a population have a historical range of occurrence that is endemic (normal) for a specific population, timeframe, and location. We call the upper end of that normal range an **epidemic threshold**, which is established after multiple periods have produced endemic ranges of disease over time. Once the level of a specific disease surpasses the normal level of disease, and exceeds the epidemic threshold, only then do we refer to this increased level as an epidemic. Consequently, the number of disease occurrences that constitute an epidemic can vary dramatically. For example, since smallpox has been eradicated from human populations, the epidemic threshold has been established at zero, so even one occurrence of smallpox infection is considered an epidemic. On the other hand, the common cold has a very high rate of normal disease, so it will take a very large number of common colds in a population before we would declare that there is an epidemic of common colds.

Another term referring to an epidemic of a disease is **pandemic**. A pandemic is also an epidemic, but a pandemic is considered to be geographically widespread. The difference between a pandemic and an epidemic is becoming harder to determine with the highly mobile global world in which we live. Traditionally, an epidemic that occurs in more than one continent was referred to as a pandemic.

As long as there have been civilizations, there have been records of epidemic (or pandemic) disease. Some examples include the plague of Athens (430-427 and 425 BC) and the outbreak of plague in China in the 1330s that spread to Italy and the rest of Europe and resulted in 25 million deaths (one-third the population of Europe) in just under five years. In more recent times, the Spanish flu outbreak of 1918-1919 spread to all continents and eventually infected one-third of the world's population. HIV, the virus that causes AIDS, is currently a pandemic, with infection rates as high as 25% in southern and eastern Africa. AIDS could kill 31 million people in India and 18 million in China by 2025, according to projections by population researchers of the United Nations, and the AIDS death toll in Africa may reach 90-100 million by 2025.

epidemic threshold: upper end of the normal endemic level of infections

pandemic: an epidemic that has become geographically widespread

HISTORICAL MILESTONES IN EPIDEMIOLOGY

There are many examples of how diseases were controlled using research methods even before science had caught up with identifying the responsible agent. Edward Jenner (1749-1823) developed a vaccine against smallpox using cow pox 160 years before the virus was identified. John Snow (1813-1858) described the association between dirty water and cholera 44 years before the suspect bacterium, *Vibrio cholerae*, was identified. Ignaz Semmelweis (1818-1865) described the association between childbed fever, a life-threatening infection contracted by a woman during or shortly after childbirth, and physicians' unclean hands 32 years before a causal agent was discovered. James Lind (1716-1794) conducted an experiment showing that scurvy, a disease common among sailors on long voyages with no access to fresh fruits or vegetables, could be treated and prevented with limes, lemons, and oranges 175 years before ascorbic acid was discovered. In 1915, Joseph Goldberger

(1874-1927) proved that pellagra, a disease characterized by diarrhea, dermatitis, dementia, and death, was not infectious but nutritional in origin and could be prevented by increasing the amount of animal products in the diet and by substituting oatmeal for corn grits. This finding occurred 10 years before the cause of pellagra, a deficiency of vitamin B_3 or niacin, was discovered. Throughout this text, references to historic milestones will be presented as they apply to the topic under discussion.

ETHICS IN EPIDEMIOLOGY

There are several important reasons to study ethics and to use ethical principles when conducting epidemiologic studies. This field differs from other disciplines in regard to ethical issues because epidemiology is the study of human populations and involves individuals. The subjects who participate in these studies often derive no direct benefit, even though the results of the studies are relevant to society in general. Even when the subjects' names are not collected, information on other personal identifiers such as address, Social Security number, or other identifier may be collected and could be used to identify a particular person. Studies to explore the health of a population are often funded from public sources, and following ethical standards ensures that the studies are fairly conducted and that all subjects in the target population have an opportunity to be included and that their individual information will remain confidential.

What constitutes "**human subjects** research"? It is defined as any research activity involving people. This would include original research where information is collected from subjects directly by questionnaires or indirectly by a search of existing medical or health records. For example, if you collect data from a classroom and ask students to report their exercise behavior and then match that data with academic records (grades), this would be an example of a study that must be reviewed by an oversight committee to protect the rights of the human subjects. Secondary data analysis of census or health data published by federal agencies does not fall under the "human subjects research" umbrella because individuals cannot be identified. Examples include studies of public data files such as housing values and crime statistics by Zip code. In these cases, no individual person can be identified, so there would be no need for a human subjects review.

human subject: any person that is observed for purposes of research

History

The need for a code of ethics to guide all research involving human subjects developed because of numerous scientific abuses by many countries. One particular example includes Nazi human experimentation on large numbers of prisoners in concentration camps mainly in the early 1940s. Prisoners were coerced into participating: they did not willingly volunteer, nor did they provide informed consent. Typically, the experiments resulted in death, disfigurement, or permanent disability and were examples of medical torture. This type of experimentation led

Historical Note 1-2

Dr. Joseph Goldberger

Joseph Goldberger (1874-1929) was born in Hungary and came to the United States in 1883. He received an M.D. from Bellevue Hospital Medical School in New York in 1895. He became interested in a disease that affected poor southern shareholders. This disease, pellagra, caused many symptoms and eventually resulted in death. At the time, most physicians thought that pellagra was caused by a germ, similar to other diseases known at that time. However, Goldberger suspected that pellagra was the result of a dietary deficiency. He came to this conclusion after observing that prisoners were affected by pellagra, whereas the prison workers who came in close contact with the prisoners were not affected. He was even more convinced that pellagra was not caused by germs when he, along with his laboratory assistants and his wife, injected themselves with blood from pellagra patients and none of them developed pellagra. Although he did not know the particular dietary deficiency responsible, he suspected that it was a result from eating tainted corn, a staple of southern diet. He tried various modifications to the diet but was not totally successful in identifying the preventive element of the diet. In the process of his investigation, Goldberger had prisoners volunteer for his dietary study with a promise of early release. Eventually, he found that adding yeast or providing a diet of meat and vegetables prevented this disease, even though the actual cause of pellagra (vitamin B_3 deficiency) was not identified until 10 years later. Goldberger's experiments occurred many years prior to established ethical guidelines, but he did allow prisoners to volunteer and to receive some benefit for their participation.

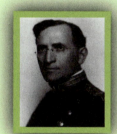

Courtesy of Centers for Disease Control and Prevention Public Health Image Library (PHIL): http://phil.cdc.gov/Phil/details.asp

informed consent: the subject understands the scope of the study and can make an informed decision to participate

to the development in 1948 of the Nuremberg Code, which forms the basis for the ethical rules of conducting research that we use today. One of the important concepts from the Nuremberg Code is that of **informed consent**, which means that the subject understands the scope of the study and can make an informed decision to participate. The major components of the Nuremberg Code are shown and described in Table 1-3.

TABLE 1-3 Key Elements of the Nuremberg Code

Element	Application
Voluntary consent	All subjects must agree to participate, and they must understand the scope of the study.
Yield fruitful results	The research must be expected to provide useful results.
Based on animal studies and natural history	The study's design must be based on previous work that provides a biological basis.
Avoid all unnecessary physical and mental suffering	The subjects should be protected from all unnecessary pain.
No "a priori" reason to believe harm will occur	The research should not be conducted if harm is expected.
Degree of risk never outweighs benefit	The risk of the research should never be more than the benefit.
Provide proper facilities, preparation, and equipment	Facilities and equipment should be safe.
Conducted by scientifically qualified persons	All research staff should be trained.
Subjects can always "quit"	Subject always has the right to stop participation.
Scientist must always be willing and able to end study	Researchers must agree to stop the study if conditions warrant.

Based on the Nuremberg Code: http://ohsr.od.nih.gov/guidelines/nuremberg.html

In 1978, the U.S. Department of Health and Human Services (HHS) revised and expanded its regulations for the protection of human subjects in a report entitled, "Ethical Principles and Guidelines for the Protection of Human Subjects of Research." This report was named the Belmont Report, for the Belmont Conference Center, where the committee met when first drafting the report.

The Belmont Report identifies three fundamental ethical principles for all human subject research—respect for persons, beneficence, and justice. Those principles remain the basis for the HHS human subject protection regulations. Today, the Belmont Report continues as an essential reference for oversight committees that evaluate research proposals involving human subjects, in order to ensure that the research meets the ethical foundations of the regulations. The three major ethical principles of the Belmont Report are shown and described in Table 1-4.

TABLE 1-4 Elements, Components, and Application of the Belmont Report

Element	Key Components	Application
Respect for persons	Autonomy; protection for those with diminished autonomy (e.g., children, people with some psychiatric conditions or dementia, prisoners)	Use informed consent so that subjects understand what is expected of them, what the study entails, their rights to stop participating at any time, and the researchers' assurance of confidentiality of all data collected.
Beneficence	Do no harm; maximize benefits, minimize harm	Favorable risk/benefit assessment
Justice	Those who will receive the benefits of research should share its burden.	Fair procedures in the selection of research subjects—this involves selecting subjects from the target population that will eventually benefit from the research and protects vulnerable populations such as minors, pregnant women and fetuses, cognitively impaired persons, and prisoners.

Based on the Belmont Report: http://ohsr.od.nih.gov/guidelines/belmont.html#top

Requirements for Training

All researchers, even students, are required to complete training in research ethics. If a student is conducting a study at a university, there are procedures in place for proper training and study review prior to collecting data. Training is also required when an external organization funds the research. Because of the importance of maintaining ethical standards for research studies, as of October 2000, the U. S. National Institutes of Health has required education on the protection of human research participants for all investigators submitting applications for grants or proposals for contracts or receiving new or non-competing awards for research involving human subjects. It is important to recognize that not only do the principal investigators need to be properly trained, but all staff associated with the research (data collectors, study coordinators, data analysts, etc.) must also undergo training appropriate for the level of involvement.

Ethical and Practical Obligations

Based on the ethical guidelines developed over time, it is important to be aware of these six key elements necessary to conduct ethically sound research:

1. Risks to study participants are minimized.

2. Risks are reasonable in relation to anticipated benefits.

3. Selection of study participants is equitable.

4. Informed consent is obtained and documented for each participant.

5. Adequate monitoring of data collection is required to ensure the safety of study participants.

6. Privacy of participants and confidentiality of data are protected.

Confidentiality

One of the most important elements of the research code is the need to keep the information collected on individuals confidential. The confidential aspects of all data collected should be spelled out in the "informed consent" document that the subject reads, signs, and keeps a copy of for future reference. To ensure that personal information (such as name, Social Security number, address, date of birth) is not used incorrectly, the investigator must store data records in a safe place such as a locked file cabinet. Only the investigator should have access to the personal information, and all research staff should be trained in the importance of maintaining confidentiality. One way to ensure privacy of personal information is to create and use study numbers, rather than using names or Social Security numbers on all forms and computerized data sets. At the end of the study, all data with individual identifying information should be destroyed. The publications resulting from the research should use combined data only so that individual persons cannot be identified. If breaches of confidentiality occur, the repercussions can range from loss of grant funding to criminal prosecution.

Research Misconduct

In addition, there are other issues that impact research integrity. One of these is fabrication or falsification of data. Although falsifying data results is ethically unacceptable, this can happen when a researcher mistakenly believes that showing positive results will lead to additional funding to continue research projects. Falsification of data is a direct violation of research ethics, and sanctions can include fines, criminal prosecution, removal of funding, and retraction of published articles.

Plagiarism (using ideas of others as your own) can occur in many contexts. Using text, tables, or other materials from any published source, even your own work, is considered plagiarism. To avoid problems, it is possible to obtain permission from the original source to use a specific piece of information (such as a table), then to cite the permission and the source in the new work. Aside from this, all work must be revised such that it becomes new material that is distinct from the original source. If a publication is in the public domain (which means it is not copyrighted and may be used freely), the source must still be cited. Using written or electronic resources (even if in the public domain) without proper referencing is considered plagiarism. Each school has a policy on plagiarism. It is important to review that policy and understand the definition.

plagiarism: using ideas of others as your own

Misconduct issues related to authorship include failing to give credit to those who participated in the work (either as an author or through acknowledgments), as well as including people as authors if they have not met the criteria for authorship. Generally, to be considered as a co-author in a journal manuscript, the criteria include participation in at least one of the following: conception of the study; development of the methods, study protocol, or analysis plan; interpretation of the data; and writing or editing of the manuscript. However, each journal has specific criteria that should be followed when submitting reports of the study to that particular journal.

Other examples of research misconduct include bias in conducting the research or in reviewing the research of other scientists. Avoiding this bias or appearance of bias is important for the credibility of the field, as well as for personal credibility. It is up to the researcher to ensure that the products of the research are scientifically and ethically sound. To avoid misconduct, use these four steps for ethical decision making:

1. Follow regulations from the institution, state, and federal government;

2. Use guidelines from journals, professional societies, and institutional policies;

3. Follow standards and common practice; and

4. Use ethical decision making that includes reasoned argument, consistent principles, and critical thinking skills.

Summary

In this chapter, we learned the meaning of epidemiology and how it is used. The historical origin of the field was described. In addition, there was a discussion of the epidemiology method and its role in conducting effective research studies. The diversity of the field was highlighted by describing the many content areas that epidemiologists study. We also learned about ethical guidelines and how important it is to learn and adhere to these guidelines when conducting research with human subjects. Finally, we discussed research misconduct, including plagiarism and its ramifications during academic studies and throughout a professional career.

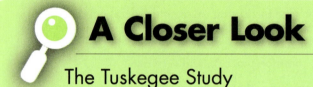

A Closer Look

The Tuskegee Study

During World War II, human experimentation in Nuremberg outraged the rest of the world and led to the 1947 development of the Nuremberg Code, which establishes a set of ethical principles regarding the treatment of medical subjects. However, one of the most serious breaches of medical ethics occurred in the United States through a study widely known as the Tuskegee Study. From 1932-1972, the U.S. Public Health Service conducted an experimental study to monitor the natural progression of untreated syphilis. At the start of the study, there were no known treatments for syphilis; but before the study ended in 1972, penicillin had become available and widely used to treat syphilis. However, this drug was withheld from the participants of the study.

Background

Syphilis is a sexually transmitted disease caused by the bacterium *Treponema pallidum* (see more detailed information on syphilis in Chapter 8). The primary stage of syphilis is usually marked by the appearance of a single sore that heals without treatment. However, if adequate treatment is not administered, the infection progresses to the secondary stage, which may include a skin rash and lesions. The signs and symptoms of secondary syphilis will resolve with or without treatment, but if not treated the infection will progress to the latent and possibly late stages of disease. This latent stage can last for years. Syphilis is easy to cure in its early stages. A single intramuscular injection of penicillin, an antibiotic, will cure a person who has had syphilis for less than a year. Additional doses are needed to treat someone who has had syphilis for longer than a year. There are no home remedies or over-the-counter drugs that will cure syphilis. Because syphilis presented in many forms, scientists in the early part of the twentieth century were very interested in studying its natural history, or the course of a disease if left untreated. A study in Oslo, began in 1909 and published in 1928, evaluated the natural history of untreated syphilis in 2,000 white subjects. Because no treatment was available, the point of that study was to document the characteristics of primary and secondary syphilis and to see if age or gender had an effect on subsequent cause of death (Clark & Danbolt, 1955).

The Tuskegee Study

The U.S. medical specialists suspected that the disease would probably follow a different course in African American males, which led to the development of the Tuskegee syphilis experiment. The major purpose of this study, conducted between 1932 and 1972 in Tuskegee, Alabama, by the U.S. Public Health Service, was to study the natural progression of untreated syphilis. Investigators enrolled a total of 399 impoverished, African American sharecroppers from Macon County, Alabama, who had contracted syphilis before the study began. For participating in the study, the men were given free medical care, meals, and free burial insurance. They were never told they had syphilis, nor were they ever treated for it. The men were told they were being treated for "bad blood," a local term used to describe several illnesses, including syphilis, anemia, and fatigue.

At the time the study began, there was no effective treatment for syphilis, but in the early 1940s, penicillin had been shown to cure the disease and, by 1947, had become the standard treatment for syphilis. Rather than treating all the Tuskegee subjects and closing the study, or splitting off a control group for testing with penicillin, the scientists continued the study without treating *any* participants. In addition, the scientists prevented participants from accessing syphilis treatment programs available to others in the area. Despite concerns raised over the years, the study continued until 1972 when a leak to the press eventually resulted in its termination.

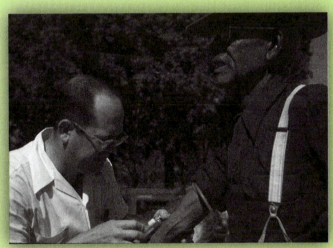

Participant in the Tuskegee Syphilis Study
National Archives of the United States: http://arcweb.archives.gov

Aftermath

By the end of the study in 1972, only 74 of the test subjects were alive. Of the original 399 men, 28 had died of syphilis, 100 had died of related complications, 40 of their wives had been infected, and 19 of their children were born with congenital syphilis. The Tuskegee Syphilis Study led to the 1979 Belmont Report and the establishment of federal laws and regulations requiring Institutional Review Boards for the protection of human subjects in studies.

Review Questions

1. In one sentence, define *epidemiology.*

   _____

2. Analysis of disease by time, place, and demographics is known as:
   a. Distribution
   b. Determinants

3. Physical, biological, social, cultural, and behavior factors that influence health are:
   a. Distribution
   b. Determinants

4. Who was known as the First Epidemiologist?

   _____

5. **True or False** All epidemiologists have the same training and can cover the same content areas, if needed.

6. Which of the following are examples of plagiarism? (Circle all that apply.)
   a. Using one paragraph, word-for-word, from a paper you had previously written and submitted.
   b. Using one paragraph, word-for-word, from a paper you had previously written and submitted, but cited as to the source.
   c. Writing new material based on several published sources, with appropriate citations.
   d. Copying a methods section from a published source because you are using the same data set and there is no other way to describe it.

7. **True or False** Modifying study results can sometimes be justified if the end product provides benefits for society.

8. Which of the following ethical guidelines for the protection of human subjects did the Tuskegee Study violate?
   a. Voluntary consent
   b. Degree of risk never outweighs benefit
   c. Scientist must always be willing and able to end study
   d. All of the above

9. **True or False** One of the important steps in conducting epidemiologic research includes developing a testable hypothesis.

10. Discuss each of the following situations and describe if the situation requires a human subjects review. Why or why not?
    a. A clinical trial comparing two experimental drugs
    b. A retrospective review of medical charts
    c. A simple "no risk" questionnaire (e.g., student attitudes toward lectures vs. small group learning)
    d. Secondary analysis of aggregate census or health data published by a federal agency

11. **For Deeper Thought** Three students are working on a group project for a class in criminology. One of the students has previously done work in this area and has suggested that the group use a portion of his previous project for the current group project. Because over 75% of the project will be new and the work was originally done by one of the students, one of the students thinks this practice is plagiarism, whereas the other two do not. Explain why or why not this is considered plagiarism.

Website Resources

Find the Belmont Report and the Nuremberg Code at the National Institutes of Health Office of Human Subjects Research. Click on "Regulations and Ethical Guidelines" tab: http://ohsr.od.nih.gov

Bioethics resources on the web can be found at the National Institute of Health: http://bioethics.od.nih.gov

For more information on research misconduct: http://grants.nih.gov/grants/research_integrity/research_misconduct.htm

For more information on plagiarism: http://www.plagiarism.org

For more information on syphilis, visit the CDC website's information on "Sexually Transmitted Diseases": http://www.cdc.gov

References

Belmont Report. Retrieved from: http://ohsr.od.nih.gov/guidelines/belmont.html#top

Clark, E. C., & Danbolt, N. (1955). The Oslo study of the natural history of untreated syphilis: An epidemiologic investigation based on a restudy of the Boeck-Bruusgaard material–A review and appraisal. *Journal of Chronic Diseases, 2,* 311-344. doi:10.1016/0021-9681(55)90139-9

http://en.wikipedia.org/wiki/List_of_epidemics

http://grants.nih.gov/grants/research_integrity/research_misconduct.htm

http://www.cdc.gov/std/syphilis/STDFact-syphilis.htm

National Institute of Health. Bioethics resources on the web. Retrieved from: http://www.nih.gov/sigs/bioethics

Nuremberg Code: http://ohsr.od.nih.gov/guidelines/nuremberg.html

Porta, M. (Ed.) (2008). *Dictionary of epidemiology* (5th ed.). New York: Oxford University Press.

Chapter 2

FUNDAMENTALS OF EPIDEMIOLOGY

Learning Objectives

Upon completion of this chapter, you should be able to:

1. Describe the concept of natural history of disease.
2. Explain the model of disease known as the epidemiology triangle.
3. Describe disease occurrence in terms of person, place, and time.
4. List the guidelines used to assess causality in epidemiological studies of infectious and noninfectious diseases.
5. Explain the difference between primary, secondary, and tertiary prevention.

Key Terms

causality
cause
clinical
dependent variable
descriptive epidemiology
direct cause
epidemiologic triangle
exposure
incubation period
independent variables

indirect cause
Koch's postulates
latency period
levels of prevention
morbidity
mortality
nonclinical
outcome
positive predictive value

preclinical
primary prevention
screening test
secondary prevention
sensitivity
specificity
study population
subclinical
tertiary prevention

Chapter Outline

INTRODUCTION

This chapter deals with certain fundamental ideas that are important to explore because they provide the foundation for the study of epidemiology. The practice of epidemiology is enhanced with a background in biology to provide a basic understanding of how a body works. This chapter will build on that background and touch on concepts of health and discuss how diseases develop and progress with and without intervention. The importance of measuring disease status and understanding the various stages of disease are introduced. The concept of **causality** (or determining the cause of a disease) as it is used in epidemiology is presented, along with guidelines to use for studying both infectious and noninfectious diseases. Although one of the main goals of epidemiology is to prevent diseases from occurring, it is also important to understand how to prevent complications once a disease is present. Another issue in epidemiology has to do with evaluating a **screening test**, a test that is given to people who have no symptoms to check for the presence of a particular disease. The assessment and use of screening tests are also included in this chapter.

> **causality:** refers to determining the cause of a disease
>
> **screening test:** a test given to people who have no symptoms to check for the presence of a particular disease

NATURAL HISTORY OF DISEASE

Diseases have always been around, many in the same form as we see them today. For example, heart disease and cancer are leading causes of death today, but they have existed for many years. Before the discovery of antibiotics, many people did not live long enough to develop heart disease and died of other causes instead. After antibiotics were routinely used for treatment of infectious diseases and life expectancy increased, heart disease rose in importance, although it had always been present in the population. As mentioned in Chapter 1, the natural history of a disease refers to its course if it is left untreated. Several characteristics of the natural history of a disease include understanding how the disease is spread (more about how diseases spread can be found in Chapter 8, Infectious Diseases), the **latency period** or the **incubation period** (the time from the start of the disease process or infection until signs and symptoms appear), and the clinical features of the disease.

When studying the epidemiology of a disease, it is important to know what stage of the disease to study. Many diseases are not recognized until the **clinical** stage or when signs and symptoms appear. However, the disease processes may have begun much earlier. There are also **nonclinical** stages of disease (when no signs or symptoms are present). Diseases in this stage can be **preclinical** because signs and symptoms are not yet present or **subclinical** because symptoms will not ever become apparent. Finally, diseases can also be nonclinical after signs and symptoms have improved during their convalescent phases. Most diseases have a preclinical stage, and, depending on the disease, this stage can last seconds, days, months or years, whereas other diseases are subclinical, and the presence of disease can only be determined by biopsy, culture, or similar means. Clinical disease also has various stages as shown in Figure 2-1. The course of the disease can lead to recovery, **morbidity** (illness), disability, or **mortality** (death). Even recovery may be only temporary as in the case of persistent conditions such as hypertension. And finally, a person may be a carrier, which means that person does not appear to be ill but could harbor the infection and pass it on to others. When studying the epidemiology of a disease, it is important to know what stage of the disease to study. Many diseases are not recognized until the clinical stage or when symptoms appear. However, the disease processes may have begun much earlier.

latency period: the time from the start of a disease process until signs and symptoms appear

incubation period: the time between infection and clinical disease

clinical: the stage of disease when signs and symptoms appear

nonclinical: the stage of disease when clinical signs and symptoms are not present

preclinical: nonclinical disease because signs and symptoms are not yet present

subclinical: nonclinical disease because signs and symptoms will not become apparent

morbidity: any departure from a state of physiological or psychological well-being

mortality: resulting in death

EPIDEMIOLOGY TRIANGLE

epidemiologic triangle: a graphic demonstration of the relationship between the agent, environment, and individual as a function of time

One of the key concepts of epidemiology is the traditional **epidemiologic triangle**, a graphic demonstration of the relationship between the agent, environment, and individual as a function of time. The triangle (Figure 2-2A) is composed of three parts: *agent* (what causes the disease), *host* (personal characteristics of those affected by the disease), and *environment* (external factors that cause or allow the disease to

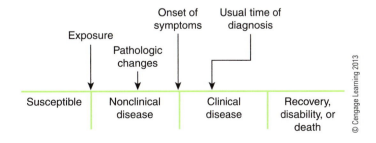

FIGURE 2-1 Natural History of Disease Schematic

© Cengage Learning 2013

spread). Time is another important part that ties into the elements of the triangle and is crucial in understanding disease transmission. The traditional epidemiology triangle is most appropriate for the study of infectious diseases and is discussed further in Chapter 8.

To reflect the different characteristics of noninfectious diseases, the traditional epidemiology triangle can be modified and is shown in Figure 2-2B, labeled the "modern epidemiologic triangle." The time element is still present, but the modern epidemiologic triangle includes groups of *populations* (instead of "person"), *causative factors* (instead of "environment"), and *risk factors* (instead of "agent"). Note that the risk factors (characteristics associated with disease development) can include physiological, as well as environmental, behavior, and cultural elements. The major purpose of these triangles is to describe how various characteristics influence the occurrence of disease and its spread. The triangle also serves as a model for prevention because interrupting any leg of the triangle can be critical in controlling the disease.

Agents are a key component of the triangle. From studying the epidemiology of most infectious diseases (such as influenza), one finds that the agents are microbes such as bacteria or viruses. From studying the epidemiology of noninfectious diseases (such as heart disease or cancer), one finds that the agents are risk factors such as smoking, high blood pressure, or exposure to chemicals or

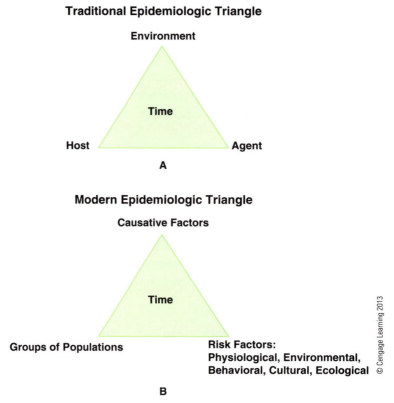

FIGURE 2-2 Traditional and Modern Versions of the Epidemiologic Triangle

radiation. Breaking this leg of the triangle involves avoiding or limiting exposure to agents.

Hosts are organisms, usually humans or animals that are exposed to and harbor a disease. The host can be the organism that gets sick, or an organism that transmits an infection, but may or may not get sick. Also note that different people (hosts) may have different reactions to the same agent. For example, adults infected with the virus *varicella* (chickenpox) are more likely than children to develop serious complications. Other characteristics of hosts that may affect disease susceptibility are age, gender, race or ethnicity, occupation, immune status, and behaviors such as alcohol or drug use and having multiple sexual partners. These host characteristics are still present when we refer to groups of populations. To break this leg of the triangle is to prevent exposure to agents and encourage immunization.

The "environment" refers to the favorable surroundings and conditions external to the host that cause or allow the disease to be transmitted. Some diseases live best in dirty water whereas others survive in human blood. Still others thrive in warm temperatures but are killed by high heat. Environmental characteristics that have been shown to promote diseases are weather, population density, and geography. Environment factors also include the season of the year. For example, in the United States, the peak of the flu season is between November and March. In the modern epidemiologic triangle, causative factors can include genetic effects or family history.

In the center of the triangle is time. Most infectious diseases have an incubation period—the time between when the host is infected and when disease symptoms occur. This time can be a few hours to a few days or weeks, depending on the disease. For chronic diseases, this time between exposure and symptoms is called the latency period, which can range from a few months to many years. Time may also describe the duration of the illness or the amount of time a person is sick before death or recovery occurs.

The mission of epidemiology is to break the triangle to prevent disease completely or to control the spread of disease. This is done by understanding what causes disease, which groups are likely to get the disease, and what geographical factors are conducive to the spread of disease. For example, if we want to prevent measles, we need to understand what causes measles, which individuals or groups are likely to get measles, and conditions in the environment that support the spread of measles. To be effective, we do not need to entirely eliminate the disease cause, but we can interrupt the triangle at any point. If we cannot avoid exposure to the measles virus (the agent), we can immunize children (hosts) so that if exposed, they will not develop measles. For other types of infectious diseases that do not have vaccines, environmental issues could be addressed by isolating people with certain diseases to prevent spread among the general population. This conceptual tool is used to reduce the spread of disease in a population even though not everything is known about the specifics of the disease. For chronic diseases, the triangle can be broken most easily through identification and control of risk factors.

DISEASE OCCURRENCE

descriptive epidemiology: the pattern of disease occurrence from the perspectives of person, place, and time

outcome: refers to a particular disease under study

dependent variable: something that we are studying, usually called an "outcome"

exposure: also known as a "risk factor" or an "independent variable"

independent variables: risk factors or exposures that we think might affect the outcome

Every disease has its own pattern, usually described by who is affected, where this takes place, and when it takes place. Much can be learned from a disease by studying its pattern from the perspectives of person, place, and time. This is typically referred to as **descriptive epidemiology** and is typically the first process in understanding the impact of a particular disease on a population. There are a few other important terms to become familiar with. When looking at a particular disease, we often use the term **outcome**. It is important to know that outcome can refer to a particular disease under study or another kind of event, such as an injury. Specifically, an outcome is the **dependent variable** or something that we are studying and that we think might change depending on the effect of risk factors (also called **exposures**). These risk factors or exposures represent **independent variables** or something that we think might affect the outcome.

Person

study population: refers to the group of individuals being studied

The field of epidemiology deals with groups of people, whereas the field of medicine deals with one person at a time. Because of this, "people" in epidemiological studies are often referred to as the **study population**, or the group of individuals being studied. A study population can be defined as a group of women, adolescents, or everyone in a county or in an entire country. Every study must define a study population. Although this can vary from study to study, it is important for a particular study to be clear about who is being studied so that the results can be applied to similar populations.

Place

The place of a study is generally meant to imply the geographical location. However, it could also be a particular school, a worksite, or another location. This might be very important when studying environmental exposures such as radiation that may affect certain locations. There is an important concept in epidemiology that refers to a geographic location where a particular disease occurs frequently. We may call an area "endemic for cholera," for example. This means that this area has a consistent occurrence of this disease, whereas surrounding areas do not.

Time

Another important part of descriptive epidemiology is the notion of time. This could apply to seasonal patterns, such as seen with flu seasons, or it could refer to trends over time. Understanding how disease occurrence changes over time can be important in assessing unusual increases or decreases. Using time can also help identify an epidemic, or a disease that occurs at a greater than expected frequency. For example, if there were many cases of flu in the United States, looking at seasonal patterns may help determine if the number of cases observed were normal for that time of year or if there were many more cases than would be expected (epidemic).

CAUSALITY

When the term **cause** is used in epidemiology, it refers to something that brings about an effect or result. For example, it is important to know that cigarette smoking causes many conditions, including lung cancer and respiratory problems. Understanding that cigarette smoking is a risk factor provides a way to control or prevent these diseases by eliminating smoking behavior. However, it may appear that a risk factor is causally associated with a disease when in fact it is not. For example, in the nineteenth century, it was thought that cholera was associated with altitude because deaths from cholera occurred more frequently at lower altitudes than at higher altitudes. However, clean water was less available at lower altitudes; so in this case, it was the exposure to contaminated water that was the cause of cholera rather than the altitude. These examples demonstrate two types of causes: direct and indirect. In the case of **direct cause** (e.g., a car accident causes a broken leg), it is clear which factor causes the problem without any intermediate steps. In the case of **indirect cause**, the factor may cause the problem, but with an intermediate factor or step (e.g., alcohol causes the car accident that causes the broken leg). Because alcohol itself does not cause the leg to break, it is considered an indirect cause.

cause: something that brings about an effect or a result

direct cause: refers to a factor that causes a problem without any intermediate steps

indirect cause: refers to a factor that may cause a problem, but through an intermediate step

Causality of Infectious Diseases: Koch's Postulates

How do we know what causes a particular disease? Determining those causes is complex, and because of this, it is important to have a set of guidelines to consider. For most infectious diseases, it is usually straightforward to determine cause by using postulates that Robert Koch developed in 1890. At the time, Koch was studying tuberculosis and anthrax, and understanding what caused these diseases was critical to controlling their spread. In an attempt to define what an infectious disease actually is, he formulated **Koch's postulates** or four rules that establish the causal relationship between an infectious agent and a particular infection. Basically, if (1) an organism can be isolated from a host suffering from the disease, AND (2) the organism can be cultured in the laboratory, AND (3) the organism causes the same disease when introduced into another host, AND (4) the organism can be reisolated from that host, THEN the organism is the cause of the disease and the disease is an infectious disease. These postulates led to the four criteria (see Table 2-1) that Koch established to identify the causative agent of a particular disease.

Koch's postulates: four rules that establish the causal relationship between an infectious agent and a particular infection

TABLE 2–1 Koch's Criteria

1. The microorganism or other pathogen must be present in all cases of the disease.

2. The pathogen can be isolated from the diseased host and grown in pure culture.

3. The pathogen from the pure culture should cause the disease when inoculated into a healthy, susceptible laboratory animal.

4. The pathogen must be reisolated from the new host and shown to be the same as the originally inoculated pathogen.

© Cengage Learning 2013

Since these criteria were initially developed, they have been modified to reflect new knowledge. For example, it is now known that some organisms cannot be grown in pure culture. It is also known that different pathogens cause the same disease with the same symptoms and that some pathogens can cause several diseases. Nevertheless, in spite of these limitations, Koch's postulates are still a useful benchmark in judging whether there is a cause-and-effect relationship between a bacteria (or any other type of microorganism) and a clinical disease.

Historical Note 2-1

Robert Koch, 1843–1910, was one of the most important and influential bacteriologists in history. He is credited with developing many innovative and fundamental laboratory techniques—some of which are still used today—and proving that microorganisms caused anthrax, cholera, and tuberculosis. His work was essential in proving the germ theory of disease and in establishing that such diseases were contagious. Koch was also instrumental in applying the germ theory to public health and hygiene practices in order to prevent disease in his native Germany and elsewhere. He won the Nobel Prize for Physiology or Medicine in 1905 and received many other medals and honors during his lifetime and after his death.

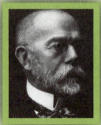

Images from the History of Medicine (IHM): www.ihm.nlm.gov

Causality of Noninfectious Diseases: Bradford Hill

For noninfectious diseases, the process of establishing causality is more complicated. Reasons for this include a long latency period (some diseases occur long after exposure to the agent that starts the process) and the possibility that there may be multiple causes for the same disease. To help epidemiologists sort through many scientific studies, some of which are contradictory, Sir Austin Bradford Hill, a British medical statistician, developed a list of elements to consider. These guidelines were originally presented as a way of determining the causal link between a specific factor (e.g., cigarette smoking) and a disease (such as emphysema or lung cancer). The principles that Hill set forth (shown in Table 2-2) form the basis of evaluation used

TABLE 2-2 Causality Based on Hill's Aspects

Temporal Relationship	Exposure (agent or risk factor) always precedes the outcome.
Strength	This is defined by the size of the association as measured by appropriate statistical tests.
Dose-Response Relationship	An increasing amount of exposure increases the risk.
Consistency	The association is consistent when results are repeated in studies in different settings using different methods.
Plausibility	The findings agree with currently accepted understanding of pathological processes.
Consideration of Alternate Explanations	In judging whether a reported finding is causal, it is always necessary to consider multiple hypotheses before making conclusions about the causal relationship between any two items under investigation.
Experiment	The condition can be altered (prevented or ameliorated) by an appropriate experimental regimen.
Specificity	This is established when a single putative cause produces a specific effect.
Coherence	The association should be compatible with existing theory and knowledge.

in all modern epidemiological research. Although these aspects provide a framework for assessing causality, no single aspect is sufficient, and the only one necessary is temporality. Instead, these aspects are useful when thinking about a problem and looking for explanations.

LEVELS OF PREVENTION

levels of prevention: refers to three types of prevention: primary, secondary, and tertiary

primary prevention: avoids the initial occurrence of a disease

secondary prevention: limits the effect of a disease by early detection and treatment

tertiary prevention: reduces the impact of a disease that has already developed by preventing complications

Another important concept integral to the study of epidemiology is that of **levels of prevention**, a term that specifically defines three types of intervention stages: primary, secondary, and tertiary (see Figure 2-3). Ideally, health scientists would opt for **primary prevention** or preventing diseases from occurring at all. Some examples include: if fewer people were smokers, many cases of lung cancer could be prevented; if all children were immunized for measles, none would develop the disease. If primary prevention is not possible, then the next choice would be **secondary prevention**, or to diagnose diseases in an early stage where treatment or lifestyle modifications can divert the natural course of the disease. This is most easily done by screening for early disease and treating it in the nonclinical stage before symptoms are present. An example would be mammography for breast cancer: a technique that could identify suspicious lesions before the woman has symptoms and before the disease spreads to other parts of her body. Even after a disease has developed, there is room for **tertiary prevention**, meaning to prevent further complications and disability. For example, if a person with diabetes adheres to a proper diet and maintains blood sugar balance, the serious complications often seen with this disease, such as amputations and blindness, would be minimized. These concepts will be explored in subsequent chapters dealing with screening and disease-specific applications.

SCREENING TESTS

People may have a disease that has not yet been diagnosed. Identifying diseases prior to the clinical stage means that prevention efforts can begin immediately. Because the disease is already present, this is an example of secondary prevention. Using screening tests, a disease can be discovered in a very early stage when it is treatable. This type of secondary prevention may reduce the complications of the disease and improve overall survival.

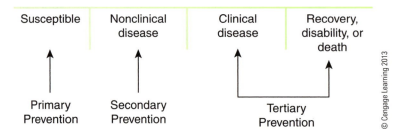

FIGURE 2-3 Levels of Prevention

Historical Note 2-2

James Lind (1716–1794) observed the effect of time, place, weather, and diet on the spread of disease by comparing sick persons to well persons. During his time, a debilitating disease called scurvy was common among sailors who were on long voyages and who had no access to fresh fruits and vegetables. This disease occurred over a few months and could be fatal. Lind's most notable scientific finding was how to prevent scurvy on British ships. In 1753, he conducted a clinical trial with 12 sailors. He divided the sailors into groups of two and put each group on a separate diet. He observed that the group who received citrus fruit daily recovered from scurvy in 6 days. Continuing his experiments, he discovered that sailors who received citrus fruit daily did not develop scurvy. His findings led to the practice of providing limes aboard all British ships to prevent this disease and to the nickname "Limey" for British sailors. This is an example of primary prevention (the disease of scurvy did not occur). Note that epidemiologic methods led to prevention of the disease even though the biological cause of scurvy (lack of vitamin C) had not yet been discovered.

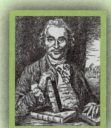

Courtesy of Wikipedia Commons: http://en.wikipedia .org/wiki/James_Lind

Sensitivity and Specificity

sensitivity: the probability that a test defines a person as having a disease when the person does have the disease

specificity: the probability that a test defines a person as NOT having a disease when the person actually does NOT have the disease

There are two concepts that apply to screening tests for diseases: **sensitivity** refers to the probability that the test correctly identifies a person as having a disease when the person does have the disease, whereas **specificity** is the probability that a test correctly identifies a person as *not* having a disease when the person actually does NOT have the disease. A screening test is used when it is not practical for people without symptoms to undergo a clinical diagnostic examination. However, if a noninvasive screening test can identify people who are likely to have a disease, then they will be referred to a clinician for a diagnostic examination. If they are identified as unlikely to have the disease, there may be no follow-up. For these reasons, it is important for a screening test to be as accurate as possible so people who do not have the disease will not have to undergo unnecessary testing and so people who may have the disease are identified in time for an early diagnosis.

To assess the sensitivity and specificity of a screening test, a standard format, such as the one shown in Table 2-3, is used to display test results in the columns and true status of the person being tested in the rows. To set up this table, one must

TABLE 2-3 Basic Table Layout to Assess Sensitivity and Specificity

Test Results

True Status	Positive (+)	Negative (−)
Disease (+)	a	b
No Disease (−)	c	d

© Cengage Learning 2013

know the true clinical status of the person and his or her score on the test. These two numbers are compared.

If the test correctly identifies most of the people who actually have the disease, then the number in cell "a" will be high, meaning the sensitivity of the test is good. However, if the test does not identify most of the people who have the disease, then the number in cell "b" will be high and the sensitivity of the test is poor. Likewise, if the test correctly identifies most of the people who do not have the disease as being disease-free, the number in cell "d" will be high, whereas if the test incorrectly identifies the people who have the disease as not having the disease, the numbers in cell "c" will be high. Using numbers and a simple calculation will make this easy to see. The formulas for calculating sensitivity and specificity are as follows:

$$\text{Sensitivity} = \frac{a}{a + b}$$

$$\text{Specificity} = \frac{d}{c + d}$$

Using some typical numbers, the following data shown in Table 2-4 can be used to calculate actual values for sensitivity and specificity. As you can see, of the

TABLE 2-4 Results for Breast Cancer (Mammogram) Compared to the Actual Clinical Diagnosis

Mammogram Test Results

Diagnosis of Breast Cancer	Positive (+)	Negative (−)	
Yes (+)	622	161	783
No (−)	185	182,166	182,351
	807	182,327	183,134

© Cengage Learning 2013

183,134 women tested, 783 had a clinical diagnosis of breast cancer, and 161 of these women were not found to have breast cancer based on the mammogram. Based on these numbers, the sensitivity of the test is 0.79, but it is typically multiplied by 100 to convert it to a percentage. So we can say that the sensitivity of the test is 79%. The specificity of the test, on the other hand, was 99%; 185 women who screened positive for breast cancer did not actually have the disease. These numbers are considered acceptable for a screening test.

Predictive Values

Another way to assess screening results is to evaluate the **positive predictive value** of a test, defined as the proportion of people who test positive for a disease who actually have the disease. Although this measure is important clinically, its value is dependent on the prevalence of the disease, which may vary. This value may be artificially high if the prevalence of the disease is high. In this case, using the sensitivity or specificity of the test may be a better measure. Referring to Table 2-4, the formula for calculating positive predictive values is:

$$\text{Positive Predictive Value} = \frac{a}{a + c}$$

Applying this formula to the data in Table 2-4, we can calculate a positive predictive value of 0.77 or 77% after multiplying it by 100 to get a percentage. This value indicates that of all the women who test positive for breast cancer based on mammography, 77% actually have the disease.

Examples of screening that are important for prevention of disease include mammograms for women to discover breast cancer before their symptoms lead to clinical diagnosis. The opportunities for effective treatment and long-term survival are better when breast cancer is diagnosed at an early stage. Other screen modalities that have been associated with early effective treatment are available for prostate cancer, colorectal cancer, and cervical cancer.

positive predictive value: the proportion of people with positive test results who are correctly diagnosed

Summary

In this chapter, information is presented about the natural history of disease and the epidemiology triangle that includes the important concepts of person, place, and time. The subject of causality was introduced as a method to determine what factors may be either directly or indirectly causing a particular infectious or noninfectious disease. Another key concept in epidemiological studies, levels of prevention, was introduced and examined in the context of both infectious and noninfectious diseases. Finally, the interpretation of sensitivity, specificity, and predictive value, tools applied by epidemiologists to evaluate screening tests, were discussed.

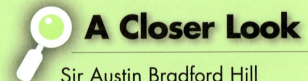 **A Closer Look**

Sir Austin Bradford Hill

Austin Bradford Hill is considered a brilliant statistician. Although he is well known for his work in developing guidelines for establishing causality for studies of noninfectious diseases, his other contributions to the field of epidemiology and statistics are remarkable. Understanding how his early career path was changed because of illness gives context to his outstanding accomplishments.

Background

Austin Bradford Hill ("Tony" to his family and friends) was born in 1897 to Sir Leonard Erskine Hill, a distinguished physiologist in London. Tony had planned to study medicine, but the First World War intervened. While a pilot with the Royal Air Force (RAF), he contracted tuberculosis, which at that time was literally a death sentence. After four years of hospitalization and convalescence, he survived but was unable to pursue a medical degree. Instead, he completed a degree in economics by correspondence at London University.

An Unexpected Career

Armed with a degree in economics, a field in which he had no intention of working in, Hill was able to obtain a grant from the Medical Research Council (MRC) with the help of Major Greenwood, a long-time family friend. Through this grant, he investigated the reason for the high mortality of young adults, and this research enabled him to attend statistics courses. The success of his research enabled him to obtain further appointments with the MRC's industrial health research board. He remained a member of the board's scientific staff until 1933 when he was given a position in epidemiology and vital statistics at the London School of Hygiene and Tropical Medicine, where Major Greenwood was Chair of Medical Statistics. In 1945, he succeeded Greenwood as Chair and also became the Director of the MRC's statistical research unit. In this dual capacity, he rapidly came to be accepted as one of the most respected medical statisticians in the English-speaking world—a remarkable achievement for a man who held no degree in either medicine or statistics.

In this role, Hill's major accomplishment was the effect his teaching had on the way medical research developed in the two decades after the World War II. Specifically, his innovative ideas included developing epidemiological methods for investigating the causes of noninfectious diseases and his introduction of randomization when conducting clinical trials. He emphasized the need for epidemiologists to compare "apples with apples" (not oranges) to avoid potential sources of bias and to allow for chance, but, unlike statisticians of this era, Hill specified that the procedures needed to be explained in plain language, not formulas. In this way, Hill was instrumental in getting researchers to present their research results both logically and quantitatively.

Using this approach and relying on logic enabled Hill to design epidemiological studies and to assess their results in such a way that it was possible to conclude not only that an observed association was real, but also that it did, or did not, imply cause and effect (see Table 2-1). His logical analysis was first applied effectively to the study of the causes of lung cancer in 1948, which he began with the assistance of a young physician, Richard Doll, later Sir Richard Doll. The study was initiated at the request of the MRC, which had been alerted to the great increase in mortality attributed to lung cancer and sought to determine what environmental exposures or behavioral factors more clearly distinguished patients with or without the disease admitted to 20 London hospitals. In discussion of the results, Hill set out clearly—for the first time—the various possible explanations of an observed association that had to be taken into account (bias, confounding, chance, and cause and effect) and the characteristics that would enable a conclusion to be reached that the disease was a result of cause and effect. To verify the conclusions drawn from the hospital study, Hill designed the first large-scale study of people with defined exposures by obtaining information about the smoking habits of some 40,000 British physicians. The results of this study found that smoking also caused myocardial infarction, chronic obstructive lung disease, and many other diseases.

Hill's professional appointments speak to the breadth and depth of his knowledge. He served on the research and experimental department of the Ministry of Home Security and in the medical directorate RAF during World War II; he maintained his relationship with the RAF as an honorary civil consultant in medical statistics and as a member of its flying personnel research committee until 1978. He also served as dean of the London School of Hygiene and Tropical Medicine from 1955–57, as civil consultant to the RN from 1958–77, as a member of the committee on safety of medicines from 1964–75, and as secretary of the Royal Statistical Society from 1940–50, being president from 1950–52. He was clearly one of the great leaders in the field and set the stage for the methods that have become the foundations of epidemiology.

Review Questions

1. **True or False** It is not possible to prevent disease until all aspects of its etiology are known.

2. Of the three levels of prevention, which one includes the process of screening for early detection of disease?
   a. Primary
   b. Secondary
   c. Tertiary

3. **True or False** After a disease has developed, there is no longer any reason to consider prevention aspects.

4. The traditional epidemiologic triangle has which of the following elements?

   a. Environment, host, agent, time
   b. Environment, host, agent, diagnosis
   c. Time, energy, prevention, agent
   d. Subclinical disease, environment, host, time
   e. None of the above

5. The modern epidemiologic triangle has which of the following elements?

   a. Environment, host, populations, time
   b. Agent, time, causative factors
   c. Behavior, time, causative factors, groups
   d. Host, populations, culture, agent
   e. None of the above

6. According to studies by James Lind, what was related to quick recovery from scurvy?

   a. Beer
   b. Citrus fruit
   c. Salt pork
   d. Fresh vegetables

7. Although many guidelines exist to help assess causality, which of the following is the only one that is required?

   a. Consistency
   b. Strength of association
   c. Biological plausibility
   d. Temporality

8. **True or False** A risk factor is something that increases the likelihood of developing a disease.

9. According to the modern epidemiologic triangle, which of the following elements are associated with disease?

   a. Behaviors
   b. Time
   c. Physiological factors
   d. Culture
   e. All of the above

10. **True or False** If all of Bradford Hill's guidelines for causality are not met, there is no basis for establishing a causal relationship between the exposure and outcome.

11. The specificity of a measurement or a screening test is the ability of a test to:
    a. Correctly identify those that have a disease
    b. Be done many times in a row
    c. Identify confounding
    d. Correctly identify those that do not have a disease

12. A screening test for breast cancer was administered to 400 women with biopsy-proven breast cancer and to 400 women without breast cancer. The test results were positive for 100 of the proven cases and for 50 of the women without breast cancer. What is the sensitivity of the test?
    a. 88%
    b. 67%
    c. 25%
    d. 33%
    e. 12%

13. Using the example from above, what is the specificity of the test?
    a. 88%
    b. 67%
    c. 25%
    d. 33%
    e. 12%

14. **For Deeper Thought** There were unusually high levels of influenza in City A last month. Nearby City B is concerned about the spread of influenza among its citizens. Discuss some cost-effective ways to ensure that the epidemic occurring in City A does not spread unnecessarily to City B.

Website Resources

For information on cancer screening, see: http://www.cancer.org

References

Doll, R., & Hill, A. B. (1964). Mortality in relation to smoking; ten years' observations of British doctors. *British Medical Journal, 1*, pp. 1399–1410, 1460–1467.

Hill, A. B. (1937). *Principles of Medical Statistics.* London: Lancet (updated 15 times until his death in 1991).

Hill, A. B. (1965). The environment and disease: Association or causation? *Proceedings of the Royal Society of Medicine, 58*, pp. 295–300. Retrieved from http://www.edwardtufte.com/tufte/hill

Chapter 3

MEASURING DISEASE OCCURRENCE AND EXPOSURE

Learning Objectives

Upon completion of this chapter, you should be able to:

1. Describe measures used to describe disease states.
2. Describe the difference between proportions and rates.
3. Explain the difference between the incidence of a disease and its prevalence.
4. Give one example of an adjusted rate and how it is used.
5. Explain how the incidence and the prevalence of a disease are related.

Key Terms

adjusted rate	incidence	prevalence proportion
case	incidence rate	proportion
case definition	period prevalence	rate
case severity	person time	specific rate
contingency table	point prevalence	suspect case
crude rate	prevalence	2 × 2 table

Chapter Outline

INTRODUCTION

Why do we have a chapter on "how to count"? Counting should be easy, and it does not take much explanation. All epidemiologists know that although counting is easy, what to count and how to use the numbers counted are not so easy. Epidemiologists need to count everything when we use data or perform a study. We need to know how many people are in our study, how many records we have, how many people have missing information, how many people are ill or injured, how many people are exposed to risk factors, how many people died, how many were born: we could fill the rest of this chapter with the things we need to count in epidemiology. However, the fundamental things we need to count in epidemiology are who has the disease we are interested in and who has the exposure that we are interested in. But counting is not easy until we know the exact definitions of what to count and how to represent our "counts." In epidemiology, we call counting a means of *measuring disease or exposure occurrence.*

One of the first steps in studying disease distribution and determinants is to understand how to measure disease states and related exposures. This chapter will lay the groundwork for understanding key aspects and terminology used in measuring the health of populations. Basic information on the types of measures and the calculation of rates that are used to compare population subgroups will also be introduced. Throughout the chapter, the terms "disease" and "outcome" will be used interchangeably, even though in some studies, the outcome may not be a disease, but a behavior or a characteristic. Also, we will refer to any illness, condition, or injury that is the outcome of interest as a "disease."

DISEASE AND EXPOSURE OCCURRENCE

What could be simpler, counting the number of people with a particular disease? The same question could be asked about counting an exposure; what is so hard about counting the number of people that, say, smoke cigarettes? Of course it is easy to do, but difficult to be done correctly and even more difficult to do when the purpose is to compare the things that you count.

Consider some examples of things that are counted in epidemiology. A commonly counted characteristic is gender. Generally counting gender is a simple thing to do when an investigator has direct access to individual subjects, but it becomes harder to do correctly when the investigator has to rely on information from other methods (see Chapter 7, Accuracy). Consider counting the number of deaths among a group of people. Although it is simple to know who to count as dead and who to count as alive, it is more difficult to count those who died as a result of a specific cause (see Chapter 4, Data Sources). An example of counting a typical exposure would be counting cigarette smoking. Think about who should be counted as a "smoker." Does smoking one cigarette a day qualify a person as a "smoker"? How about smoking several cigarettes a day, but not every day? Does that qualify a person to be counted as a smoker? What if a smoker does not smoke the entire cigarette each time? What if the subject has been smoking for 15 years and just quit last week? Should that person be counted as a smoker?

One last example is counting the occurrence of an outcome that is a process, such as a stress fracture of the tibia. Tibial stress fractures develop over a period of weeks. In the beginning of the process, most investigators would not count the subject as having a stress fracture. But as the injury process continues, more and more investigators would count the subject as having a stress fracture. However, there is often disagreement on each case as to when to count the stress fracture. So although counting may be easy, counting correctly can be difficult.

Case Concepts

To measure disease occurrence, it is important to understand case concepts such as case and case definition. A **case** is a person in the population or study group identified as having the particular disease, health disorder, or condition under investigation. In epidemiology, the term "case" is often synonymous with disease or outcome of interest. But a case is very specific to a particular surveillance effort or study, and a person who is called a case in one study is not necessarily a case in another study. By definition, the disease or condition used to identify a case is determined by the hypothesis. So if, for example, an investigator is studying the risk of smoking cigarettes and lung cancer, a case is a person in the study who has lung cancer.

The most important aspect of measuring or counting disease occurrence is adopting a very simple, clear, and useable definition of who to count as a case. A **case definition** is the characteristics or condition of an individual who will be considered a case for the purposes of surveillance or research. A good case definition includes

case: refers to a person in the population or study group identified as having the particular disease, health disorder, or condition under investigation

case definition: characteristics or condition of an individual who will be considered a case for the purposes of surveillance or research

person, place, time, and condition. However, although a case definition needs to be established before data collection, and rigidly followed, in some situations, it is important to allow the case definition to evolve. For example, in an outbreak scenario (see Chapter 9, Outbreak Investigations), the date of onset is a very important part of the case definition. As more information becomes available, the date of onset can be redefined, which would result in the number of cases changing. To be useful and successful, a case definition must be very clearly described so that different people would interpret the case status the same way, time after time.

In some circumstances, it may be necessary to develop a definition for a suspect case. A **suspect case** is defined as a subject who meets all of the characteristics and symptoms of a case but does not have a formal diagnosis. For example, consider a food borne illness that is being investigated from a restaurant during a one-week period. Anyone who ate at that restaurant and had vomiting and diarrhea during that week could be considered a suspect case even if the person had not gone to the physician. Not all outcomes need to have a definition for a suspect case, but once a suspect case is identified, a decision must be made how to count these subjects.

With some case definitions, a measure of severity will also be important to define. **Case severity** can be identified by measuring results such as length of hospital stay, number of follow-up visits, recovery time, disability, or death. Case severity can bring added information to a study by allowing more than just a "yes or no" answer to the outcome information. In addition, case severity may also be used when doing studies looking at the cost of a specific disease.

> **suspect case:** a subject who meets all of the characteristics and symptoms of a case but does not have a formal diagnosis
>
> **case severity:** a measure of adverse events resulting from the disease that can be identified by measuring results such as length of hospital stay, number of follow-up visits, recovery time, disability, or death

Disease Stages

Understanding disease stages is also important to identifying and counting of cases. As noted in Chapter 2, most of the time, diseases are identified when the symptoms appear. Each disease has a diagnostic set of signs, symptoms, and laboratory results that clinicians look for to make a determination about an individual's illness or injury. As long as an investigator knows the correct signs, symptoms, and laboratory results for a disease, it is relatively easy to count clinical disease occurrence.

It is more difficult to measure disease occurrence when a disease is not clinically apparent. As mentioned in Chapter 2, nonclinical disease is the stage of disease when clinical signs and symptoms are not present. Diseases in this stage can be preclinical because signs and symptoms are not yet present or subclinical disease because symptoms will not ever become apparent. Subclinical diseases can be identified through cultures. Finally, diseases can also be nonclinical after signs and symptoms have improved during the convalescent phase of the disease. When measuring a disease with a nonclinical stage, the case definition must include criteria for whether to count disease only when it is clinical or to count it during a nonclinical stage.

Acute and Chronic Disease

Another important aspect to measuring disease occurrence is to recognize that some diseases are acute and some are chronic. Although acute disease is usually easy to identify, because it is often of short duration, the timing of a study will affect the ability to count acute diseases through direct case detection. Consider an investigation of a food borne illness outbreak. In these types of investigations, it is critical to count cases as the outbreak is occurring because these types of illnesses are very acute and usually happen only hours after the event, while resolving within a day or two. If acute diseases such as this are not measured in "real time," then it becomes more difficult to get an accurate count of the problem.

On the other hand, chronic diseases are diseases that persist for an extended period of time, generally more than three months. Chronic diseases can be clinical or nonclinical for long periods of time and, depending on the disease stage, may be difficult to count.

Exposure Occurrence

Like counting disease, counting exposure is equally dependent on good definitions of the characteristics being measured for each subject. However, the concept of exposure occurrence first depends on identifying the characteristics that will be classified as exposures for any given study or data collection. Pretty much any characteristic, behavior, or even disease can be included as an exposure to be measured in the hypothesis of a study. The investigator should determine the lists of exposures and the criteria for their measurement before beginning any data collection. For example, as discussed previously, if an investigator determines that one of the exposures will be cigarette smoking, then criteria must be determined for classifying a subject as a "smoker" versus a "nonsmoker," or whether there is going to be varying classifications of smoking defined by quantity, frequency, and duration. An example of a disease being an exposure might be a stress fracture, because in many cases, an athlete who suffers a stress fracture is often at greater risk of another injury. So a study looking at injuries in runners as an outcome may also wish to include previous injuries in the list of exposures.

Although many investigators understand the need for a good case definition for their disease, they often forget to develop equally clear and consistent definitions for their exposure variables. This is a dangerous oversight that can affect the quality of a data set or study. There are usually many more exposure variables or risk factors to be collected from study subjects; and if these are not counted correctly, the results of the study will be questionable and possibly even wrong.

Denominators

Counts of the occurrence of disease or exposures can be referred to as numerator data, because it simply compiles the numbers of subjects or occurrences that meet the definitions. However, arguably more important than numerator data is the group of subjects or populations that the numerator comes from, the denominator. It is the denominator that truly determines the scope of a problem or that enables numerator data to be compared. Without knowing the denominator, measuring disease or exposure occurrence is only partially helpful and very often misleading. For example, simply knowing that you have 15 cases of diabetes from your study is not helpful unless you know how many subjects were in the study—were there only 15 subjects or 150 subjects?

Denominator data can be difficult, not so much from the need to count it, but from the need to ensure that it is appropriate for the numerator. If an investigator has a study with 150 subjects, of whom 15 subjects have diabetes, then the denominator for the 15 subjects is 150. However, if the group from which the cases of diabetes were counted is not so easily defined, then the denominator can be more challenging. As a rule, the denominator should be the population or group that the cases (or numerator) came from. In addition, the numerator should include all of the cases from a given denominator. For example, consider a study investigating the number of cases of respiratory illness in a school by reviewing the records from the school nurse. Although some of the cases of respiratory illness from the school will report to the school nurse, other cases will not come to school and instead be seen by their private health care providers. To use the entire population of the school as the denominator for the number of cases seen by the school nurse would be misleading. One last important criteria is that population included in the denominator must have the chance to be able to be counted in the numerator if they were to become a case. For example, if the numerator is the number of pregnancies, it would be inappropriate to include men in that denominator.

Population Size

Another aspect of a denominator that must be considered is that the size of a population often changes over time. People are born and people die. People move into an area and people move out of an area. Many procedures are available to be considered for determining an appropriate denominator when the size changes. One option is to consider designating one point in time and determining the number at that time. One common convention is to use the number in a population at the midpoint in a time period, such as the midpoint in a year. It is also possible to use numbers for the beginning or end of a time period as well. Another option is to calculate an average population over a period of time, such as getting the number of persons in a population on each day and then dividing by the total number of days in the time period. A popular option is to calculate a value for the denominator made up of person time.

Person time is a measure that combines the number of people multiplied by a unit of time. For example, if 150 people are followed for 1 year, that would result in 150 person-years. Person time can be accumulated for a population with varying numbers of people or length of time period. If 150 people are followed for 1 year and 50 people are followed for 2 years, the total would be 250 person-years. A denominator of person time provides a very valuable tool for investigators wishing to compare disease occurrence because two different numerators using person-years as a denominator are able to be directly compared as a proportion per person-years.

person time: a measure that combines the number of people multiplied by a unit of time

One other key area in the determination of a denominator to be considered is when the numerator is made up of deaths. If the numerator is death as a result of any cause, or a specific cause, it helps to determine what the appropriate denominator ought to be. One way to look at the rate of death is with the denominator being the entire observed population, and another way to look at the rate of death is with the denominator being just the people with the specific disease, whether they died or not. These two denominators make rates with very different meanings. A rate of death with a denominator of the total observed population provides information about the impact of the cause of death on the population (example is death rate as a result of cancer in the entire population). A rate of death with a denominator of the total number of people with the same condition as the cause of death provides information about the severity of that specific cause of death (example is death rate as a result of cancer among all people diagnosed with cancer). Rates with both of these kinds of death rates are discussed in Chapter 4, Data Sources.

PROPORTIONS AND RATES

To use and compare the numerator and denominator data in epidemiology, it is important to review proportions and rates. Proportions and rates are the fundamental measures used in describing the distribution of disease, and they enable the comparisons necessary to identify determinants of disease.

Proportions

A **proportion** is the representation of a numerator as a fraction of a denominator. As shown in Figure 3-1, a proportion is presented in several ways. The proportion can simply be presented in its raw form as the number in the numerator over the number in the denominator. A proportion can also be presented as a decimal that results from dividing the numerator by the denominator. But most commonly a proportion is represented by multiplying the decimal by a standard number, such as 100, to get a percentage. The standard number that is used to report a proportion is often decided based on the size of the numerator compared to the denominator. Although many people are used to hearing proportions represented as a percentage,

> **proportion:** the representation of a numerator as a fraction of a denominator

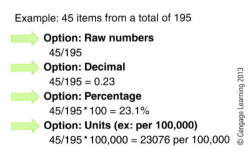

Example: 45 items from a total of 195

Option: Raw numbers
45/195
Option: Decimal
45/195 = 0.23
Option: Percentage
45/195 * 100 = 23.1%
Option: Units (ex: per 100,000)
45/195 * 100,000 = 23076 per 100,000

© Cengage Learning 2013

FIGURE 3-1 Presentation of a Proportion

many population samples in epidemiology are often presented per 100,000. This is largely due to the fact that most individual diseases are rare in human populations (generally less than 1 percent), and investigators prefer to present proportions as whole numbers. For example, many people have a difficult time conceptualizing 0.001 percent (or per 100), but they may feel more comfortable representing that same proportion as 1.0 per 100,000.

Rates

A **rate** is a proportion measured over a period of time. In its simplest form, a rate can be presented as a proportion in a designated period of time, such as 10 per 100,000 per year. This form indicates that during a year, 10 people of every 100,000 have a particular disease. However, a rate is not often presented in its simplest form and can be interpreted as an instantaneous potential during the time period. For example, a very common rate is miles per hour (mph) on your car speedometer. If you are traveling down the road at 35 mph and you look down at your speedometer, you are not actually traveling 35 miles at the moment. But if you keep going at that same rate, then you will travel 35 miles in one hour. So the moment you look at the speedometer, you are reading a potential to travel 35 miles if you maintain that rate of speed for the next hour. Rates in epidemiology are interpreted the same way. A rate of disease in one year means that although there may not be that many cases of disease at any one moment during the entire year, there will be that many cases after a year.

Another aspect of a rate is that it does not have to represent a constant potential. Just as in driving a car, during an hour, the rate of speed may vary, but at the end of that hour, the distance traveled will determine the overall rate for the hour. The same may occur with rates in epidemiology, so over a period of time, the number of cases that are counted may differ from time to time, but the total number for the period is observed at the end.

> **rate:** a proportion measured over a period of time

Crude, Specific, and Adjusted Rates

All rates can be represented as three types: (1) crude, (2) specific, and (3) adjusted. So for example, a mortality rate can be calculated as a: (1) crude mortality rate, (2) specific mortality rate, and (3) adjusted mortality rate. Each of these types provides a different use for any rate, and each of the three types requires more information to determine. The main value of these types of rates is the ability to compare one rate to another. In general, a crude rate is easy to determine, but is not easily compared to other rates. Whereas, the adjusted rate is much more complicated to determine, but allows direct comparison to other similarly adjusted rates.

> **crude rate:** also referred to as a raw rate, a rate from the entire population under observation, consisting of a numerator that is all events from the population and a denominator that is the entire population under observation

Crude Rates

A **crude rate**, also referred to as a raw rate, is a rate from the entire population under observation and consists of a numerator that is all events from the population and a denominator that is the entire population under observation. As long as the events have a good definition and the population is defined, a crude rate is simple to determine. Because of this simplicity, a crude rate is useful for describing the distribution of a disease or an exposure in the defined population, and it provides one overall rate. However, unless another rate uses the same exact people in the denominator, at the same time, it is not appropriate to compare crude rates.

Consider an example of a study to determine the rate of tuberculosis in Crestview Elementary School of 750 students. After screening the entire student population, the investigator finds that 47 students have tuberculosis. The crude rate of tuberculosis in Crestview at the time of the study is $47 / 750 \times 100 = 6.27\%$. This information can help educators and health department officials determine the impact of tuberculosis on Crestview Elementary School, but that is the limit of the use of this crude rate. If investigators want to compare this rate of tuberculosis to another elementary school, it is not appropriate to make direct comparison with the crude rate from another school unless that other school has the exact same population of students (which is not possible). This is true even if the other school has the exact same number of students in the school. In order to be comparable, a rate of tuberculosis from another school must have a denominator that matches the characteristics of the student body of Crestview Elementary School. This is because the student populations in the two schools may differ with respect to characteristics that could influence the amount of tuberculosis in each school. The two schools could simply differ with respect to the grades and ages or gender distribution. There could be differences in ethnic characteristics and family sizes of the children. The schools could differ in the number of students recently transferring to or from the schools, as well as many other characteristics.

The problem with comparing crude rates becomes even more apparent when rates are from large populations such as cities or counties. Then the large size and diversity of these populations make direct comparison with other cities and counties difficult to justify. Consider two cities of approximately 500,000 people each, but the first city's population has an average age of 35-years-old, and the second city's population has an average age of 65-years-old. Any disease being studied related to age (which includes most diseases) would produce crude rates that would not be directly comparable in the 500,000 people in the first city and the 500,000 people in the second city.

Specific Rate

specific rate: a rate comprised of a numerator and denominator that is a subset of the population under observation. The subsets can be variables that may affect the outcome being measured, such as age.

To make crude rates more useful and comparable, portions of the numerator and denominator of the crude rates can be separated to make rates that have more defined characteristics. A **specific rate** is a rate comprised of a numerator and denominator that is a subset of the population under observation. The subset can be based on any variable that the investigator believes is important to the outcome. For example, the most common specific rate is an age-specific rate. An age-specific rate is developed by counting the numerator and denominator from a very narrow age category, such as 15-20-year-old subjects. This type of specific rate provides the ability to make a comparison with other rates of 15-20-year-old subjects if the only concerning characteristic is age. Specific rates can be developed for many characteristics and are easy to identify because most of the time, they are labeled with the word "specific" in them. Other examples include gender-specific rates, race-specific rates, occupation-specific rates, and cause-specific rates. In addition, specific rates can be based on the subset of several characteristics at the same time, such as age/gender-specific rate. An example of an age/gender-specific rate would be a rate among 15-20-year-old males. The disadvantage of theses specific rates with multiple categories is that they can be cumbersome to develop beyond more than one or two characteristics.

Adjusted Rate

The problem with specific rates is that, although they are comparable, they only provide information about a small group of a population. If an entire population were to be described using specific rates, it would take many rates to do it. So it would be helpful for epidemiologists to have a rate that is a summary for the entire observed population and one that is comparable with respect to the characteristics of the population. The good news is that there is a type of rate that does both, but the bad news is that type of rate can be very difficult (and scary to novices) to develop. This good news/bad news type of rate is called an **adjusted rate**, a rate that is mathematically transformed to provide a summary rate for an observed population after differences in specified characteristics are removed. An adjusted rate is also known as a *standardized rate*.

The definition of an adjusted rate has a number of key points to highlight. An adjusted rate provides a "summary rate for the observed population," which is good news because it provides one rate for the entire population. The adjusted rate is "mathematically transformed," which means that the resulting rate is an estimated value. This estimated value may be the same as or different than the crude rate. There are multiple mathematical procedures to transform these rates (several of these are discussed in Chapters 6 and 7). Finally, the definition of adjusted rates states that "differences in specified characteristics are removed." In order to adjust rates, the investigator must identify a set of characteristics that may have an effect on morbidity or mortality. Once these characteristics are identified, the mathematical procedures will remove the differences in those characteristics in the populations that are to be compared. The term "removed" in this definition can also be interpreted as making the characteristics the same. For more discussion and examples of adjusted rates, see Chapter 6, Using Rates and Ratios.

> **adjusted rate:** a rate that is mathematically transformed to provide a summary rate for an observed population after differences in specified characteristics are removed

MORBIDITY: PREVALENCE AND INCIDENCE

In order to measure and use morbidity information, it is important to recognize that disease needs to be classified as either new or existing morbidity. As described earlier, for the purposes of the discussion of morbidity, the term "disease" will also be used as an indication of an illness, condition, or injury. There is a basic difference between new morbidity and existing morbidity for several reasons. Most importantly, it is because investigators know more about new disease than they do about existing disease. This is similar to a paradigm that everyone learns when taking driver's education that is referred to as the "stale green light." A stale green light is a green light that you are approaching that was green when you first see it. For example, you come around a bend, and the first moment you see the traffic signal, it is a green light, referred to as a stale green light. We all know the feeling when we approach a stale green light; we feel apprehensive about what the situation is, we do not know when it turned green, and we do not know if it is about to turn yellow. We are not sure if we should speed up or slow down. We basically do not have all the information about a stale green light. However, if we approach a traffic signal and we see it turn green, we know that for the immediate future, we can comfortably proceed through the intersection; we also know the traffic signal is working. Measuring existing disease in epidemiology is very similar to the stale green light—we are missing crucial information about that disease. Conversely, measuring new disease is like approaching an intersection and actually seeing the light turn green.

In epidemiology, we refer to existing cases of disease as **prevalence** and to new cases of disease as **incidence**. A **prevalence proportion** is the number of existing cases of disease at a given time divided by the observed population in the same time period.

$$\frac{\text{Number of existing cases}}{\text{Total observed population}} \times 100$$

Many times a prevalence proportion will be referred to as a prevalence rate. However, prevalence is generally assessed at a point in time and not during a time period. So it is better to assume that prevalence is a proportion.

An **incidence rate** is the number of new cases of disease in a given time (usually one year) divided by the population "at risk" to develop the disease over that same time.

$$\frac{\text{Number of new cases of disease in time period}}{\text{Population at risk of the same disease in same period}} \times 100$$

prevalence: the number of existing cases of disease

incidence: the number of new cases of a disease in a specified time frame

prevalence proportion: the number of existing cases of disease divided by the population

incidence rate: the number of new cases of disease in a specified time (usually one year) divided by the population "at risk" to develop the disease

Like all rates, incidence rates can be presented in three types: crude, specific, and adjusted. In addition, prevalence proportions can be presented in the same three types. Very often these morbidity measures will be stratified into subsets such as an age-specific prevalence proportion for 10-14-year-old subjects or a gender-specific incidence rate for males. It is also common to adjust prevalence proportions and incidence rates. Both of these measures are frequently age-adjusted by standardizing them to a reference population for comparison with other similarly standardized rates (see Chapter 6, Using Rates and Ratios).

Although the distinction between prevalence and incidence may seem straightforward, it is a very complex concept to implement in real life. Even investigators who have been working in epidemiology for many years have a difficult time distinguishing between prevalence and incidence in some cases.

Prevalence

The number of existing cases of disease is very often easier to identify than new cases. Armed with a good case definition, an investigator can count prevalent cases in a short period of time and often by using existing records or databases. However, even measuring prevalence can have difficulties such as identifying all the existing cases or accessing records that use a different case definition from that of the investigator. Also, the identification of the appropriate denominator for a prevalence proportion can be difficult. Consider the situation of measuring prevalence of disease using a hospital population. The denominator for that prevalence measure should be everyone that would use that hospital, not just the patients in the hospital. So determining the denominator for a hospital-based prevalence proportion is one example that is often challenging.

Prevalence can also be measured using various time frames. The prevalence referred to above can also be referred to as a **point prevalence** because it is a count of existing cases of disease at a specific point in time. This point prevalence makes most sense to people, but it is a difficult concept to implement. If one considers measuring point prevalence in a large population, it may take a period of time to actually count the existing cases. If the counting process takes six months, many wonder if this is truly only a point in time. In fact, some individuals may not have disease when you start counting, but by the time you get around to counting them, they now have the disease. In this case, are you still counting prevalence, or are you now counting incidence? Also, the situation could exist that some individuals have the disease when you start counting, but by the time you get around to counting them, they no longer have the disease. The answer to both these questions is that regardless of how long it takes to count disease, if the goal is point prevalence, the individuals are counted as "yes or no" only at the moment they are counted.

Another time frame in which prevalence can be measured is over a period of time. A **period prevalence** is the number of existing cases during a specified time period. The time period is often a year in length but can be any time period. The criteria for an existing case during the time period are that if someone has the disease at any time during the time period, they would be counted. The ascertainment of cases during a period prevalence should be an ongoing process, or at least have the ability to determine whether anyone in the observed population had the disease during the time period. So unlike point prevalence, a disease should be counted as a case if the person had the disease during the time period even if he or she did not have it at the moment the counting takes place. Also, period prevalence can be confused with incidence during the same period because a person may not get the disease until the end of the time period. The distinction between period prevalence and incidence during the same period is that to truly be counted as incidence, the investigator must have a method to determine that everyone in the population is actually disease-free at the beginning of the time period. If there is not a process to ensure that the population is disease-free at the beginning of the period, then those with disease during the time period must be counted as period prevalence because it cannot be certain that they are new cases.

point prevalence: the count of existing cases of disease at a specific point in time

period prevalence: the number of existing cases during a specified time period

Both point prevalence and period prevalence are indications of burden of disease in a population. Prevalence information can be used to determine the needs for health care services, the economic cost of a disease, or the impact of a disease on the population. However, the problem with prevalence is that the duration of the disease confuses it. Prevalence is the "stale green light" of measuring disease occurrence. Consider a disease that has a long duration such as cancer. Although it might be easy enough to count the numbers of cancer for a point prevalence, it would be a mistake to consider all of those with existing disease have the same economic or health care impact because some of the prevalent cases could be recently diagnosed and others may have had the disease for years. Also, when measuring a period prevalence, some investigators may be tempted to refer to it as a prevalence "rate"; however, for consistency, it is better to label all prevalence as a proportion.

Incidence

As epidemiologists, we much prefer incidence data to prevalence data. Incidence is the number of new cases of a specific disease during a time period. By definition, incidence must be from a time period; so there is no such thing as "point incidence." Although it is acceptable to use the term "period incidence," it is redundant because all incidence data must come from a period of time. The reason that all incidence data must come from a time period is that counting incidence requires a minimum of two assessments: (1) establishing and counting a disease-free population and (2) follow-up counting of new cases of disease. There may be more than one follow-up count, and an ideal method would be to have ongoing assessments to identify new cases as they occur. The period of time is often a year but can be defined as any time period that makes sense for the specific disease. In contrast to a period prevalence, in order to count incident cases in a time period, there must be a mechanism to ensure that the observed population is entirely disease-free at the beginning of the time period to count incidence as new cases. This may seem like an insignificant difference, but it is a very important distinction between the two measures of morbidity. This criterion of needing to certify a population as disease-free at the beginning of the time period often makes measuring disease incidence very difficult to do in a large, diverse population; so true incidence information usually comes from enrolled subject populations or smaller communities.

Another aspect of incidence is that when it is presented as a rate, the denominator has more strict criteria that many other rates. The denominator should only include individuals who were "at risk" to be included in the numerator count. Initially, this may not seem different than other population-based rates, but the difference is that the denominator of the incidence rate should not include people who may have already had a disease that subjects can only get once or those who are immune to the disease of interest. Further, it would not be appropriate to include in a denominator of an incidence rate subjects with no opportunity for the outcome, such as an outcome of adverse pregnancy events should not include males in the denominator. One additional aspect of the denominator of an incidence rate is that over the time period, the "at risk" population may change as a result of the subjects getting a disease. So an investigator needs to decide if they should remove people from the denominator as they get the disease and are counted in the numerator. This is usually not a concern if there is just one follow-up count, but if there are multiple follow-up counts, it may be necessary to provide a separate rate for each follow-up because the denominator may be decreasing as the numerator increases.

An aspect of measuring disease incidence that an investigator also needs to consider is whether to count individuals with the disease or the number of cases of the disease. Some diseases can occur multiple times in individuals. So if a single subject gets two respiratory diseases during the time period, should that be counted as one person with a new disease or two new diseases during the period? The answer to what to do in this situation is very dependent on the type of the disease and the purpose of the study.

Prevalence versus Incidence

Understanding the relationship between prevalence and incidence is very important to understanding morbidity in a population. The typical illustration used in epidemiology to demonstrate the relationship between incidence and prevalence is by using a sink. As shown in Figure 3-2, the prevalence of a disease in a population is the water level in the sink. The incidence in the population is the water coming out of the faucet. The water leaving the sink through the drain is made up of those that recover from the disease or die. Using this illustration, you can see that the water level of the sink (prevalence) is dependent on the volume coming out of the faucet (incidence) and on the volume leaving through the drain (duration of disease). The water level in the sink can rise by either turning the faucet on to a high volume or closing the drain, or both. Conversely, the level in the sink can decrease either by turning down the faucet or opening the drain or both.

Continuing the sink analogy, prevalence equals incidence multiplied by duration of disease ($P = I \times D$). This means that prevalence is related to incidence by the

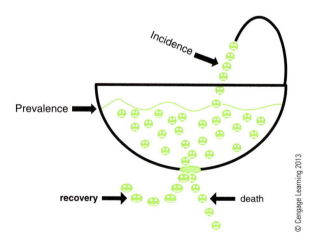

FIGURE 3-2 The "Sink" of Prevalence

duration of disease. So if the duration is very short, the prevalence will simply be the same level as the level of incidence. This would be the result in the sink if the drain was very large so that as soon as water entered the sink, it would leave the drain. An example of a short-duration disease would either be a condition like a seizure, which usually only lasts minutes, or a serious heart attack from which most people die immediately. Both of these conditions would result in a very short duration of disease, and the prevalence would be about the same as the incidence. On the other hand, if the disease is of a long duration, the prevalence would be much higher than the incidence because cases would accumulate in the population. This would be the result if the drain in the sink were stopped or slowed dramatically. Of course the prevalence in the population can be affected by increasing the incidence (turning up the faucet) such as in an epidemic, but most often the level of prevalence is dependent on the duration of the disease (size of the drain).

Another critical comparison between prevalence and incidence is in the application of each measure. As described previously, epidemiologists prefer incidence as a measure of disease because we have complete information about new cases. However, the big concept is that incidence is an estimate of the future risk of a disease. For example, if the incidence rate of disease in the previous year is 8.0%, the expectation is that the incidence rate in the following year will also be 8.0%. It is not appropriate to make the same expectation with prevalence proportion. So we say that the risk of disease in a future time period is expected to be the same as the incidence rate from the previous time period.

Summary

In this chapter, we learned about counting diseases and exposure information, including what to count, how to count, and when to count. We also learned some of the key measures used to assess disease occurrence, including the concepts of incidence and prevalence. This chapter laid the groundwork for understanding key concepts and terminology to use when assessing and evaluating population data. The basic measures and rates used to identify disease occurrence and exposure were introduced, along with information needed to compare population subgroups and to organize data sets for later use.

A Closer Look

Introduction to 2 × 2 Tables

The discussion about measuring disease and exposure would not be complete without introducing the **2 × 2 table**, a method to organize and present measures of disease and exposure in an observed population. This type of table is used extensively in every area of epidemiology to organize data for analysis and interpretation.

Mechanics of Creating 2 × 2 Tables

In order to use a 2 × 2 table, the data for both disease and exposure must be categorized into two groups each such as with or without disease and with or without exposure. So with two categories of outcome and exposure, the resulting table will have two columns and two rows as shown in Figure 3-3.

A standard convention for arranging a 2 × 2 table is to label the columns as disease status and to label the rows with exposure. The four numbers inside the table are referred to as "cells," and the numbers around the outside of the table are called "margins." The margins combine the two numbers in the corresponding row or column, and the margin at the bottom right corner of the table is the total number of subjects represented by the entire table. The internal cells of

	Outcome	No Outcome	**Total**
Exposed	**a**	**b**	**a + b**
Not exposed	**c**	**d**	**c + d**
Total	**a + c**	**b + d**	**a + b + c + d**

© Cengage Learning 2013

FIGURE 3-3 The 2 × 2 Table

2 × 2 table: a method to organize and present measures of disease and exposure in an observed population

the table are labeled with the lowercase letters, "a", "b", "c", and "d." The interpretation of the fours cells is:

a = subjects with disease and with exposure
b = subjects without disease and with exposure
c = subjects with disease but without exposure
d = subjects without disease and without exposure

The nature of a 2 × 2 table is that you do not actually need all the information for every cell and margin to be able to completely fill it out and use the table to assess a hypothesis. For example, if you know one cell and its corresponding margin, you can determine the missing cell through subtraction. If you know both internal cells in a row, you can determine that row margin by addition. The internal cells of a row or column can be determined by only knowing the margin total and the rate. For example, in Figure 3-3, if you know that the total number of subjects with the exposure is 100 people, and you know that the rate of disease is 30% in the exposed group, then you can determine that the "a" cell is 30 and the "b" cell is 70.

Using 2 × 2 Tables

Examining the table in Figure 3-3, it is apparent that the organization of a 2 × 2 table easily assists with the completion of rates. For example, the rate of disease for the entire population represented in a 2 × 2 table is the bottom margin of the column for those with disease divided by the number in the bottom right corner of the table (total population). In addition, the rate of exposure for the entire population represented in a 2 × 2 table is the right-side margin of the exposure row divided by the bottom right corner of the table (total population).

But even more important is the concept that a 2 × 2 table allows the identification of rates that can be compared between study groups whether comparing the exposed to the nonexposed, or the diseased to the nondiseased. Examine the 2 × 2 table in Figure 3-4. This table represents the results of a study of the relationship between eating salt in the diet and high blood pressure. The outcome is classified as high blood pressure and normal blood pressure; the exposure is classified as eating salt and not eating salt. The study is performed in 200 total subjects over 1 year. The total rate of high blood pressure in this observed population is 48 / 200 × 100 = 24%. It is also easy to see that the rate of high blood pressure in just those that eat salt is 30 / 100 × 100 = 30%. Further, it can be seen that the rate of high blood pressure among just those that do not eat salt is 18 / 100 × 100 =18%. In Chapter 6, Using Rates and Ratios, we will discuss how these specific rates can be compared to draw conclusions about the relationship between eat salt and high blood pressure.

	High BP	Normal BP	
Eat salt	30	70	100
No salt	18	82	100
	48	152	200

BP = Blood Pressure

© Cengage Learning 2013

FIGURE 3-4 Results of a Study Investigating the Relationship between Salt in the Diet and High Blood Pressure

Continues

Additional Features

It is important to realize that a 2 × 2 table can be expanded to tables with more than two rows and two columns. A table in epidemiology that arranges numbers to allow the comparison of exposure and outcome is called a **contingency table**. A 2 × 2 table is a contingency table when the data for exposure and outcome are classified in only two categories each. However, if either the exposure or the outcome is classified into more than two categories, the table can be expanded to have the number of rows or columns to accommodate the additional categories of the variables. For example, an investigator may want to study an outcome such as such as blood pressure in three categories: (1) high blood pressure; (2) normal blood pressure; and (3) low blood pressure. In this situation, we could construct a table that has three columns. Similarly, if an investigator is studying an exposure that is classified in four categories, then we could construct a table that has four rows. So although a contingency table can have any number of rows and columns, the most common contingency table used in epidemiology is the 2 × 2 table.

contingency table: a table in that it arranges data, allowing the comparison of exposure and outcome. A special case of a contingency table is a 2 × 2 table, which has just two rows and two columns.

Review Questions

1. Examples of prevalence proportion(s) include the:
   a. Number of sore throat episodes suffered by a 3-year-old per year
   b. Number of new cases of prostate cancer per year per 100,000 males
   c. Number of cases of multiple sclerosis in a high school
   d. Total number of cases of diabetes per 100,000 population in 1996
   e. All of the above

2. When a new treatment is developed that prevents death but does not produce recovery from a disease, the following will occur:
   a. Prevalence of the disease will decrease.
   b. Incidence of the disease will increase.
   c. Prevalence of the disease will increase.
   d. Incidence of the disease will decrease.
   e. Incidence and prevalence of the disease will decrease.

3. New cases of this disease occur every day. If the disease results in death on the same day that it is acquired, which of the following statements is true? (Circle all that apply.)
   a. The single-day incidence will be greater than prevalence.
   b. The single-day incidence will be less than prevalence.
   c. The single-day incidence will be the same as prevalence.
   d. The one-week incidence will be greater than the prevalence at the end of the week.

4. What information would you want to have if you are doing a study regarding the long-term effects of smoking?

    a. Number of cigarettes smoked per day
    b. Age when started to smoke
    c. Number of cigarettes smoked when drinking alcohol
    d. Number of years of smoking cigarettes
    e. Exercise patterns

5. **True or False** A clinical case and a preclinical case are both considered cases for an epidemiological study.

6. Match the following terms in Column A with their corresponding terms in Column B.

Column A	**Column B**
Number of cases of a disease	Denominator
Number of people exposed to an event	Numerator
Total number of study subjects	
Average population for one year	

7. **True or False** If 200 people are followed for 1 year and 500 people are followed for 6 months, the total person-years would be 450.

8. Which measure would give you a rate that can most easily be compared to a population with a different age structure?

    a. Crude rate
    b. Age-specific rate
    c. Age-adjusted rate
    d. Gender-specific rate
    e. All of the above

9. Which of the following are characteristics of point prevalence?

    a. All subjects meet the case definition at the time they are interviewed.
    b. It is a good method to obtain incidence data.
    c. It is a measure of the burden of disease in a population.
    d. A and C only
    e. All of the above

10. **True or False** Incidence is affected by the prevalence of a disease and its duration.

11. **True or False** The prevalence proportion of an area can be lowered by access to effective medical treatment.

12. **True or False** A contingency table has the same use as a 2 × 2 table, but it includes more than two rows or more than two columns.

13. **For Deeper Thought** If your class was assigned a project to collect information on the occurrence of colds during the fall semester, describe which type of measure you would choose (incidence, prevalence, point prevalence, period prevalence) and justify your choice.

Website Resources

For information on rates of disease, visit the Centers for Disease Control and Prevention website, http://cdc.gov, and search for the "National Center for Health Statistics."

Chapter 4

DATA SOURCES

Learning Objectives

Upon completion of this chapter, you should be able to:

1. List at least three common data sources used to obtain health information in the United States.
2. List one advantage and one disadvantage of using vital records to obtain health information of U.S. residents.
3. Calculate and interpret common mortality rates.
4. Explain the benefits of having a standardized classification for diseases.
5. Describe at least one issue related to data quality.

Key Terms

age-specific mortality rate

cause-specific mortality rate

crude birth rate

crude mortality rate

fetal death rate

infant mortality rate

International Classification of Disease (ICD)

neonatal mortality rate

public health surveillance

registry

reportable (or notifiable) disease/ condition

research data

surveillance data

World Health Organization (WHO)

Chapter Outline

INTRODUCTION

This chapter focuses on various ways to obtain health data and discusses the accuracy and scope of systems currently in place to track and monitor the health status of a population. Population health characteristics are assessed by calculating and comparing rates over time. Rates are calculated using data on births or deaths for the numerator and census data, collected every 10 years, for the denominator. Surveillance (or tracking) systems using standardized records provide for regular monitoring of diseases, conditions, or risk factors. Trends observed over time allow public health workers to identify reductions in diseases or risk factors or emerging epidemics.

There are some key issues to remember regarding data sources. Most data sources discussed in this chapter are based on ongoing surveys used to assess population trends (also called **surveillance data**) rather than on studies that focus on finding risk factors for a particular disease (also called **research data**). It is important to distinguish between these two data sources to correctly interpret published studies on health. Other points to note include the importance of statistical sampling. Because we cannot assess the health status of every individual in the population, estimates for such things as cancer incidence are made from statistically valid samples of a portion of the population. Although surveys and tracking systems usually represent a geographical area (e.g., whole nation, state, county, community), data collected for research studies can define a different target population, for example, a cohort of all people born in a particular year. And, finally, the related issues of the accuracy of data systems are discussed.

surveillance data: ongoing surveys used to assess population trends

research data: studies that focus on finding risk factors for a particular disease

Although most data systems discussed in this chapter are U.S.-based, every country should have data systems in place to track the health of its population. When the same data elements are collected in different countries, it may be possible to compare health status and trends between countries, especially if a standardized classification system is used. However, international data comparisons are often limited by completeness of the data and inconsistency of the data collection efforts. The particular problems involved in collecting and maintaining data sources in developing countries will be discussed in Chapter 15: The Practice of Epidemiology in Developing Countries.

VITAL RECORDS

The purpose of vital records is to monitor key indicators of the health of a population. All developed countries have record-keeping systems to track vital events, including (at least) births, deaths, and fetal deaths. Because of the advantages of comparing key health indicators across countries, many times the same data items are collected and processed in the same way.

Historical Note 4-1

John Graunt

John Graunt (1620–1674) was instrumental in vital statistics development. He was one of the first demographers, though by profession he was a haberdasher. Born in London, Graunt, along with William Petty, developed early human statistical and census methods that later provided a framework for modern demography. He is credited with producing the first life table, giving probabilities of survival to each age. Graunt is also considered as one of the first experts in epidemiology because his writings were focused mostly on public health statistics. His book *Natural and Political Observations Made upon the Bills of Mortality* (1662) analyzed the mortality rolls in early modern London by systemically recording age, sex, cause, location, date of death, and type of death (acute or chronic). In this way, Graunt was able to learn how many persons per year died of what kind of event or disease. Officials in London wanted him to create a system to warn of the onset and spread of bubonic plague in the city. Unfortunately, he died at the age of 53 and his work was discontinued.

National Vital Statistics System

In the United States, the National Vital Statistics System (NVSS) is monitored by the National Center for Health Statistics (NCHS) and includes information related to births, deaths, fetal deaths, marriages, and divorces. Using these data, it is possible to compare basic birth and death rates between areas of the country or to compare rates over time. By itself, the vital records system provides numerator data only. These data are very useful for planning purposes. For example, the number of deaths in a specific age group or as a result of various diseases can help to plan for future health care resources or for the needs of an aging population. The numbers of births each year, along with the age of the mothers, can help agencies to plan for schools and other public services. However, to understand what these numbers (numerators) mean in terms of rates and trends, we need to know how many people are in the United States (denominator) at a given time. Every 10 years since 1790, the U.S. government has conducted a census to count its residents (http://www.census.gov/). These census data provide denominators used to calculate rates. Typically the same census year (2000, for example) is often used for age-adjustment so that the resulting rates can be compared over time. Using statistical methods, one can estimate the U.S. population for years between the census years.

Figures 4-1 and 4-2 display copies of birth and death certificates, as revised in 2003, that are used to obtain numerator data for calculating information on births and deaths. Data that comprise the Vital Records system occurs individually with the 50 states, two cities (Washington, DC, and New York City), and five territories (Puerto Rico, the Virgin Islands, Guam, American Samoa, and the Commonwealth of the Northern Mariana Islands). These reports are collected and processed by NCHS, which provides summary data and makes files available online for processing by the public (NVSS, 2010). The advantage of using vital records is that the data represent the entire United States, but the collection of these events depends on the cooperation of the various states and territories. Cooperation is enhanced because federal funding is allocated based on population size.

However, there are frequently problems with the accuracy and completeness of birth and death certificates. Although there is a lot of information requested on the birth certificate (smoking, education, and occupation of the parents, for example), many times these fields are not completed. Also, many birth defects are not apparent at delivery and are not noted in the birth certificate. For death certificates, the attending physician may record the cause of death, but the underlying causes or health conditions may not be known or recorded. All causes of death are coded to obtain summary statistics, but the person assigning the code may not have access to all the medical information to make an informed decision.

Commonly Used Rates Derived from Vital Records

The rate is the cornerstone of the way epidemiologists organize and represent epidemiologic data. Although there are literally thousands of rates that are used in epidemiology, some are used often enough that there is a commonly accepted "label" or name for them. There are some common themes for the labels. If the label includes

U.S. STANDARD CERTIFICATE OF LIVE BIRTH

LOCAL FILE NO.

BIRTH NUMBER:

CHILD

1. CHILD'S NAME (First, Middle, Last, Suffix)	2. TIME OF BIRTH (24 hr) / 3. SEX / 4. DATE OF BIRTH (Mo/Day/Yr)
5. FACILITY NAME (If not institution, give street and number)	6. CITY, TOWN, OR LOCATION OF BIRTH / 7. COUNTY OF BIRTH

MOTHER

8a. MOTHER'S CURRENT LEGAL NAME (First, Middle, Last, Suffix)	8b. DATE OF BIRTH (Mo/Day/Yr)
8c. MOTHER'S NAME PRIOR TO FIRST MARRIAGE (First, Middle, Last, Suffix)	8d. BIRTHPLACE (State, Territory, or Foreign Country)
9a. RESIDENCE OF MOTHER-STATE / 9b. COUNTY	9c. CITY, TOWN, OR LOCATION
9d. STREET AND NUMBER	9e. APT. NO. / 9f. ZIP CODE / 9g. INSIDE CITY LIMITS? ☐ Yes ☐ No

FATHER

10a. FATHER'S CURRENT LEGAL NAME (First, Middle, Last, Suffix) / 10b. DATE OF BIRTH (Mo/Day/Yr) / 10c. BIRTHPLACE (State, Territory, or Foreign Country)

CERTIFIER

11. CERTIFIER'S NAME: _____
TITLE: ☐ MD ☐ DO ☐ HOSPITAL ADMIN. ☐ CNM/CM ☐ OTHER MIDWIFE
☐ OTHER (Specify)_____

12. DATE CERTIFIED
____ / ____ /
MM   DD   YYYY

13. DATE FILED BY REGISTRAR
____ / ____ /
MM   DD   YYYY

INFORMATION FOR ADMINISTRATIVE USE

MOTHER

14. MOTHER'S MAILING ADDRESS: ☐ Same as residence, or: State: ___   City, Town, or Location:
Street & Number: Apartment No.:   Zip Code:

15. MOTHER MARRIED? (At birth, conception, or any time between) ☐ Yes ☐ No
IF NO, HAS PATERNITY ACKNOWLEDGEMENT BEEN SIGNED IN THE HOSPITAL? ☐ Yes ☐ No

16. SOCIAL SECURITY NUMBER REQUESTED FOR CHILD? ☐ Yes ☐ No

17. FACILITY ID. (NPI)

18. MOTHER'S SOCIAL SECURITY NUMBER:

19. FATHER'S SOCIAL SECURITY NUMBER:

INFORMATION FOR MEDICAL AND HEALTH PURPOSES ONLY

MOTHER

20. MOTHER'S EDUCATION (Check the box that best describes the highest degree or level of school completed at the time of delivery)	21. MOTHER OF HISPANIC ORIGIN? (Check the box that best describes whether the mother is Spanish/Hispanic/Latina. Check the "No" box if mother is not Spanish/Hispanic/Latina)	22. MOTHER'S RACE (Check one or more races to indicate what the mother considers herself to be)
☐ 8th grade or less	☐ No, not Spanish/Hispanic/Latina	☐ White
☐ 9th - 12th grade, no diploma	☐ Yes, Mexican, Mexican American, Chicana	☐ Black or African American
☐ High school graduate or GED completed	☐ Yes, Puerto Rican	☐ American Indian or Alaska Native (Name of the enrolled or principal tribe)_____
☐ Some college credit but no degree	☐ Yes, Cuban	☐ Asian Indian
☐ Associate degree (e.g., AA, AS)	☐ Yes, other Spanish/Hispanic/Latina	☐ Chinese
☐ Bachelor's degree (e.g., BA, AB, BS)	(Specify)_____	☐ Filipino
☐ Master's degree (e.g., MA, MS, MEng, MEd, MSW, MBA)		☐ Japanese
☐ Doctorate (e.g., PhD, EdD) or Professional degree (e.g., MD, DDS, DVM, LLB, JD)		☐ Korean
		☐ Vietnamese
		☐ Other Asian (Specify)_____
		☐ Native Hawaiian
		☐ Guamanian or Chamorro
		☐ Samoan
		☐ Other Pacific Islander (Specify)_____
		☐ Other (Specify)_____

FATHER

23. FATHER'S EDUCATION (Check the box that best describes the highest degree or level of school completed at the time of delivery)	24. FATHER OF HISPANIC ORIGIN? (Check the box that best describes whether the father is Spanish/Hispanic/Latino. Check the "No" box if father is not Spanish/Hispanic/Latino)	25. FATHER'S RACE (Check one or more races to indicate what the father considers himself to be)
☐ 8th grade or less	☐ No, not Spanish/Hispanic/Latino	☐ White
☐ 9th - 12th grade, no diploma	☐ Yes, Mexican, Mexican American, Chicano	☐ Black or African American
☐ High school graduate or GED completed	☐ Yes, Puerto Rican	☐ American Indian or Alaska Native (Name of the enrolled or principal tribe)_____
☐ Some college credit but no degree	☐ Yes, Cuban	☐ Asian Indian
☐ Associate degree (e.g., AA, AS)	☐ Yes, other Spanish/Hispanic/Latino	☐ Chinese
☐ Bachelor's degree (e.g., BA, AB, BS)	(Specify)_____	☐ Filipino
☐ Master's degree (e.g., MA, MS, MEng, MEd, MSW, MBA)		☐ Japanese
☐ Doctorate (e.g., PhD, EdD) or Professional degree (e.g., MD, DDS, DVM, LLB, JD)		☐ Korean
		☐ Vietnamese
		☐ Other Asian (Specify)_____
		☐ Native Hawaiian
		☐ Guamanian or Chamorro
		☐ Samoan
		☐ Other Pacific Islander (Specify)_____
		☐ Other (Specify)_____

Mother's Name | Mother's Medical Record No.

26. PLACE WHERE BIRTH OCCURRED (Check one)	27. ATTENDANT'S NAME, TITLE, AND NPI	28. MOTHER TRANSFERRED FOR MATERNAL MEDICAL OR FETAL INDICATIONS FOR DELIVERY? ☐ Yes ☐ No
☐ Hospital	NAME: _____ NPI: _____	IF YES, ENTER NAME OF FACILITY MOTHER TRANSFERRED FROM:
☐ Freestanding birthing center	TITLE: ☐ MD ☐ DO ☐ CNM/CM ☐ OTHER MIDWIFE	
☐ Home Birth: Planned to deliver at home? ☐ Yes ☐ No	☐ OTHER (Specify)_____	_____
☐ Clinic/Doctor's office		
☐ Other (Specify)_____		

REV. 11/2003

Continues

FIGURE 4-1 Certificate of Live Birth
Centers for Disease Control and Prevention: http://www.cdc.gov/nchs/vital_certs_rev.htm

MOTHER

29a. DATE OF FIRST PRENATAL CARE VISIT	29b. DATE OF LAST PRENATAL CARE VISIT	30. TOTAL NUMBER OF PRENATAL VISITS FOR THIS PREGNANCY
___/___/___ □ No Prenatal Care M M D D YYYY	___/___/___ M M D D YYYY	_____ (If none, enter ʌ0".)

31. MOTHER'S HEIGHT _____ (feet/inches)	32. MOTHER'S PREPREGNANCY WEIGHT _____ (pounds)	33. MOTHER'S WEIGHT AT DELIVERY _____ (pounds)	34. DID MOTHER GET WIC FOOD FOR HERSELF DURING THIS PREGNANCY? □ Yes □ No

35. NUMBER OF PREVIOUS LIVE BIRTHS (Do not include this child)		36. NUMBER OF OTHER PREGNANCY OUTCOMES (spontaneous or induced losses or ectopic pregnancies)	37. CIGARETTE SMOKING BEFORE AND DURING PREGNANCY For each time period, enter either the number of cigarettes or the number of packs of cigarettes smoked. IF NONE, ENTER ʌ0".	38. PRINCIPAL SOURCE OF PAYMENT FOR THIS DELIVERY

35a. Now Living
 	
Number _____
 	
□ None
	35b. Now Dead
	
	Number _____
	
	□ None
		36a. Other Outcomes
		
		Number _____
		
		□ None
			Average number of cigarettes or packs of cigarettes smoked per day.
			         # of cigarettes # of packs
			Three Months Before Pregnancy _____ OR _____
			First Three Months of Pregnancy _____ OR _____
			Second Three Months of Pregnancy _____ OR _____
			Third Trimester of Pregnancy _____ OR _____
				□ Private Insurance
				□ Medicaid
				□ Self-pay
				□ Other
				  (Specify) _____

35c. DATE OF LAST LIVE BIRTH ___/___ MM YYYY	36b. DATE OF LAST OTHER PREGNANCY OUTCOME ___/___ MM YYYY	39. DATE LAST NORMAL MENSES BEGAN ___/___/___ MM D D YYYY	40. MOTHER'S MEDICAL RECORD NUMBER

MEDICAL AND HEALTH INFORMATION

41. RISK FACTORS IN THIS PREGNANCY (Check all that apply)

Diabetes
- □ Prepregnancy (Diagnosis prior to this pregnancy)
- □ Gestational (Diagnosis in this pregnancy)

Hypertension
- □ Prepregnancy (Chronic)
- □ Gestational (PIH, preeclampsia)
- □ Eclampsia

- □ Previous preterm birth

- □ Other previous poor pregnancy outcome (Includes perinatal death, small-for-gestational age/intrauterine growth restricted birth)

- □ Pregnancy resulted from infertility treatment-If yes, check all that apply:
  - □ Fertility-enhancing drugs, Artificial insemination or Intrauterine insemination
  - □ Assisted reproductive technology (e.g., in vitro fertilization (IVF), gamete intrafallopian transfer (GIFT))

- □ Mother had a previous cesarean delivery
  If yes, how many _____

- □ None of the above

42. INFECTIONS PRESENT AND/OR TREATED DURING THIS PREGNANCY (Check all that apply)

- □ Gonorrhea
- □ Syphilis
- □ Chlamydia
- □ Hepatitis B
- □ Hepatitis C
- □ None of the above

43. OBSTETRIC PROCEDURES (Check all that apply)

- □ Cervical cerclage
- □ Tocolysis

External cephalic version:
- □ Successful
- □ Failed

- □ None of the above

44. ONSET OF LABOR (Check all that apply)

- □ Premature Rupture of the Membranes (prolonged, ∃12 hrs.)
- □ Precipitous Labor (<3 hrs.)
- □ Prolonged Labor (∃ 20 hrs.)
- □ None of the above

45. CHARACTERISTICS OF LABOR AND DELIVERY (Check all that apply)

- □ Induction of labor
- □ Augmentation of labor
- □ Non-vertex presentation
- □ Steroids (glucocorticoids) for fetal lung maturation received by the mother prior to delivery
- □ Antibiotics received by the mother during labor
- □ Clinical chorioamnionitis diagnosed during labor or maternal temperature ≥38°C (100.4°F)
- □ Moderate/heavy meconium staining of the amniotic fluid
- □ Fetal intolerance of labor such that one or more of the following actions was taken: in-utero resuscitative measures, further fetal assessment, or operative delivery
- □ Epidural or spinal anesthesia during labor
- □ None of the above

46. METHOD OF DELIVERY

A. Was delivery with forceps attempted but unsuccessful?
 □ Yes □ No

B. Was delivery with vacuum extraction attempted but unsuccessful?
 □ Yes □ No

C. Fetal presentation at birth
- □ Cephalic
- □ Breech
- □ Other

D. Final route and method of delivery (Check one)
- □ Vaginal/Spontaneous
- □ Vaginal/Forceps
- □ Vaginal/Vacuum
- □ Cesarean
  If cesarean, was a trial of labor attempted?
  - □ Yes
  - □ No

47. MATERNAL MORBIDITY (Check all that apply) (Complications associated with labor and delivery)

- □ Maternal transfusion
- □ Third or fourth degree perineal laceration
- □ Ruptured uterus
- □ Unplanned hysterectomy
- □ Admission to intensive care unit
- □ Unplanned operating room procedure following delivery
- □ None of the above

NEWBORN INFORMATION

NEWBORN

Mother's Name | Mother's Medical Record No.

48. NEWBORN MEDICAL RECORD NUMBER

49. BIRTHWEIGHT (grams preferred, specify unit)
_____ 9 grams 9 lb/oz

50. OBSTETRIC ESTIMATE OF GESTATION:
_____ (completed weeks)

51. APGAR SCORE:
Score at 5 minutes: _____
If 5 minute score is less than 6,
Score at 10 minutes: _____

52. PLURALITY - Single, Twin, Triplet, etc.
(Specify) _____

53. IF NOT SINGLE BIRTH - Born First, Second, Third, etc. (Specify) _____

54. ABNORMAL CONDITIONS OF THE NEWBORN (Check all that apply)

- □ Assisted ventilation required immediately following delivery
- □ Assisted ventilation required for more than six hours
- □ NICU admission
- □ Newborn given surfactant replacement therapy
- □ Antibiotics received by the newborn for suspected neonatal sepsis
- □ Seizure or serious neurologic dysfunction
- □ Significant birth injury (skeletal fracture(s), peripheral nerve injury, and/or soft tissue/solid organ hemorrhage which requires intervention)
- 9 None of the above

55. CONGENITAL ANOMALIES OF THE NEWBORN (Check all that apply)

- □ Anencephaly
- □ Meningomyelocele/Spina bifida
- □ Cyanotic congenital heart disease
- □ Congenital diaphragmatic hernia
- □ Omphalocele
- □ Gastroschisis
- □ Limb reduction defect (excluding congenital amputation and dwarfing syndromes)
- □ Cleft Lip with or without Cleft Palate
- □ Cleft Palate alone
- □ Down Syndrome
  - □ Karyotype confirmed
  - □ Karyotype pending
- □ Suspected chromosomal disorder
  - □ Karyotype confirmed
  - □ Karyotype pending
- □ Hypospadias
- □ None of the anomalies listed above

56. WAS INFANT TRANSFERRED WITHIN 24 HOURS OF DELIVERY? 9 Yes 9 No IF YES, NAME OF FACILITY INFANT TRANSFERRED TO: _____	57. IS INFANT LIVING AT TIME OF REPORT? □ Yes □ No □ Infant transferred, status unknown	58. IS THE INFANT BEING BREASTFED AT DISCHARGE? □ Yes □ No

Rev. 11/2003
NOTE: This recommended standard birth certificate is the result of an extensive evaluation process. Information on the process and resulting recommendations as well as plans for future activities is available on the Internet at: http://www.cdc.gov/nchs/vital_certs_rev.htm.

FIGURE 4-1 (Continued)

U.S. STANDARD CERTIFICATE OF DEATH

LOCAL FILE NO.   STATE FILE NO.

NAME OF DECEDENT — For use by physician or institution

To Be Completed/ Verified By: FUNERAL DIRECTOR

1. DECEDENT'S LEGAL NAME (Include AKA's if any) (First, Middle, Last) | 2. SEX | 3. SOCIAL SECURITY NUMBER

4a. AGE–Last Birthday (Years) | 4b. UNDER 1 YEAR — Months / Days | 4c. UNDER 1 DAY — Hours / Minutes | 5. DATE OF BIRTH (Mo/Day/Yr) | 6. BIRTHPLACE (City and State or Foreign Country)

7a. RESIDENCE-STATE | 7b. COUNTY | 7c. CITY OR TOWN

7d. STREET AND NUMBER | 7e. APT. NO. | 7f. ZIP CODE | 7g. INSIDE CITY LIMITS? ☐ Yes ☐ No

8. EVER IN US ARMED FORCES? ☐ Yes ☐ No | 9. MARITAL STATUS AT TIME OF DEATH ☐ Married ☐ Married, but separated ☐ Widowed ☐ Divorced ☐ Never Married ☐ Unknown | 10. SURVIVING SPOUSE'S NAME (If wife, give name prior to first marriage)

11. FATHER'S NAME (First, Middle, Last) | 12. MOTHER'S NAME PRIOR TO FIRST MARRIAGE (First, Middle, Last)

13a. INFORMANT'S NAME | 13b. RELATIONSHIP TO DECEDENT | 13c. MAILING ADDRESS (Street and Number, City, State, Zip Code)

14. PLACE OF DEATH (Check only one: see instructions)

IF DEATH OCCURRED IN A HOSPITAL: ☐ Inpatient ☐ Emergency Room/Outpatient ☐ Dead on Arrival | IF DEATH OCCURRED SOMEWHERE OTHER THAN A HOSPITAL: ☐ Hospice facility ☐ Nursing home/Long term care facility ☐ Decedent's home ☐ Other (Specify):

15. FACILITY NAME (If not institution, give street & number) | 16. CITY OR TOWN , STATE, AND ZIP CODE | 17. COUNTY OF DEATH

18. METHOD OF DISPOSITION: ☐ Burial ☐ Cremation ☐ Donation ☐ Entombment ☐ Removal from State ☐ Other (Specify): | 19. PLACE OF DISPOSITION (Name of cemetery, crematory, other place)

20. LOCATION-CITY, TOWN, AND STATE | 21. NAME AND COMPLETE ADDRESS OF FUNERAL FACILITY

22. SIGNATURE OF FUNERAL SERVICE LICENSEE OR OTHER AGENT | 23. LICENSE NUMBER (Of Licensee)

ITEMS 24-28 MUST BE COMPLETED BY PERSON WHO PRONOUNCES OR CERTIFIES DEATH | 24. DATE PRONOUNCED DEAD (Mo/Day/Yr) | 25. TIME PRONOUNCED DEAD

26. SIGNATURE OF PERSON PRONOUNCING DEATH (Only when applicable) | 27. LICENSE NUMBER | 28. DATE SIGNED (Mo/Day/Yr)

29. ACTUAL OR PRESUMED DATE OF DEATH (Mo/Day/Yr) (Spell Month) | 30. ACTUAL OR PRESUMED TIME OF DEATH | 31. WAS MEDICAL EXAMINER OR CORONER CONTACTED? ☐ Yes ☐ No

To Be Completed By: MEDICAL CERTIFIER

CAUSE OF DEATH (See instructions and examples)

32. PART I. Enter the chain of events--diseases, injuries, or complications--that directly caused the death. DO NOT enter terminal events such as cardiac arrest, respiratory arrest, or ventricular fibrillation without showing the etiology. DO NOT ABBREVIATE. Enter only one cause on a line. Add additional lines if necessary.

Approximate interval: Onset to death

IMMEDIATE CAUSE (Final disease or condition ------> resulting in death)   a._____ Due to (or as a consequence of): _____

Sequentially list conditions, if any, leading to the cause listed on line a. Enter the UNDERLYING CAUSE (disease or injury that initiated the events resulting in death) LAST   b._____ Due to (or as a consequence of): _____
c._____ Due to (or as a consequence of): _____
d._____

PART II. Enter other significant conditions contributing to death but not resulting in the underlying cause given in PART I | 33. WAS AN AUTOPSY PERFORMED? ☐ Yes ☐ No | 34. WERE AUTOPSY FINDINGS AVAILABLE TO COMPLETE THE CAUSE OF DEATH? ☐ Yes ☐ No

35. DID TOBACCO USE CONTRIBUTE TO DEATH? ☐ Yes ☐ Probably ☐ No ☐ Unknown | 36. IF FEMALE: ☐ Not pregnant within past year ☐ Pregnant at time of death ☐ Not pregnant, but pregnant within 42 days of death ☐ Not pregnant, but pregnant 43 days to 1 year before death ☐ Unknown if pregnant within the past year | 37. MANNER OF DEATH ☐ Natural ☐ Homicide ☐ Accident ☐ Pending Investigation ☐ Suicide ☐ Could not be determined

38. DATE OF INJURY (Mo/Day/Yr) (Spell Month) | 39. TIME OF INJURY | 40. PLACE OF INJURY (e.g., Decedent's home; construction site; restaurant; wooded area) | 41. INJURY AT WORK? ☐ Yes ☐ No

42. LOCATION OF INJURY: State: City or Town: Street & Number: Apartment No.:   Zip Code:

43. DESCRIBE HOW INJURY OCCURRED: | 44. IF TRANSPORTATION INJURY, SPECIFY: ☐ Driver/Operator ☐ Passenger ☐ Pedestrian ☐ Other (Specify)

45. CERTIFIER (Check only one):
☐ Certifying physician-To the best of my knowledge, death occurred due to the cause(s) and manner stated.
☐ Pronouncing & Certifying physician-To the best of my knowledge, death occurred at the time, date, and place, and due to the cause(s) and manner stated.
☐ Medical Examiner/Coroner-On the basis of examination, and/or investigation, in my opinion, death occurred at the time, date, and place, and due to the cause(s) and manner stated.

Signature of certifier:_____

46. NAME, ADDRESS, AND ZIP CODE OF PERSON COMPLETING CAUSE OF DEATH (Item 32)

47. TITLE OF CERTIFIER | 48. LICENSE NUMBER | 49. DATE CERTIFIED (Mo/Day/Yr) | 50. **FOR REGISTRAR ONLY**- DATE FILED (Mo/Day/Yr)

To Be Completed By: FUNERAL DIRECTOR

51. DECEDENT'S EDUCATION-Check the box that best describes the highest degree or level of school completed at the time of death.
☐ 8th grade or less
☐ 9th - 12th grade; no diploma
☐ High school graduate or GED completed
☐ Some college credit, but no degree
☐ Associate degree (e.g., AA, AS)
☐ Bachelor's degree (e.g., BA, AB, BS)
☐ Master's degree (e.g., MA, MS, MEng, MEd, MSW, MBA)
☐ Doctorate (e.g., PhD, EdD) or Professional degree (e.g., MD, DDS, DVM, LLB, JD)

52. DECEDENT OF HISPANIC ORIGIN? Check the box that best describes whether the decedent is Spanish/Hispanic/Latino. Check the "No" box if decedent is not Spanish/Hispanic/Latino.
☐ No, not Spanish/Hispanic/Latino
☐ Yes, Mexican, Mexican American, Chicano
☐ Yes, Puerto Rican
☐ Yes, Cuban
☐ Yes, other Spanish/Hispanic/Latino (Specify) _____

53. DECEDENT'S RACE (Check one or more races to indicate what the decedent considered himself or herself to be)
☐ White
☐ Black or African American
☐ American Indian or Alaska Native (Name of the enrolled or principal tribe) _____
☐ Asian Indian
☐ Chinese
☐ Filipino
☐ Japanese
☐ Korean
☐ Vietnamese
☐ Other Asian (Specify) _____
☐ Native Hawaiian
☐ Guamanian or Chamorro
☐ Samoan
☐ Other Pacific Islander (Specify) _____
☐ Other (Specify) _____

54. DECEDENT'S USUAL OCCUPATION (Indicate type of work done during most of working life. DO NOT USE RETIRED).

55. KIND OF BUSINESS/INDUSTRY

REV. 11/2003

FIGURE 4-2 Certificate of Death
Centers for Disease Control and Prevention: http://www.cdc.gov/nchs/vital_certs_rev.htm

death, it will generally include the word "mortality." If the label applies to a certain part of the population, it will include the word "specific." Many of the labels will simply be the same as the group counted in the numerator. Also, notice that the denominator of many of them is listed as the "midyear" population. The midyear population is just one option for measuring the population under observation. That population can be represented a number of ways, but the midyear is often chosen. Of course, if the rate was over a time period different than a year, then the denominator would change to match the time frame of that rate. Remember that a rate is a proportion over time, and a proportion can be represented by any "units" that you chose. So by multiplying the rate times 100, the rates are percentages, but if you chose to represent the rates with other units, that is at the discretion of the investigator.

The **crude mortality rate** represents the number of all individuals dying from all causes in the observed population during a time period, usually 12 months. This rate is considered a crude rate, but a mortality rate can be presented in subsets of the population for an **age-specific mortality rate**. This rate is often adjusted to make it more comparable to other observed populations. Most commonly this rate is adjusted for the age of the population, resulting in an age-adjusted mortality rate. A **cause-specific mortality rate** is the number of deaths from a specified cause in the total observed population during the time. A cause-specific mortality rate is different from an overall mortality rate because it is a subset of the entire number of deaths specifically for one illness or injury. This rate acts as a crude rate, but is also clearly a specific rate. It can be further specified by other characteristics such as age, which would result in an age-specific, cause-specific mortality rate. The cause-specific mortality rate can also be adjusted for any variables deemed important by the investigator for comparison with other cause-specific mortality rates. It is also important to notice that because of the denominator being a total population, this rate provides an indication of how the specific cause impacts in the death rate in the entire population.

One of the important indicators of a country's overall health system is how few infants die. There are several rates used to measure this health indicator. The **infant mortality rate** represents the number of deaths of live born children less than 1 year old divided by all live births in the same 12-month period. This rate is considered a crude rate even though it is a subset of the entire population because it is targeted just at infants. This rate can be adjusted, obviously not for age, but by demographic variables such as gender or ethnic category for comparison with other populations. The infant mortality rate is often used as an indication of such things as health care access, economic status, and geographic differences in environment. The **neonatal mortality rate** is the number of deaths in newborn infants less than 28 days old among all live births in the same time. This rate is similar to an infant mortality rate except that number of deaths is only among the very youngest newborns. This rate can also be an indication of health care access and economic status. The **fetal death rate** is the number of deaths of unborn fetuses among the total number of fetal deaths, plus live births in the same 12-month period. This rate is generally considered a crude rate; however, like an infant mortality rate, it can be presented as a specific or an adjusted rate.

A **crude birth rate** is calculated by the number of births in a period of time divided by the total population during that same time. Similar to infant mortality

crude mortality rate: (same as crude death rate) the number of deaths in a period of time divided by the total midpoint population during that same time (multiplied by 1,000 or 100,000)

age-specific mortality rate: death (mortality) rates for specific age groups calculated by the number of deaths in a particular age group divided by the midpoint population in that age group (multiplied by 1,000 or 100,000)

cause-specific mortality rate: the number of deaths as a result of a specific disease divided by the total midpoint population (multiplied by 1,000 or 100,000)

infant mortality rate: the number of deaths among infants less than one year of age divided by the total number of live births (multiplied by 1,000)

neonatal mortality rate: the number of deaths among infants less than 28 days old divided by the total number of live births (multiplied by 1,000)

fetal death rate: the total number of fetal deaths divided by the total number of live births, plus the total number of fetal deaths (multiplied by 1,000)

crude birth rate: the total number of live births divided by the total midpoint population (multiplied by 1,000 or 100,000)

rates, a birth rate can be presented for subgroups of the population by demographic characteristics. Examples of these rates are shown in Table 4-1.

As shown in Table 4-1, many health indicators can be derived from data contained in vital records. Most important are the birth and death rates as these are typically used to track the health of a country. The numerator data from the birth and death certificates are combined with census data to provide population statistics. Usually

TABLE 4-1 Selected Information Calculated Using the Vital Records System

Name	Numerator	Rate/Percent	Calculation*
Births	Number of Live Births	Crude Birth Rate	$\dfrac{\text{Total Live Births}}{\text{Total Midpoint Population}} \times 1000^{**}$
	Number of Live Births to Women Aged 15-49 Years	Age-Specific Birth Rate	$\dfrac{\text{Live Births to Mothers of Specific Ages}}{\text{Female Population of Same Specified Age}} \times 1{,}000^{**}$
	Number of Infants Born Weighing less than 2,500 Grams	Percentage of Infants Born with Low Birth Weight	$\dfrac{\text{Infants Born Weighing less than 2,500 Grams}}{\text{Total Live Births}} \times 100^{**}$
Deaths	Number of Deaths	Crude Mortality (Death) Rate	$\dfrac{\text{Total Deaths}}{\text{Total Midpoint Population}} \times 1{,}000^{**}$
	Number of Deaths in a Specific Age Group	Age-Specific Mortality (Death) Rate	$\dfrac{\text{Deaths for Specific Age Group}}{\text{Population for Same Specific Age Group}} \times 1{,}000^{**}$
	Number of Deaths due to a Specific Cause	Cause-Specific Mortality (Death) Rate	$\dfrac{\text{Deaths Due to a Specific Cause}}{\text{Total Midpoint Population}} \times 100{,}000^{**}$
	Number of Infant Deaths	Infant Mortality (Death) Rate	$\dfrac{\text{Total Deaths Among Infants Under One Year of Age}}{\text{Total Live Births}} \times 1{,}000^{**}$
	Number of Neonatal Deaths	Neonatal Mortality (Death) Rate	$\dfrac{\text{Total Deaths Among Infants under 28 Days Old}}{\text{Number of Live Births}} \times 1{,}000^{**}$
Fetal Deaths	Number of Fetal Deaths	Fetal Mortality (Death) Rate	$\dfrac{\text{Total Fetal Deaths}}{(\text{Total Live Births} + \text{Total Fetal Deaths})} \times 1{,}000^{**}$

Based on Centers for Disease Control and Prevention, National Vital Statistics System: http://www.cdc.gov/nchs/nvss/about_nvss.htm

*The numerator and denominator for all rates refer to a specific time period, usually a year.

**These units are typically used for interpretation but may be changed as needed.

the time frame for these rates is a specific year. Vital statistics also provide data on marriages and divorces, which gives information on the social health of a country.

REPORTABLE DISEASES AND CONDITIONS

One goal of public health is to protect people from diseases and conditions that are preventable and to alert officials of an emerging problem that needs to be addressed. Because of the need to rapidly assess potential health problems, the national government developed a list of **reportable or notifiable diseases/conditions**. When any of these diseases/conditions occur, each U.S. state health department sends a report to the CDC (either monthly or as otherwise noted), and these reports are summarized nationally and published weekly in the Mortality and Morbidity Weekly Report (MMWR: http://www.cdc.gov/mmwr/). Each year, the list of reportable diseases/conditions is updated. The reporting period can be extremely urgent (within 4 hours of identification of a case), urgent (within 24 hours of identification of a case), or standard (during the next reporting period—usually one week) (CDC Nationally Notifiable Conditions, 2011). See Table 4-2 for a sample list of selected reportable diseases/conditions and their reporting timeline for 2011. Some of these reports are

reportable (or notifiable) disease/condition: a disease/condition that requires reporting to a public health agency

TABLE 4-2 Examples of Selected Notifiable Diseases, 2011

Infectious	Report Timing (next reporting cycle unless noted)
Anthrax, unknown source	Extremely urgent (4 hours)
Anthrax, naturally-occurring or occupational	Urgent (24 hours)
Botulism	Extremely urgent (4 hours)
Chlamydia trachmatis infection	Standard
Dengue virus infections	Standard
Diphtheria	Urgent (24 hours)
Giardiasis	Standard
Gonorrhea	Standard
Haemophilus influenza, invasive disease	Standard
Hansen disease (leprosy)	Standard

Hepatitis (A, B, and C) acute or chronic	Standard
HIV infection	Standard
Lyme disease	Standard
Malaria	Standard
Measles	Urgent (24 hours)
Mumps	Standard
Pertussis	Standard
Plague, suspected intentional	Extremely urgent (4 hours)
Plague, not suspected intentional	Urgent (24 hours)
Poliomyelitis, paralytic	Extremely urgent (4 hours)
Poliomyelitis, non-paralytic	Urgent (24 hours)
Rabies in a human	Urgent (24 hours)
Salmonellosis	Standard
Smallpox	Extremely urgent (4 hours)
Syphilis	Standard
Tetanus	Standard
Toxic-shock syndrome	Standard
Tuberculosis	Standard
Typhoid fever	Standard
Yellow fever	Urgent (24 hours)
Non-infectious	
Cancer	Standard (at least annually)
High blood lead levels	Standard (quarterly for children and twice a year for adults)

Based on Centers for Disease Control and Prevention, Nationally Notifiable Diseases Surveillance System: http://www.cdc.gov/osels/ph_surveillance/nndss/phs/infdis2011.htm

used to track outbreaks of food borne illnesses (e.g., salmonella) or diseases that should be under control (e.g., measles). The MMWR is available online and is used often by state and local health agencies.

NATIONAL HEALTH SURVEYS

In addition to the collection and dissemination of vital statistics, the NCHS coordinates a variety of population-based health surveys. These are listed in Table 4-3. There are several strengths of these surveys. First, because they are population-based, the sampling technique used can provide prevalence estimates for different areas of

TABLE 4-3 Health Surveys Sponsored by the Centers for Disease Control and Prevention through the National Center for Health Statistics

Name	Population	Years	Topics
National Health and Nutrition Examination Survey (NHANES)	Children and adults, age included depends on questions asked	Early 1960s to present	Health and nutritional status
National Health Care Surveys (NHCS)	Hospitals, emergency rooms, physician offices, nursing homes	1973 to present	Answers key questions of interest to health care policy-makers, public health professionals, and researchers
National Health Interview Survey (NHIS)	Civilian non-institutionalized population of adults age 17 and older and children	1957 to present	Principal source of information on health status
National Immunization Survey (NIS)	Children between the ages of 19 and 35 months	1994 to present	Produces timely estimates of vaccination coverage rates for all recommended childhood vaccinations
National Survey of Family Growth (NSFG)	Women 15-44 years of age Men 15-44 years of age	1973 to present 2002 to present	Provides data on marriage, divorce, contraception, infertility, and the health of men, women, and infants
Longitudinal Studies of Aging (LSOA)	Persons 55 years and older in 1984; persons 70 years and older in 1994	1984 to present	Assesses disability and health behaviors as persons age

Based on Centers for Disease Control and Prevention, Survey and Data Collection Systems: http://www.cdc.gov/nchs/surveys.htm

the country, as well as for demographic characteristics. Second, the surveys use standard questions, many of which have been asked in generally the same way for years. Third, these surveys are repeated on a regular basis (annually, or every few years) so that tracking of health status is possible.

As you can see from the information in Table 4-3, all aspects of the population are covered including infants, children, adults, and older people. These surveys are used to guide public policy and inform prevention programs. They are also useful for planning medical care, social services, hospital services, and nursing home needs.

Because prevention of risk factors is important to prevent development of diseases in the future, there are surveys that focus primarily on risky behaviors and can provide data for a state or region of the country (see Table 4-4). The largest one is the Behavioral Risk Factor Surveillance System, which has been operational since 1984. This survey is developed and coordinated by the Centers for Disease Control and Prevention (CDC) but is administered by each state by phone to a statistically sampled group of adults aged 18 and older. Because it is administered by phone, only individuals with landline phones are eligible to be included. This methodology excludes data collection from low-income or homeless individuals, as well as from adults who do not maintain a landline (primarily young adults). Another problem has to do with the low number of people who respond to the survey. Fewer people are favorable to completing surveys on the phone, and innovative methods are being discussed for obtaining this information in the future. Some of the strategies being discussed include using website resources.

The source of risk factor information for adolescents in grades 9-12 is based on the Youth Risk Behavior Surveillance System (YRBSS). This survey is administered in a school setting to a statistically selected sample of schools in the United States, and estimates are made for the entire country. Students who are not in school on the day of the administration and those who have dropped out of school are not eligible to be included, thus missing an important group of adolescents who may have particularly risky behaviors.

TABLE 4-4 National Risk Factor Surveillance Systems Sponsored by the Centers for Disease Control and Prevention

Name	Population	Years	Topics
Behavioral Risk Factor Surveillance System (BRFSS)	Adults aged 18 and older with land phone lines	1984 to present	Smoking, physical inactivity, and other risk behaviors
Youth Risk Behavior Surveillance System (YRBSS)	Adolescents in grades 9-12	1991 to present	Smoking, physical inactivity, and other risk behaviors

Based on Centers for Disease Control and Prevention, Youth Risk Behavior Surveillance System (YRBSS): http://www.cdc.gov/brfss/ and http://www.cdc.gov/HealthyYouth/yrbs/index.htm

INTERNATIONAL HEALTH SURVEYS

World Health Organization (WHO): the coordinating authority for health within the United Nations system of 193 member countries

Although all countries have one or more centralized health data systems, one of the best sources of international health data is from the **World Health Organization (WHO)**, the coordinating authority for health within the United Nations system of 193 member countries (http://www.who.int). Among other things, WHO is responsible for providing leadership on shaping the global health research agenda, setting norms and standards, and monitoring and assessing population health trends worldwide. Although international standards for causes of death have been in place since the 1890s, not all countries consistently used them, nor were they updated on a regular basis.

Historical Note 4-2

William Farr

William Farr (1807–1883), a British epidemiologist, is also known as one of the founders of the field of medical statistics. When he was asked to collect "cause of death" information on the residents of England and Wales, he found the system currently used to classify diseases had not been revised to allow for the advances of medical science. In addition, the information was not standardized and could not be used for statistical purposes. For example, the same disease could have several different names, and practitioners filling out the Bills of Mortality (death certificates) used their own terminology. Farr urged the adoption of a uniform system as follows:

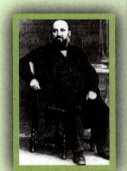

Courtesy of Wikipedia Commons: http://en.wikipedia.org/wiki/File:Farr_william1870.gif

> The advantages of a uniform statistical nomenclature, however imperfect, are so obvious, that it is surprising no attention has been paid to its enforcement in Bills of Mortality. Each disease has, in many instances, been denoted by three or four terms, and each term has been applied to as many different diseases: vague, inconvenient names have been employed, or complications have been registered instead of primary diseases. The nomenclature is of as much importance in this department of inquiry as weights and measures in the physical sciences, and should be settled without delay.

Sources: http://www.who.int/classifications/icd/en/HistoryOfICD.pdf; http://en.wikipedia.org/wiki/File:Farr_william1870.gif

Because the classification of disease varied from country to country and even within a country from year to year or from provider to provider, one major responsibility of the World Health Organization (WHO) in 1948 was to take over the support of an **International Classification of Disease (ICD)** system that could be used worldwide for assigning mortality codes. For assigning morbidity (such as hospital diagnoses), a clinical modification was added (ICD-CM). The ICD (and ICD-CM) is updated regularly, and the latest version (tenth revision: ICD-10 and ICD-10-CM), which has been available for use since 1994, will become the standard in 2013. Up until then, the ICD-9 and ICD-9-CM will be used.

In addition to this important role, WHO collects and publishes data on health statistics using standard questions for the purposes of comparison, as well as provides technical expertise to countries that want to develop their own data systems. Most of the international health comparison data that is published comes from one of the many WHO publications and is also available online at no cost. The annual World Health Statistics reports present the most recent international health statistics and are a valuable source of comparison and trend data.

Examples of nationwide health surveys from other countries include the Australian National Health Survey, which tracks the health status of the country and includes up-to-date data on diseases and risk factors. This survey, along with related census data (denominator data) is collected by the Australian Bureau of Statistics (http://www.abs.gov.au). For Canada, nationwide statistics from various surveys are published through Health Reports from Statistics Canada (http://www.statcan.gc.ca). For Great Britain, general health statistics for the country and different regions are collected, summarized, and reported by the Office for National Statistics (http://www.statistics.gov.uk).

> **International Classification of Disease (ICD):** a standardized format for recording deaths and diseases; revised periodically (last revision, ICD-10, in 1994)

OTHER SOURCES OF DATA

Sometimes it is not possible to answer a particular health question using the routinely collected data sets just discussed. In this situation, it may be necessary to develop a special-purpose study or to obtain data from other sources. Depending on the question that needs to be answered, there are many opportunities to get information from existing data in a number of settings.

Registries

> **registry:** a listing containing information from people with a particular condition or risk factor

A **registry** in its simplest form is a listing of information. CDC defines a registry as: "an organized system for the collection, storage, retrieval, analysis, and dissemination of information on individual persons who have either a particular disease, a condition (e.g., a risk factor) that predisposes to the occurrence of a health-related event, or prior exposure to substances (or circumstances) known or suspected to cause adverse health effects" (NCVHS, 2010). There are several registries that collect public health data as shown in Table 4-5.

TABLE 4-5 Public Health Registries

National Exposure Registry	The National Exposure Registry, operated by the Agency for Toxic Substances and Disease Registries, is designed to identify and enroll persons who may have been exposed to a hazardous environmental substance and to conduct follow-up monitoring of these persons.
The Metropolitan Atlanta Congenital Defects Program	The purpose of this registry, operated by CDC, is to monitor the occurrence of serious malformations in a defined population for changes in trends and unusual patterns that may suggest avoidable risk factors and to maintain a case registry for epidemiologic and genetic studies.
Immunization Registries	Immunization registries, supported by both federal and state funds, are currently established in many states. These registries are computerized systems that will consolidate and record vaccination histories of numerous individuals—and that will have information for an entire community—on the basis of information provided from a large number of health care providers.
Surveillance, Epidemiology, and End Results (SEER) Program	The SEER Program, supported by the National Cancer Institute, collects cancer data on a routine basis from designated population-based cancer registries in the United States.
Insulin-dependent Diabetes Mellitus Registries	Currently there are over 20 insulin-dependent diabetes mellitus (IDDM) registries in the United States and throughout the world. The purpose of these registries is to determine the incidence of IDDM in defined populations and to identify persons for subsequent enrollment in case-control studies and other research projects.
The United States Eye Injury Registry (USEIR)	The United States Eye Injury Registry, a nonprofit organization sponsored by the Helen Keller Eye Research Foundation, is a federation of state eye registries that uses a standardized form to obtain voluntarily reported data on eye injuries and to obtain six-month follow-up information.
Rare Diseases Registries	There are over a dozen registries listed on the Internet in the Organizational Database maintained by the National Organization for Rare Disorders.

Based on National Committee on Vital and Health Statistics: http://www.ncvhs.hhs.gov/9701138b.htm

The most common type of registry used for health studies is a cancer registry. In the United States, the Surveillance, Epidemiology, and End Results (SEER: http:// seer.cancer.gov/) Program of the National Cancer Institute (NCI) provides information on cancer incidence and survival in the United States. SEER currently collects data on patient demographics, primary tumor site, tumor morphology and stage at diagnosis, first course of treatment, and follow-up for vital status. From these data, cancer incidence and survival data statistics are published annually. The SEER registry provides estimated incidence data for the whole United States by statistically summarizing information received from population-based cancer registries covering approximately 28% of the U.S. population. Mortality data reported are provided by NCHS for the entire country, and the population data used in calculating cancer rates are obtained periodically from the Census Bureau. To address the quality of the reports received from the area registries, NCI staff work with the North American Association of Central Cancer Registries (NAACCR) to ensure data content and compatibility acceptable for pooling data and improving national estimates.

Local information for a state or a county can often be obtained using state-based cancer registries. All registries can take advantage of using standard data collection information provided by NAACCR.

Hospitals, Clinics, Physician Offices, Laboratories

It would seem that the best records about disease conditions would come from hospitals, clinics, and related laboratories where patients are diagnosed and treated. There are several problems with this approach. First of all, not all diseases are severe enough to require hospitalization or to be reported to a central agency by physician offices or laboratories. Another problem is that individuals may be seen at several locations, which may lead to overcounting. The choice of health providers varies with location, and insurance issues are such that people in the same neighborhood may get their health care and diagnoses at different locations, which makes defining a geographic area (denominator) difficult. The best use of data from these sources is to supplement ongoing data registries or to confirm diagnoses for reporting specific diseases. Many of the notifiable diseases (see Table 4-2) are reported directly from these sources (hospitals, clinics, and laboratories).

USING DATA SOURCES FOR SURVEILLANCE

public health surveillance: a system for monitoring health events in a defined population

Surveillance involves measuring diseases and risk factors over time to understand the scope of a problem, to allocate resources to control emerging problems, and to monitor the success of interventions. **Public health surveillance** is a system designed to assess and control problems that affect the population. There are several necessary steps for conducting an effective public health surveillance system. These include collecting, analyzing, and interpreting data, then disseminating the results to relevant agencies. The key elements of a surveillance system includes a data source (or multiple data sources) for a defined area (assume an entire country), a standardized set of items that can be repeated on a regular basis (annually, for example), and feedback to the responsible health agencies.

Issues that require surveillance arise from problems identified by health care workers or the public, and these problems usually spread easily or indicate an emerging health problem. Once a problem is defined, existing data systems are used (if possible) to track the problem. Effective surveillance systems make use of multiple data sources to obtain a complete picture of the problem and lead to potential interventions. For example, surveillance of risk factors, such as smoking, has been used to monitor smoking initiation among adolescents. Regular reports are generated and analyzed. The interpretation of these results is summarized and presented to the relevant agencies for action. Once this information is received, health agencies can make decisions as how to best implement control measures, whether the problem is an infectious disease, a chronic disease, or a risky behavior. Over time, the surveillance system continues to track the same problem to see if intervention efforts have been successful, or, if necessary, the system is modified to track a new problem. Refer to Figure 4-3 and the example of childhood obesity to see how these elements form a loop.

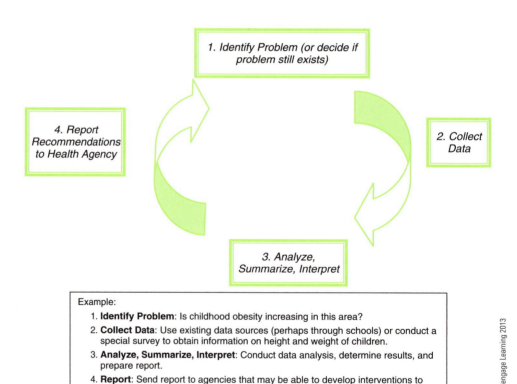

1. Identify Problem (or decide if problem still exists)

2. Collect Data

3. Analyze, Summarize, Interpret

4. Report Recommendations to Health Agency

Example:
1. **Identify Problem**: Is childhood obesity increasing in this area?
2. **Collect Data**: Use existing data sources (perhaps through schools) or conduct a special survey to obtain information on height and weight of children.
3. **Analyze, Summarize, Interpret**: Conduct data analysis, determine results, and prepare report.
4. **Report**: Send report to agencies that may be able to develop interventions to control problem.

FIGURE 4-3 Information Loop for Public Health Surveillance

Summary

In this chapter, we learned about existing health data systems and their use in monitoring the health status of people both in the United States and in other parts of the world. We also learned about data systems used for surveillance and research studies. Advantages and disadvantages of these various systems were explored. The benefits of monitoring health and risk factors were discussed.

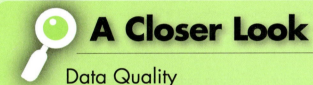

A Closer Look

Data Quality

The analysis of health data is only as good as the quality of the data collected, and several factors can affect that quality. These factors can include incomplete information, coding errors or misclassifications, and data processing errors.

Incomplete Information

Although standardized forms (such as birth and death certificates) are important and very useful, many times the information listed on the certificate may not be complete. This happens for a number of reasons. For death certificates, the person recording the items may not know the details of the decedent's personal history to correctly record risk factors as listed on the certificate (e.g., smoking, occupation). Likewise, for birth certificates, some of the information requested on the form is not available prior to the form being sent forward for inclusion in the national database. Examples are birth defects that are not identified until later. Although birth and death certificates are collected within days of the event and submitted so that statistics are available in a few months, changes or alterations to the certificates or additional data items that were not completed initially can be sent later. Some data sets, such as cancer registries, may not have the complete information on a subject (including pathology reports and initial treatment) available until several months after the diagnosis.

Misclassification

In addition to the completeness of the data, other factors may play a role in affecting the quality of the data. Misclassification of the cause of death can happen when the recorder transcribes the handwritten notes of the physician (or whoever filled out the death certificate) into a standardized coding system (such as the ICD-10). There are over 14,000 possible codes with many subtle differences that may be hard to evaluate. For example, if the cause of death was melanoma (cancer) of the eye, the death certificate may specify eye disease and would not be coded as cancer of the eye. Another misclassification issue has to do with the underlying cause of death. For example, if a person dies of heart disease, the fact that a person has diabetes may not be recorded as one of the underlying causes. This could occur when the person filling out the death certificate is not familiar with the medical history of the patient.

Continues

Data Processing Errors

Errors can creep into a data file from many different sources from simple typos to misunderstanding the question being asked. Data processing errors can also come into play when data are sent from many different locations (such as cancer registries) to a central area in similar but not identical formats. One way to pick up on this type of error is to spot check a dozen or so records, comparing the electronic information to the original document. Another way to identify data processing errors is to pay careful attention to the out-of-range values. Although it might be easy to pick up large errors (e.g., ages and dates that are out of range), subtle errors may go unnoticed. Computer-assisted data entry has been useful in reducing the number of errors that make their way into a completed data set. This approach involves programming a computer to verify each entry before it can be saved. If this is done while the person is being interviewed, conflicting information can be corrected immediately. If it is done afterwards, the investigator can make decisions as to how to handle conflicting information.

Wrap-Up

These are just examples of issues to be aware of when working with data collected from multiple sources and helps to explain why collecting and maintaining a quality data set is an expensive proposition, but worth the effort. Taking care of the errors that can be identified from manipulating the data files is called "cleaning the data," an important first step before any analysis can begin. The old computer saying "Garbage In = Garbage Out" applies here.

Review Questions

1. List one of the data systems used to track the health status of a community.

    _____

2. Which of the following statements are true of using vital health records? (Check all that apply.)
    a. You can obtain standard information for the whole United States.
    b. Information obtained is timely.
    c. Not all U.S. states and territories report through the vital status system.
    d. Accuracy of the data may be limited because of missing information.

3. **True or False** It is easy to use data systems to compare health status between countries.

4. Which data source(s) would you use to look for trends in health behaviors among youth?

    _____

5. **True or False** There are data files to use for assessing health trends and behaviors in the United States over the past 50 years.

6. **True or False** Using the International Classification of Disease system assists in comparing data over time and between data systems.

7. Which of the following data systems would be useful in finding new cases of a specific disease, such as cancer?
   a. Hospital admission records
   b. University researchers
   c. Cancer registry
   d. National Health Interview Survey

8. Match the list in the left column with the appropriate letter from the list in the right column. (Letters from the right column may be used more than once.)

____Numerator of infant mortality rate	a. midyear population
____Denominator of infant mortality rate	b. # of deaths < 1 year of age
____Denominator of cause-specific mortality rate	c. # of live births
____Denominator of age-specific mortality rate	d. # of deaths from a particular disease
____Numerator of cause-specific mortality rate	e. deaths in persons aged 1-14
____Numerator of age-specific mortality rate	f. # deaths in total population
	g. midyear population aged 1-14

9. **For Deeper Thought** State funding for a childhood injury prevention program has just become available. To gather baseline data on childhood injuries, the staff is discussing whether to conduct a survey or to establish a surveillance system. Discuss the advantages and disadvantages of these two approaches.

Website Resources

Australian Health Survey: http://www.abs.gov

Birth/Death Certificates: http://www.cdc.gov

Census data: http://www.census.gov

Health Statistics Great Britain: http://www.statistics.gov.uk

Health U.S.A., 2009: http://www.cdc.gov/nchs/data

Mortality MMWR: http://www.cdc.gov/mmwr

NCHS Trend data: http://www.cdc.gov. Search for "National Center for Health Statistics." Click on "Publications" for up-to-date reports and health briefs.

Reportable Diseases: http://www.cdc.gov. Search for "National Notifiable Diseases Surveillance System" (NNDSS).

Vital Statistics online data: http://www.cdc.gov. Search for "National Vital Statistics System" (NVSS) to visit the homepage.

WHO: http://www.who.int

References

Centers for Disease Control and Prevention. (2011). Nationally Notifiable Conditions. Retrieved from http://www.cdc.gov/osels/ph_surveillance/nndss/phs/files/NNC_2011_Notification_Requirements_By_Category.pdf

Centers for Disease Control and Prevention. (2010). About the National Vital Statistics System. Retrieved from http://www.cdc.gov/nchs/nvss/about_nvss.htm

National Cancer Institute. (2010). Surveillance Epidemiology and End Results (SEER). Retrieved from http://seer.cancer.gov

National Committee on Vital and Health Statistics. (2010). What Is a Registry? Retrieved from http://www.ncvhs.hhs.gov/9701138b.htm

Chapter 5

STUDY DESIGN

Learning Objectives

Upon completion of this chapter, you should be able to:

1. List and describe the goals of a study design.
2. Discuss the difference between observational versus experimental study designs and the difference between descriptive versus analytic studies.
3. Describe commonly used study designs—cohort, case control, cross-sectional, and ecological.
4. Explain the advantages and disadvantages of each of the observational study designs.
5. Explain how to interpret basic results of each study design.

Key Terms

analytic study

case control study

cohort study

confounder

cross-sectional study

descriptive study

ecological study

experimental study

follow-up period

incident cases

loss to follow-up

observational study

prevalence study

prospective cohort study

retrospective cohort study

source population

stratified random sampling

time at risk

Chapter Outline

INTRODUCTION

It is very common to see news reports about the results of studies in public health that have the findings reduced to a few "sound bites." These sounds bites are very often valid, but they can be misleading without the appropriate context for the study on which the news report is based. For example, say there was a report that women had a nine times greater risk than men of "season-ending" knee injuries in varsity athletes in a university population. Based on this sound bite, concerned athletic directors at universities all over the country would read this report and begin to wonder what they could do to protect their female athletes. But those athletic directors who had taken a basic course in epidemiology would know that they should first ask themselves three basic questions for a sound bite such as this. The questions that should be asked when interpreting the findings of any study are:

1. What is the magnitude of the hypothesized outcome?

2. What population characteristics do the findings apply to?

3. How were the data collected?

The first of these questions applies to the impact of a study's findings. Although it is true that a risk of "nine times greater than" is very strong and very likely important, the first question asked should be about how often the outcome under study occurs. So although it is very concerning that women are at such greater risk, it is possible that men may have a very low incidence of the outcome, which would also mean women have a very low incidence of outcome as well, even with nine times the risk. In other words, "nine times zero is still zero." So this first question should be asked about any study to begin to understand the true impact of a news report.

The remaining two questions that an athletic director with a basic knowledge of epidemiology would ask about the report of the study pertain to the concept of study design. Study design in epidemiology is the methodology used to determine to whom the results will refer and how to collect the data. First, many times the report will not thoroughly describe the population in which the study was performed. A basic understanding of epidemiology tells us that the characteristics of any population can easily influence the results (or misinterpretation) of a study. So if the population characteristics of a study differ from the population we are concerned about, the results may not apply. Second, reports may also not thoroughly describe how the data were collected. The methods used to collect the data for any study will strongly influence the conclusions that can be drawn from a study.

So let us find out the answers to these three questions about the news study reported above that found women were at such an increased risk for severe injury. As it turns out, the knee injury under study was in fact a career-ending injury, but this knee injury was very rare and there had been a rate of 1 per 100,000 of these knee injuries in male athletes at this university in the past 5 years. But the study found a rate of this same knee injury in women to be 9 per 100,000; but in order to get a large enough sample of women, the time period for the women was past 10 years. The data on injuries in men were collected by reviewing the athletes' medical records, but the data on injuries in women were collected by asking the women to describe their injuries over the last 10 years on a questionnaire mailed to their homes. The university conducting the study was a very small technical school that does not provide a budget for athletic training and has only one varsity sport. Finally, the study was performed in 2010, but the data covered the years 1995 through 2005. If the news report had provided these details, how many athletic directors would now be concerned about their female athletes?

Even with these very few additional pieces of information, we think differently about the results. Of the three questions asked, the last two refer to the study design. Study design affects our ability to answer research questions and our ability to apply the results of a study. Many people involved in epidemiologic studies very wisely spend a lot of time developing the methods they will use to enroll subjects and to collect their data.

A major part of study design is determining the desired characteristics of the study population and developing methods to acquire an appropriate sample. The other major part of study design is deciding how to collect data from these subjects. Throughout this chapter, the basic design methodology necessary to collect data from the desired population will be discussed, as well as the appropriate interpretation of results from the most common study designs.

GOALS OF STUDY DESIGN

Why do we perform a study? In epidemiology, the purpose of a study is usually to identify the amount of disease (distribution) or to test hypotheses about the risk factors (determinants) of disease. Another purpose of a study is to identify characteristics of disease that will be **confounders** of a hypothesis. (Confounding is discussed in more detail in Chapter 7, Accuracy.) Evaluating an intervention, such as an education program or a vaccine, may also be the target of a study to be considered.

In order to perform a study in epidemiology, we must first design it. The goal of study design is to develop the methods necessary to accomplish the goals of the study. Good study design starts with three key elements: (1) who, (2) what, and (3) when. Who is the study intended to represent? What is the disease or outcome under study? When is the risk period for the outcome? Each of these questions must be answered prior to designing a study.

For example, if a study is intended to refer to an elderly population in a retirement home (*who*), it would not be wise to collect data from a young population. Also, the disease under study (*what*) will affect the design. If the disease to be studied is a rare disease, it would not be wise to study a small group of people without knowing if there is anyone in the group with the disease. A study needs to be performed during the correct time frame (*when*) the risk period is ongoing. So it would not be wise to perform a study of the risk factors for influenza during the summer.

Once the three key elements of study design have been identified, the methods for enrolling subjects and collecting data can be developed. The overall goals of the design of a study (in no particular order) are listed in Table 5-1. An initial look at these goals recognizes that the design of the study must first follow the goals of the study.

confounder: a variable that is not the hypothesized exposure of interest or the outcome of interest but one that causes confusion or distortion of the measures of association

To illustrate, if the study is intended to test a hypothesis, then the design must be developed that will allow the hypothesis to be tested. If the study is intended to represent a specific population, such as pregnant women, then the design must be developed that will allow the results to be applied to pregnant women. Although there are general goals of study design, each study is designed with differences that are based on the goals of the study.

TABLE 5-1 Goals of Study Design
Represent desired population.
Allow appropriate determination of outcome/disease.
Eliminate and reduce bias.
Identify confounders and control for confounding.
Test hypotheses.
Find associations or evidence for causality.
Evaluate the intervention.

© Cengage Learning 2013

Represent Desired Population

The goals of study design in Table 5-1 can be achieved using a wide variety of methods. In most any scenario, the first goal listed will be addressed. Once the reference population is identified, methods for selecting subjects should be developed to enroll a study group who will represent this identified population. For example, if the goal of the study is to identify the relationship between exercise and cardiovascular disease in city bus drivers, the study would need to be sure to enroll subjects with the same characteristics as the actual city bus drivers. One way to do this is to actually enroll a group of city bus drivers as the study sample. Another way would be to learn about the characteristics of city bus drivers and then enroll a study sample with similar characteristics.

Allow Appropriate Determination of Outcome/Disease

The second goal of study design listed in Table 5-1 is to ensure that methods are chosen that will allow the appropriate determination of the outcome. Issues of outcome assessment are covered in Chapter 3, Measuring Disease Occurrence and Exposure, but it is important to develop methods that can make a valid determination whether or not the study subjects have the outcome.

In the case of the study to identify the relationship of exercise and cardiovascular disease in city bus drivers, the study design must include methods to allow the valid assessment of cardiovascular disease. For example, is it better to ask subjects whether they have cardiovascular disease, or is it better to review medical records of subjects for existing diagnosis of cardiovascular disease, or is it better to have a research physician clinically examine all subjects looking for cardiovascular disease, or is better to enroll subjects who do not have cardiovascular disease and then examine them regularly over time to see who develops cardiovascular disease? These are the kinds of decisions that need to be made when designing a study.

Eliminate and Reduce Bias and Identify Confounders

Other goals of study design include addressing issues of bias and confounding. Both of these concepts are discussed in detail in Chapter 7, Accuracy. However, when designing a study, some very important design goals are to collect valid data, recruit appropriate subjects, and collect data on the variables that may distort the results of the study (confounders). Many very simple methods address these issues.

For example, when determining the method of recruitment for a study, the choice to "knock on doors" in a neighborhood will affect the subjects contacted as potential study subjects. If the methods suggest that knocking on doors during the weekdays is the chosen method, then it should not be expected that too many people with "9 to 5" jobs will be recruited. Further, if the methods suggest that hypertension will be ascertained by asking subjects if they have high blood pressure, it can be expected that some cases of hypertension will be missed because the subjects have not recently seen a clinician, or because they have forgotten their diagnosis, or because they do not understand the term "hypertension."

Even the simplest methods can lead to dramatic and damaging systematic errors that can distort study results; so when designing a study, it is important that all methods address the concepts of bias and confounding.

Test Hypotheses

Enabling investigators to test a hypothesis, if that is the intention of performing the study, is a further goal of study design. As discussed in Chapter 1, a hypothesis is a statement of an expected relationship between an independent variable (exposure) and a dependent variable (outcome) that an investigator is trying to prove (or disprove) in a study.

In order to be able to test the hypothesis, the study must be designed to allow appropriate comparisons of subjects who have different levels of the independent variable. This appropriate comparison comes from developing methods for all aspects of the study that ensure the comparison groups are handled in the same way. If the comparison groups are handled the same, then investigators can be more confident that any differences between the comparison groups (such as risk of outcome) are true differences, not the result of improper methods.

For example, in the study about female versus male athletes and the risk of knee injuries, the knee injuries were ascertained differently for the men compared to the women. A clinician examined the men, but the women were simply asked to self-report if they had the specific knee injury. These two different methods of knee injury ascertainment would result in a different potential for error between men and women. So if there were differences in the risk of injury between men and women, the investigators could not be sure that it was NOT a result of the study design. Equally concerning would be that the risk of knee injury appears to be the same between men and women; however, with the different methods of ascertainment, the truth may be that there is a difference in risk, but the methods do not allow it to be seen. Both of these scenarios could lead to erroneous conclusions as a result of the study design. For those studies with the goal of testing a hypothesis, the study design must include the methods that allow these scientifically valid comparisons.

Find Associations or Evidence for Causality

Although similar to testing hypotheses, another goal of study design is to allow the ability to search for new associations, as well as to provide evidence toward causality by finding these associations. This goal is very often included in studies that have other goals as well.

The search for new associations may not start with a "known hypothesis." The idea may be to look for characteristics and outcomes that are related to each other in the study sample. To enable this search, methods that collect data in the most accurate way possible and in the most consistent manner possible must be developed for the study. This leads to the need to identify all of the important characteristics and variables that should be collected to search for new associations. Even the most accurately collected data, though, cannot substitute for the failure to recognize and collect information on important variables.

Many discoveries in public health have come from studies that have found new associations, but only associations from well-designed studies can be trusted.

Evaluate the Intervention

The last goal of study design in Table 5-1 pertains to those studies with the goal of evaluating an intervention such as a drug treatment, surgical procedure, vaccine, or education program. These studies are similar to those that test a hypothesis, but the investigators somehow influence the experience of the comparison groups.

For example, a study may intend to determine whether an education program can influence the behavior of members of a community. Some members receive the education program and others do not. Then the behavior of all of the members is ascertained. The study must be designed to ensure that any differences in the behavior are the result of the education program, not to other influences or poor study design.

GENERAL CLASSIFICATIONS OF STUDY DESIGNS

Study designs can be complex or simple. However, from the simplest design to the most complex, they all have one characteristic in common. Study designs are a compilation of a number of methods that determine (1) how the data will be collected and (2) the characteristics of the study sample population. So although many investigators new to epidemiology consider study design a scary concept, the reality is that study design is nothing more than a "label" for the "universe" of methods that are used to address a research or epidemiology goal. Once the study methods have been developed, investigators can apply a number of labels to the study, and these labels are based on just a few key attributes of the methods.

Before beginning to label study designs, remember this important context: no two study designs are exactly alike, but general labels are used to describe important distinctions between the designs. As an analogy, individual study designs can be like people. There are general categories for describing people such as gender, height, eye color, hair color, and so on. These general categories can be used by themselves—so if we only describe a person's gender as male, we are making no comment about his height. Conversely, if we describe a person's height as tall, we are making no comment on that person's gender. Both of these can be true about the same person. Or that person can be included in the "male" category but not included in the "tall" category and vice versa. However, when we combine these categories, we develop a better description of the individual. The following general descriptions of study design will provide large distinctions between designs, but the labels are not exclusive of each other, and a study is better described by using many of the descriptors at once.

Observational versus Experimental

One type of label for study designs is used to describe whether the study is **observational** or **experimental**. When the investigator only gathers data from the subjects, it is *observational*; when the investigator intervenes with the subjects in some way such as a drug treatment, education program, or vaccine, it is *experimental*. This label does not fully describe the entire study but does provide one general category of the study design.

An example of an observational study would be a study intended to investigate the relationship between cigarette smoking and lung cancer in which the investigator only determines each subject's smoking behavior and whether or not he or she develops lung cancer. The smoking behavior may be assessed in a variety of ways—such as self-report, a questionnaire, or direct observation—but if the investigator is only concerned with assessing the smoking behavior, without trying to influence the subject's smoking behavior, then the study design is labeled an observational study. However, if the investigator includes an attempt to influence the subject's smoking behavior through an intervention in order to determine if lung cancer risk can be reduced, then the study design is labeled as an experimental study.

observational study: study in which the investigator only gathers data from the subjects

experimental study: study in which the investigator intervenes with the subjects in some ways

Descriptive versus Analytic

Another general classification of study design refers to whether the study is **descriptive** or **analytic**. Many studies in epidemiology are intended to determine the distribution of disease in a population (*descriptive study*). These types of studies are developed to find the level of disease or risk factors in a given population. In a descriptive study, data can be collected by a variety of methods from subjects who represent the population of interest with the purpose of finding the rates and characteristics of diseases and risk factors. Descriptive studies provide valuable information about the distribution of disease in a population and are used to develop public health interventions, policies, and needs for services.

On the other hand, an *analytic study* is the label for a study that tests one or more hypotheses about the relationship between risk factors and disease, generally looking for causation. Like a descriptive study, an analytic study collects data from subjects who represent populations of interest, but, in addition, the study methods are developed to allow appropriate comparisons between groups of subjects with different characteristics of the hypothesized exposures.

> **descriptive study:** a study intended to determine the distribution of disease in a population
>
> **analytic study:** a study that tests one or more hypotheses about the relationship between risk factors and disease, generally looking for causation

THE PERSPECTIVE OF TIME IN STUDY DESIGN

Of all the ways to label a study design, the most common and most useful is based on the time frame of the study. Remember the discussion of the relationship of time in the measure of disease occurrence discussed in Chapter 3, Measuring Disease Occurrence and Exposure. Knowing whether cases of disease were new (incidence) or had already occurred and were existing (prevalence) is very important to the usefulness of a rate. This time frame is very important and useful in study design as well.

When describing the time frame of a study, the "cornerstone" of a study is the time "window" during which the investigator (or other individual) actually collects the data from the subjects for the FIRST TIME. For example, it may take an investigator 24 hours or even longer to collect the data from subjects. This means that the window of time would be the entire length of time it takes the investigator to collect the initial data from the subjects. Also, the investigator (or the individuals collecting the data) may have collected the initial data from subjects previously, say, last year. When discussing the time frame of a study, it is important to identify when the initial data were collected from the subjects.

As an example of describing the initial data collection in epidemiology, consider a study designed to investigate the relationship between cigarette smoking and lung cancer. The investigators decide to send a consent form and questionnaire to 1,000 potential study subjects. Over the next two months, subjects return the completed consent form and questionnaire to the investigators. In this scenario, the initial data collection window would be defined as the two months during which the investigators are collecting the data from the subjects. Another example would be if investigators decide to use data that their colleagues collected from subjects two years ago. The subjects were classified according to smoking behavior two years ago, which established their initial smoking behavior category. In this scenario, the initial data collection window would be two years ago when the initial data were collected from the subjects.

Why all the discussion about the definition of the initial data collection window? In epidemiology, the time frame of a study, which will be used to label

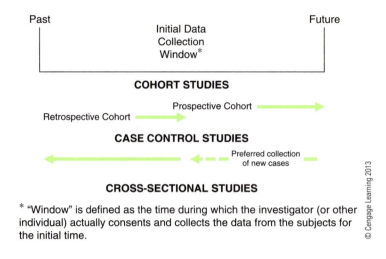

FIGURE 5-1 Observational Studies

the study design, is dependent on the appropriate definition of this window. To misunderstand or to erroneously establish the initial data collection window can lead to inappropriate use of the results from a study. It can also lead to an inappropriate classification of disease with respect to incidence or prevalence, and it has been previously discussed how important it is to get that correct. In the next several sections of this chapter, we will discuss the most common labels of study design in epidemiology, and the ability to correctly use these labels will only be achieved if the definition of initial data collection window is understood completely.

As an overview of the following sections, consider the use of the initial data collection window in Figure 5-1. In the center of the timeline is the "Initial Data Collection Window" preceded by the "Past" and succeeded by the "Future." In this figure, the definition of "window" is as described above and is the time during which the data were collected initially from the subjects. Once the time frame of the window is established, then the data collected during the study can be put into context of whether it is from the past, only from the present, or from the future. Each of these three possibilities is described in detail in the next three sections, and each determines the overall name of the study design.

COLLECTING DATA BASED ON EXPOSURE: COHORT DESIGN

The scientific "gold standard" of observational study designs in epidemiology is known as the **cohort study**. The cohort study is the only observational design that truly *measures incidence of the outcome* and by definition is the only observational design that *allows the determination of risk*. In a cohort design, the investigator gathers data on the independent variables (exposures) from the study subjects and then determines which subjects develop the hypothesized outcome of interest.

> **cohort study:** a study that compares subjects according to exposure status

The cohort study has two possible time frames: (1) following outcome-free subjects only into the future to ascertain outcome (**prospective cohort study**) or (2) utilizing exposure information of subjects from the past and then ascertaining outcome from the present (**retrospective cohort study**). However, notice that regardless of the time frame, a cohort study still *compares subjects according to their exposure status.*

The length of the cohort study time frame will either be the amount of time that a prospective cohort is followed into the future (**follow-up period**) or the amount of time back in the past that the exposure and independent variables are ascertained in a retrospective cohort design.

As displayed in Figure 5-1, the prospective cohort study *begins with the initial collection of all exposure and independent variables from the subjects at the time of data collection.* At this time, subjects are also excluded from the study if they already have the outcome of interest. Then, once this baseline information is collected, the *subjects are followed into the future.* The subjects are followed to observe who develops the outcome of interest during the follow-up period. Using this method, any outcome observed during the follow-up period is counted as incidence, or a new event. Allowing the assessment of incidence of the outcome is one of the major benefits of a prospective cohort study.

The retrospective cohort study also begins with the initial collection of the exposure and all independent variables from the subjects, but these variables are ascertained from a time in the subjects' past. Then, the *outcome information on the subjects is determined up to the current time that the data are collected.* The ability of an investigator to determine incidence data from a retrospective cohort design depends on whether the subjects were able to be established as outcome-free from the time in the past when exposure and independent variables were ascertained. If subjects can be determined to be outcome-free at the same time the initial variables are ascertained, then it can be expected that the outcomes present at the time the data are collected are new and can be called incidence. However, if it is possible that the subjects had the outcome at the time that the exposure and independent variables are ascertained, then the investigator is unable to call the outcomes "new."

Cohort studies are designed to compare those with the exposure of interest to those without the exposure of interest. That is why this study design collects data based on exposure. In fact, a key to performing a valid prospective cohort study is to ensure that any potential subjects who already have the outcome are excluded. This way, any outcome assessed during the follow-up period is in fact a new outcome. Unless all subjects are actively determined to be "outcome-free" at the beginning of the study time frame, it is impossible to know if the outcomes found during the study period are truly new. Consequently, the ideal baseline data for all subjects are only exposure data and any other independent variables that are part of the study. Then the investigators watch the subjects to see who develops the outcome. Once the study period is over, the incidence rates of outcome in the exposed and nonexposed groups are compared to determine if there is a relationship between the hypothesized exposure and outcome.

prospective cohort study: the design considered the "gold standard" of observational study designs; a study design that follows outcome-free subjects into the future to ascertain outcome; measures incidence and can determine risk

retrospective cohort study: a study design that ascertains exposure and independent variable information from the past and outcome up to the present

follow-up period: the length of time that study subjects are monitored in a prospective cohort design

Advantages of a Cohort Study Design

Some of the common advantages of a cohort study are listed in Table 5-2. As already discussed, a major advantage of a cohort study is to *accurately identify incidence data*; so it is the *only study design that can validly calculate relative risk or attributable risk*. Because incidence is necessary to determine risk, the cohort study design is the design that *allows the identification of risk and risk factors for the outcome*. Being able to identify risk factors for the same outcome contributes to the ability to establish that an exposure may be a "cause" of that outcome.

Another advantage of implementing a cohort design is that data collected are generally the *highest quality of any of the observational designs*. The reason for this is that all of the data, including both independent and dependent variables, are collected by the actual study investigators, according to a protocol designed specifically for this hypothesis. The need for consistency in the collection of any scientific data is fundamental to making valid conclusions. Further, the expectations are that in a cohort study, the individuals collecting data are trained, and the reliability of the data collected is checked. Lastly, in a cohort study, investigators can be in control of the data collection methodology and do everything possible to maintain high-quality data.

Using a cohort study allows investigators to *easily introduce an intervention into the design* if the opportunity arises. This advantage is not always important, but when the goal of a study is to evaluate an intervention, the design of choice should be a cohort design. This makes intuitive sense because it would be very difficult to evaluate an intervention by using data collected before the intervention occurred.

Cohort studies also provide the unique advantage of being able to *document the natural history of disease* (see Chapter 1). Beyond the natural history of disease, the cohort study also allows the documentation of how a disease will progress in a population even when there is treatment by health workers.

TABLE 5-2 Common Advantages of Cohort Studies
1. Allows true determination of incidence rates of outcome
2. Allows attributes associated with the outcome to be identified as risk factors
3. Enables the highest quality research data and information
4. Allows the evaluation of interventions
5. Allows the assessment and documentation of natural history of disease
6. Can assess multiple exposures and outcomes

An often overlooked advantage of a cohort study design is that investigators are *able to study multiple exposures at the same time*. The investigators can design the study to assess many exposure variables at the initial enrollment of subjects and continue to collect information on these exposures throughout the study time frame. In addition, the investigators can establish procedures that allow them to ascertain many different diseases or outcomes during the study time frame, as long as the subjects were free of that disease or outcome at the start of the study period. So a cohort study can support many different hypotheses using the exposures and outcomes that the investigators have included in their study protocol.

The cohort study also has an advantage of being *able to address changes in exposures in subjects over time* with valid information, allowing investigators to make choices about categorization of these exposures. For example, studying behaviors such as smoking cigarettes or physical activity is often "plagued" by the fact that over a period of time, these types of behaviors often change in study subjects. The changes may be dramatic and will often have an effect on the actual risk of the disease or outcome of interest. So in a well-designed cohort study, investigators will have the ability to measure and then categorize these behaviors in the subjects during the follow-up period. They can then decide how to utilize the data on the changes to more accurately reflect the true behavior experience of the subjects.

Disadvantages of a Cohort Study Design

Although cohort studies have many advantages and are generally the scientifically preferred method to investigate a hypothesis, there can be problems with the implementation of this design. Many consider the length of time and cost necessary to complete a cohort study a potential problem. However, performing a retrospective cohort study can reduce the amount of time necessary to perform the study. Another possible problem comes from the inability to keep track of the enrolled study subjects during the entire follow-up period in a prospective cohort study. There is also the possibility that only a few (or none) of the subjects will get the outcome during the designed follow-up period.

Of course, many things can go wrong with a cohort design if any of the methods are not well thought out or if they are inappropriately implemented. As with any study design, without a proper understanding of the topic, a thorough review of the literature, the appropriate consideration of bias and confounding, or the consistent handling of all comparison groups, even cohort studies can lead to inaccurate conclusions.

Enrolling Subjects in a Cohort Study

Because a cohort study is a design based on exposure, investigators must make a major decision about the process for enrollment of subjects. Consider that investigators have several options for enrolling subjects with respect to exposure category.

One option is to enroll subjects, then assess their exposure, and divide them into exposure categories. Using this method results in investigators not knowing exactly how many people will be in each exposure category. Consider a study with the hypothesis that smoking cigarettes is a risk factor for heart disease. With this enrollment option, investigators would enroll subjects, determine the subjects' smoking category, and then follow the subjects to find the incidence of heart disease in each smoking category.

Another option is to enroll subjects after identifying their exposure category. This method allows investigators to ensure that there are a prespecified number of subjects in each exposure category. Using the smoking and heart disease example, investigators would first determine potential subjects' smoking status and then enroll the predetermined number of subjects into each smoking category. The predetermined number of subjects for each category should be established such that it will make the study population referable to the desired population.

Several other options include enrolling subjects only with a specified exposure category and then using existing external groups that have known rates of outcome to be the comparison groups. The external group would not actually be enrolled in the study, but rates from the group can be used as a comparison to those measured in the enrolled group of exposed subjects. One possible comparison group would be an external group such as the "general" population that has information available about the outcome of interest during the same follow-up period. Another possible comparison group would be an external population that has information available about the outcome of interest from a past time period of similar length of time.

To continue with the smoking and heart disease example, using this enrollment option, investigators would enroll only smokers in the study population. Then the heart disease incidence in this enrolled group of smokers would be measured during the study time frame. The heart disease incidence from the enrolled group could then be compared to the heart disease incidence rate of the entire United States during the same time frame or during a previous, but equal length period of time. Of course, in the last couple of options, it must be recognized that there may be differences in the data collection methods in the comparison groups; these differences must be addressed.

Loss to Follow-Up

loss to follow-up: the number (or proportion) of enrolled subjects who cannot be followed for the entire time period of the study

An important aspect in the design of a cohort study is the method chosen to keep track of enrolled subjects over the often long study time frame. The importance of this effort cannot be overstated. **Loss to follow-up** in a prospective cohort study is defined as the number (or proportion) of enrolled subjects who cannot be followed for the entire time frame of the study. This loss may occur for known and/or unknown reasons. If the number of enrolled subjects who become lost to follow-up is too large, the ability to draw valid conclusions from the entire study can be damaged. Furthermore, if the loss to follow-up is concentrated among specific subgroups of the study group, even greater damage can occur to the study.

For example, in an extreme example, if the women in a study all decided to no longer participate before the study finished, but all the men continued to participate throughout the study period, the final results of the study would not reflect any differences (or similarities) with respect to gender.

Loss to follow-up is very important because all studies using human subjects must be voluntary, and a subject can stop participating at any time, with or without a reason. The methodology used to keep subjects in a long-term follow-up period must be initially developed and evolve to find ways to assist investigators to minimize loss to follow-up.

Some of the most successful ways to do this are to establish a sense of "community" and "purpose" within the study subjects very early in the follow-up period. Other ways to motivate subjects are to include financial incentives, health care incentives, and responsive feedback of information about the study to subjects. Depending on the length of the study period, minimizing loss to follow-up may be the most important activity in the performance of a cohort study.

Lastly, sufficient numbers of subjects should be enrolled in a cohort study so that the expected number of loss to follow-up can be accommodated without damaging the entire study.

Time at Risk

Time at risk is another important concept in a cohort study. **Time at risk** is the time that each individual accumulates between ascertaining the exposure and independent variable and developing the outcome. If the subject does not develop the outcome, then the time at risk for that individual continues to accumulate for the entire study time frame. The benefit of a cohort study is that it allows investigators to not only determine the incidence of the outcome in a population, but also to determine how much time at risk has accumulated for the entire study population. Further, investigators can also organize the time at risk into categories of the exposure of interest and compare the time at risk among those categories.

Figure 5-2 is a graphical presentation of a small prospective cohort study with 30 subjects followed for four years. Of the 30 subjects, 15 are exposed, and 15 are not exposed. The amount of time at risk for each subject is represented by a horizontal line with a length equal to the time that each subject was followed. The letter at the end of each line indicates whether the subject developed the outcome (O) or was lost to follow-up (L). If the line continues all the way to the end of the four years, that subject was followed the entire time without getting the outcome or being lost to follow-up. For example, the subject at that very top of the exposed group was followed for one year until getting the outcome.

The exposed and not exposed groups in the study presented in Figure 5-2 can be compared using the time at risk in two ways. The first way is to compare the incidence rates (discussed in Chapter 3) of both groups. In the exposed group, 9 of the 15 subjects developed the outcome before the end of the follow-up time period. In the not exposed group, 6 of the 15 subjects got the outcome before the end of the

time at risk: the time that each individual accumulates between exposure and independent variable ascertainment and getting the outcome or the end of the study

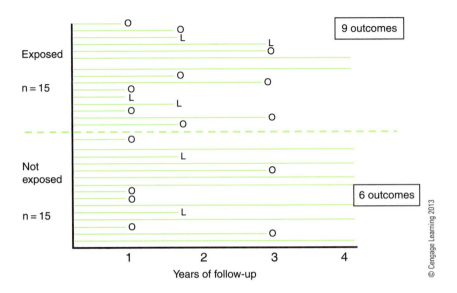

FIGURE 5-2 Diagram of Study Participants' Time in Study

follow-up period. So the risk in the exposed group is 9/15 × 100 = 60% per four years, and the risk in the not exposed group is 6/15 × 100 = 40% per four years.

The second way to compare the exposed and not exposed groups in Figure 5-2 is to use incidence densities (discussed in Chapter 3) in both groups. Add the time at risk in both groups and use it as the denominator for each group. Then, the number of new cases in each group is used as the numerator of a fraction with the time at risk as the denominator. The incidence density in the exposed group is 9 new cases in 34 person-years at risk, or 9/34 × 100 = 26.5 per 100 person-years. The incidence density in the not exposed group is 6 new cases in 42 person-years at risk, or 6/42 × 100 = 14.3 per 100 person-years.

Both the incidence rates and incidence densities are valid measures for this example, and in the next chapter, we will see how to compare these measures between the exposed and not exposed groups. However, the incidence density is used to demonstrate both the number of individuals with outcome and the amount of time at risk accumulated by the study subjects. The incidence density, by using the concept of person time discussed in Chapter 3, has the added ability to allow appropriate comparison of groups (such as exposed and not exposed) when the groups have very different sizes or different amounts of follow-up time. So in a prospective cohort study design, we not only have the ability to measure the outcome as a rate among the total number of individuals, but we also have the ability to measure the outcome as a density among the total person time at risk accumulated in the study.

Summary of a Cohort Study Design

To summarize a cohort study design, it is the study design that is the most scientifically desirable and allows an investigator to attempt to determine risk factors and "cause" for a disease. It is also the only study design that allows the true determination of the incidence of an outcome in a population. An investigator can study multiple hypotheses that include multiple exposure variables. Although the cohort design is considered a "complete" study design, it has disadvantages such as the long period of time necessary to perform the study, which usually results in increased costs. The design can also be very problematic if the disease being studied is rare because no one in the study population may get the disease during the follow-up period.

COLLECTING DATA BASED ON OUTCOME: CASE CONTROL STUDY DESIGN

In epidemiology, collecting data based on whether a subject has the outcome or not is a study design that makes sense to most people. If we are asking questions about the cause of a disease, it makes sense that those individuals with the disease will have the causative agent and that those without the disease will not have it.

The observational study design in which investigators collect data in a group of subjects with the outcome of interest, and also collect data in a group of subjects without the outcome of interest, is called a **case control study**. The case control study compares those subjects with the outcome to those without the outcome. The case control design has been traditionally also referred to as a "retrospective design" (this is not the same as the retrospective *cohort* design study), but recent changes in accepted use of this terminology argue against the similarity. The argument is that a case control study does not have to be retrospective; in other words, case control studies do not only have to rely on data from the past.

In a case control design, the investigators identify a group of potential subjects who have the outcome of interest; and if these subjects consent to participate, they become the "cases" for the study. The investigators then identify the population from which the cases came and select a sample of subjects from this source population who do not have the outcome of interest to become the "controls." There can be one or multiple controls for each case. The investigators then ascertain past information about attributes and characteristics (exposures) that are hypothesized to be related to the outcome of interest. If the exposures of the group of cases (also known as the "case series") differ from the exposures of the controls, then the investigators conclude that the exposure is associated with the outcome and that this hypothesis can be confirmed.

The time frame of a case control study can be somewhat difficult to label. In its traditional form, the case control study is a study in which all of the information collected from subjects was either from the present or from the past. So an investigator would identify a group of people with existing outcome (cases) and also identify a group of people without outcome (controls), and then ascertain all exposure and independent variable information from the past. This type of study would be retrospective in time frame. However, this retrospective case control study can lead to many biases because of the "existing" nature of the outcome and because of the possibility that the cases may have had the outcome for a long period of time. Another

case control study: a study that allows the comparison of the attributes of a group of cases (subjects with the outcome of interest) to a group of controls (subjects without the outcome of interest)

option for a case control study is to "watch" the intended population, and as new cases of the outcome occur, enroll them and at the same time enroll controls. The exposure and independent variables may be from the past but also may be after the study begins. This prospective case control study can minimize some of the problems in a retrospective case control study.

Referring to Figure 5-1, the case control study most commonly has information from the present and the past. However, the case control study ideally will have information about the exposure and independent variables from the present and past and information about those same variables and the outcome from the future. This possible multidirectional time frame of case control studies makes the interpretation of the results dependent on the actual performance of the study; however, because the comparison is between the cases and controls, there is no ability to report incidence or prevalence from a case control study. Consequently, this type of study does not allow the establishment of the risk (because risk is based on incidence) of outcome.

Advantages of a Case Control Study

However, a case control study has a number of advantages, and the more common ones are listed in Table 5-3. One of the most commonly stated advantages of a case control study is the ability to study rare diseases. This is because the case control design starts by finding a group of subjects with the disease or outcome. If designed correctly, this ensures that there will be a sufficient number of cases in the study population. In contrast, if a cohort design were used, investigators would only be able to wait and see how many individuals get the outcome during the follow-up period. If the outcome is rare, it will take a very large number of subjects or a long follow-up time period to identify sufficient subjects with the outcome. In fact, in a cohort study, it is conceivable that investigators may get no subjects at all with the

TABLE 5-3 Common Advantages of Case Control Studies

1. Best design for studying rare diseases

2. Can be performed in short period of time

3. Short performance time is generally less costly

4. Can be performed with fewer subjects than a cohort study

5. May have easy access to historical data through existing records

6. Allows the assessment of multiple independent variables (exposures)

outcome, in which case the study has been a waste of time and money. So, when the outcome of interest is known to be rare, investigators will be wise to choose a case control design and begin searching for volunteers with the disease or outcome that they plan to study.

Case control studies are also often quick and less costly to perform as compared to cohort studies. They are quick because there is no need for a follow-up period because both the outcome and the exposures have already occurred. Once the subjects are enrolled, the analysis of data can begin. Of course, there still will be a period of time involved with planning, training staff, obtaining funding, enrolling subjects, and gathering data, but these steps must be taken in any study design. There may be other cost savings because investigators can use existing data from other data sources or medical records rather than collecting new data from the participants.

A case control study also has the advantage of generally requiring fewer subjects to be enrolled in the study than is needed for a cohort study. This is fundamentally because of the ability to ensure that a large portion of the subjects have the outcome of interest (cases). Investigators are able to precisely control the number of subjects (cases and controls) that they need to enroll. Plus, because there is no time period during which subjects can be lost to follow-up, investigators do not have to collect more subjects than needed to account for the expected losses.

When high-quality data already exists on potential subjects, investigators find that the case control study is the best design to use existing historical data pertaining to both outcome and exposures. Investigators are able to enroll more subjects because of the existing data on subjects that are available without added cost or time. Of course, the advantage of using existing data can also be a big disadvantage of a case control design if the data in existing records are flawed or biased.

A case control study can only study one outcome because the subjects are enrolled based on a specific outcome category (cases and controls). However, the case control design does allow for the study of many exposures for that outcome and can investigate different hypotheses. For example, if subjects are enrolled such that those with lung cancer are cases and those without lung cancer are controls, then many different attributes and characteristics of these two groups can be ascertained—such as cigarette smoking, diet, weight, exercise, cholesterol, blood pressure, etc. Then, the investigator can perform the analyses to assess how each of these exposures is related to lung cancer.

Disadvantages of a Case Control Study

Although there are many advantages to a case control study, there are also a number of concerning disadvantages. The biggest disadvantage of a case control study is the concern over obtaining valid information. In other words, information bias is a big problem for case control designs. Although it is possible to design a case control study with little information bias, the reality is that it often requires considerably more cost and time than investigators are able to devote. Further, if time and cost are not obstacles, most choose to perform the more scientifically desirable cohort study. So in practicality, a case control study is usually affected by information bias, often to a greater extent than other study designs.

This information bias can come from many stages and parts of a case control design. If subjects are required to provide historical information about exposures, accurate memory may be an issue. Also, participants may provide incorrect information, either intentionally or unintentionally, as they may want to help the investigators by answering in a way the investigators may like. They may also answer in ways that they see as socially desirable.

These problems may affect any study design, but the nature of a case control design makes it especially prone to recall problems if the historical time frame is long. For example, dietary recall is very difficult if being asked about much longer than one or two days in the past. Smoking details, such as how many times subjects have tried to quit or the number of packs smoked per day over several years, are often difficult to remember as well. Even health care experience can be difficult to accurately recall if the information is based solely on the subjects' memory. Think about how well you would be able to recall which childhood immunizations you had and at what age you had them? Certainly, the accuracy of subjects' health information can be improved if access to their health care records is available, but many studies must rely on self-report even for medical information, and that information is not always correct.

Even information from health care records can be potentially biased for a case control study. Although there certainly can be recorded errors in the records, which obviously provide inaccurate information for investigators, other problems from existing records can affect study validity. Medical records reflect the "state of the art" for the time period during which they were recorded. As knowledge or technology changes, medical records are not usually amended to reflect an updated diagnosis. Many times medical records only reflect a suspected diagnosis, but since "treatment" was initiated and the "disease" went away, no further diagnostics were performed. Further, the need for the consistent definition of an outcome is a reason for using the technique of "watching" for future cases of the outcome for which a strict definition of the outcome can be employed.

Some outcomes require more definitive assessment when used as a research outcome compared to a diagnostic outcome. For example, many athletes have stress fractures of the tibia, an overuse injury. A skilled clinician can recognize a stress fracture often solely by the history provided by the patient. Some clinicians do not find it necessary to do many additional tests and will provide treatment and rehabilitation direction leading to recovery from the injury. However, a research study using stress fracture of the tibia as the outcome will likely determine that several additional tests are required to make a formal "research diagnosis." Medical records may not have these tests if the clinicians were treating patients but not following the study protocol. Although in most cases this difference in determining stress fractures occurrence may not result in misleading information, there is a chance that some stress fractures obtained by medical records may have been other injuries that responded equally well to the same treatment and rehabilitation.

Choosing the Control Group

In addition to the many potential information biases in case control studies, there is the potential for many selection biases as well. Several key performance issues are involved with case control studies. Arguably the most important is the selection of the control group.

Although the case group is often simply dependent on meeting the criteria of the outcome definition, the selection of the control group is dependent on many more concerns. The control group should be a sample of the reference group (population of interest) and must come from the same population as the cases. In epidemiology, the population from which the cases came from is referred to as the **source population**. The source population can be the same as the reference group but it may differ, and to be validly compared to the case group, the controls must be as similar to the cases as possible (with the exception of the exposure of interest). So, the selection of the controls should be from the source population, but first the source population must be identified. It may not be the population in close proximity to the cases. For example, if cases are selected from a referral hospital that accepts those types of cases from all over the state, the source population would be the entire state. Many times the identification of the source population is easy. Cases of upper respiratory infection from a specific elementary school would have the source population as the entire population of that same school. Once the source population is identified, it is then up to the investigators to devise a plan to sample a control group that appropriately represents the source population. One last comment on source population is that it is best to be able to enroll all cases in the source population.

Valid selection of controls from the source population also requires attention to several other issues. The controls should be as comparable to the cases as possible, with the exception of the hypothesized exposure of interest. For example, if the cases are mostly men, then it is wise to select controls that are mostly men. It is also important to select controls during a similar time frame as the cases. If cases were selected during a 12-month period, then controls should be selected during the same 12-month period. It is not a good idea to collect cases from 10 years ago, but to collect controls from the current year. It may be that technology changes or cultural changes make information collected from these two groups incomparable.

If possible, the sample of controls should be collected using random selection or other scientific selection procedures that remove any influence of the study investigators. There are many options to be used for random selection. Usually random selection procedures require establishing the parameters of the source population first. One option would then include selecting individuals from the entire population. Another option would be to make random selections of groups, such as by location, or age, or occupation, and then make random selections of individuals from the selected groups. This is known as **stratified random sampling**.

Many other randomization procedures are available, but the general idea is that the procedures for the selection of controls should be established that will eliminate the ability of individuals working with the study to make arbitrary choices about who is approached to enroll.

source population: the population from which the cases are selected

stratified random sampling: choosing subjects for the control group from random selections of randomly selected groups such as groups of subjects chosen by age, geographical location, or occupation

One other concept important to the selection of controls is that the individuals eligible for enrollment need to be "at risk" to be a participant. This means that individuals in the control group must be able to get the outcome of interest even though they do not currently have it. An obvious example would be that the control group for cases with prostate cancer should not include women, or that the control group for cases with cervical cancer should not include men.

Enrolling Subjects in a Case Control Study Design

The sequence of the collection of cases and controls can occur in one of two ways. Cases could be selected first, and then the controls would be selected. Or, cases and controls could be selected simultaneously. The decision about which of these sequences is used will depend on several considerations. First is the length of time needed to enroll the cases. If cases can be enrolled quickly, it makes most sense to enroll all cases first and then select and enroll controls. Before controls can be selected, the number of controls relative to cases must be established. The benefit of this sequence is that the attributes and characteristics of the case group can be identified, and that allows investigators to select a control group that has similar attributes and characteristics. This ability to obtain a similar control group is very important to the valid comparison of cases with controls.

If the pace of enrollment of the cases is slow, then investigators may choose to enroll cases and controls simultaneously. Another reason for simultaneous enrollment of cases and controls might be that investigators want to obtain as many cases as possible and gather all cases that occur during a long period of time. During this long period, it is advisable to gather controls at the same time to ensure that time-dependent characteristics of the control group do not differ too much from the cases. Also, the workload caused by enrolling cases may not be as busy when cases are enrolled at a slow pace. This can allow investigators the ability to enroll controls intermittently between case enrollments.

A benefit of allowing a longer period of time to enroll cases is that this allows investigators to gather cases as they happen. This is referred to as using **incident cases**. Incident cases in a case control study should not be confused with being able to calculate incidence rates from these studies. Remember, in a case control study, the investigator is designing the number of cases to be enrolled. So if the case control study is planned to have 100 cases and 100 controls, even if these cases are incident, it is not possible to calculate an incidence rate. But there are many benefits to having recently diagnosed cases. For example, because the cases are incident, the expectation is that historical information, such as exposure information, will be more recent, more easily recalled, and hopefully more accurate. Also, investigators can be more certain that the exposures preceded the outcome if the outcome has recently occurred. For example, if a subject has had a disease for a prolonged period of time, it is possible that the cases could have an exposure that has started because of the outcome. For example, if a person with lung cancer decided to stop smoking, it would be very important to know when the subject quit smoking, or the investigator may erroneously label that subject as a nonsmoker.

incident cases: cases that are enrolled as the outcome of interest occurs

Summary of a Case Control Study Design

To summarize, a case control study design makes sense to the general public because it compares those with an outcome or disease to those without the outcome. So if there are attributes or characteristics that differ between the two groups, then the expectation is that there is a relationship with the outcome. This design is very appropriate to allow the study of rare diseases, and it can be done quickly and relatively inexpensively, sometimes using existing records. The primary limitations with a case control design are that a wide variety of information biases may exist, and if controls are not selected carefully, the study may not be "referable" to the intended population.

COLLECTING DATA FOR A CROSS-SECTIONAL STUDY DESIGN

A popular method for collecting data is to design a study that looks simply at the current status of both the exposure variables and the outcome variables. A **cross-sectional study** is a study design that investigates the relationship between existing exposure characteristics and existing outcome information in a group of enrolled subjects.

Using the paradigm presented in Figure 5-1, upon enrolling them into this type of study, the subjects are assessed for all the variables existing at the time the data are collected for the study. For example, to study the hypothesis that smoking cigarettes is associated with heart disease, the information collected would be whether the subjects currently smoke cigarettes and whether they currently have heart disease. If the finding is that people who are current smokers have more heart disease than people who are not current smokers, then the hypothesis would be supported.

> **cross-sectional study:**
> a study design that investigates the relationship between existing exposure characteristics and existing outcome information in a group of subjects

Advantages of a Cross-Sectional Study Design

The cross-sectional study design has a number of advantages over its case control and cohort study design counterparts. See Table 5-4 for a summary of these advantages.

TABLE 5-4 Common Advantages of Cross-Sectional Studies
1. Relatively fast and inexpensive to conduct
2. Able to collect large numbers of subjects
3. Able to study many attributes or characteristics of subjects
4. Good for searching for potential hypotheses or risk factors

© Cengage Learning 2013

The cross-sectional study is popular mainly because of its ease, speed, and low cost. There is no follow-up period, and there is no need to search for historical records. As when using a cohort study design, investigators get the data directly from the subjects, which is good because it tends to be reliable. But unlike a cohort study, a cross-sectional study makes it impossible to determine "which came first," the exposure or the outcome.

The cross-sectional design often allows the investigators to gather data on larger numbers of subjects in a shorter period of time. In a shorter period of time, investigators can focus on larger numbers of subjects, rather than allowing time for follow-up or retrospective "look-back" for historical data on subjects. Of course, the larger study sample size may allow the investigators to make inferences to the intended reference population with more precision.

Another advantage is that this design can also allow investigators to study many attributes or characteristics of their enrolled subjects. Because this design is often used to search for potential hypotheses or new risk factors, the cross-sectional study is often used to gather larger amounts of information from subjects. This is possible because the tools that investigators often used to gather data on their subjects are questionnaires and interviews, which can be efficiently designed to obtain multiple pieces of information on the participants.

The cross-sectional design is also very popular as an initial investigation into a "new" hypothesized relationship between exposures and outcomes. So when there is limited literature available on the hypothesized relationship, many investigators will pursue a cross-sectional design as a way to gather more information before deciding to perform a more "costly" design such as a cohort or case control design.

Disadvantages of a Cross-Sectional Study Design

Although cross-sectional studies have some very important advantages, there are also some noteworthy disadvantages that often make investigators hesitant to use this design over other more scientifically desirable designs.

The most problematic disadvantage, as mentioned previously, is that the cross-sectional design does not allow investigators to determine whether the exposure occurred before the outcome or not. If nothing more is determined than the subjects have existing exposures and existing outcome, then the sequence is not clearly known. Many times, the investigator may "believe" that the exposure came before the outcome, but it is impossible to be sure when using a cross-sectional design.

Another disadvantage of the cross-sectional design is that investigators cannot know whether the prevalence of outcome/disease in their study sample is an incidence rate. This is because of only knowing that the outcome "exists" in the subjects. This lack of incidence from this design also means that risk cannot be determined from a cross-sectional study. So although the investigators can appropriately determine a prevalence rate of the outcome/disease in their study sample, it cannot be called incidence. This is the reason that the cross-sectional study is often also called a **prevalence study**. As discussed previously, it is not always necessary to determine incidence or risk from an epidemiologic study, but if knowing the incidence from

prevalence study: another name for a cross-sectional study

the study population is important to the investigator, then a cross-sectional design should not be utilized.

Cross-sectional study designs are also not a good idea for rare diseases or even for rare exposures. So although a cross-sectional design can support the enrollment of large numbers of subjects, rare outcomes or exposures may still not show up in the selected sample of subjects. Of course, investigators may be able to enroll enough subjects to ensure they will get some outcome or exposure in the study sample, but the rarer the occurrence of either, the larger numbers of subjects that will be needed.

A corresponding disadvantage of the cross-sectional study design is that it is not a good choice for outcomes that have cycles of high and low occurrences. For example, knowing that influenza outbreaks are mostly during the winter months in North America, it would not be wise to utilize a cross-sectional design only during the summer months if the outcome is influenza.

Selecting the Sample and Tools for Cross-Sectional Study Design

Two design issues are important for those choosing a cross-sectional study. One is the selection of the study sample, and the other is the choice of the tools or instrument to be used to collect the data.

The study sample for a cross-sectional study should be collected so that the study can be applicable to the intended population. Even the ability to enroll large numbers of subjects does not become an advantage if the large numbers are not selected correctly. As with all study designs, it is important to predetermine the reference population, and like all study designs, it is critical to find a study sample that can be generalized to that reference population. So although some parts of the cross-sectional study have scientific limitations, the methods needed to ensure an appropriate study sample must receive considerable attention from investigators choosing this design.

The tools used to gather information from subjects must also receive considerable attention from investigators. Many cross-sectional studies use surveys or questionnaires to gather data from subjects. The importance of scientifically valid tools cannot be understated in a cross-sectional design (as in all designs). Development of a questionnaire is a highly skilled activity, which many newer investigators may take for granted. Successful questionnaires are often researched, written, edited, pilot tested, edited, and ultimately reviewed by many external groups such as scientific protocol reviewers or institution review boards.

Summary of Cross-Sectional Study Design

In summary, the cross-sectional study design allows investigators to compare the prevalence of the outcome in groups of the exposure variables or other variables. It is often used to search for hypotheses to be investigated later using more scientifically desirable designs. But the cross-sectional study has become a very valuable method to collect data in epidemiology because it can be very useful to identify important potential risk factors.

Summary

Any time data is collected in epidemiology, there is an underlying study design. The design may be very simple or quite complex. The design may gather data (observational) or intervene with the subjects (experimental). For observational study designs, the ability to interpret the results of the data is based on the time frame during which the data were collected. The cohort study design is the most scientifically desirable design because it collects data directly from the subjects according to a study protocol and tracks subjects over time to observe which subjects develop an outcome and which ones do not. The case control design compares the historical attributes of a group of subjects with the outcome of interest to a group of subjects without the outcome. Another option for an observational study is to collect only current information about subjects for both outcome and exposure (cross-sectional study design).

To summarize the differences between study designs, consider a single hypothesis and how each of the three designs would be arranged. For illustration, the hypothesis is that regular physical activity is associated with a decline in cardiovascular disease.

To perform a cohort study, the investigators would enroll a group of subjects who can be confirmed as not having cardiovascular disease. The investigators then assess the physical activity habits of the subjects upon enrollment. Once the baseline physical activity categories are established for all subjects, the investigators then follow all subjects for a prespecified period of time to determine who develops cardiovascular disease.

To perform a case control study, the investigators would enroll a group of subjects with (preferably recent onset) cardiovascular disease and also a group of subjects who can be confirmed as not having cardiovascular disease. Then, investigators would assess the historical physical activity habits of all subjects for a prespecified period of time from the past, usually by asking subjects to self-report their physical activity.

Finally, to perform a cross-sectional study, the investigators would enroll a group of subjects. The investigators would then determine which of the subjects had cardiovascular disease and also assess their current physical activity habits. Each subject would then be categorized as to his or her current physical activity category and whether or not he or she had cardiovascular disease.

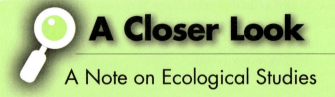

A Closer Look

A Note on Ecological Studies

There is another common study design that is used for quick comparisons of an exposure and outcome. Sometimes it is useful to evaluate the rate of exposures and outcomes in states or countries using available prevalence, incidence, or mortality data rather than collecting new data. In these studies, called **ecological studies**, the unit of analysis is a population of a community rather than an individual.

In this approach, the prevalence of an exposure (such as tobacco use) is compared to the prevalence of an outcome (such as heart disease mortality). One of the main advantages of an ecological study is its low cost (all data have already been collected) and speed (data analysis is ready to begin). This type of study is very useful in quickly generating ideas. If a strong association is found, it is logical to assume that this problem might be worth exploring further with a stronger and possibly more costly study design. Because ecological studies do not collect data on individuals, they can never be used to assess causation or to establish risk factors. For example, in spite of a strong association between a state's prevalence of cigarette smoking and its rate of heart disease mortality from an ecological study, it is not known if the people who smoke are actually the ones who die of heart disease.

ecological study: an observational study where the unit of analysis is the population of a community rather than an individual

Review Questions

1. Case control studies allow the assessment of multiple:

   a. Exposures
   b. Outcomes
   c. Both

2. Why do cohort studies have the highest quality data?

   _____

3. Which of these study designs is NOT an observational design?

   a. Cross-sectional
   b. Case control
   c. Experimental
   d. Cohort

4. Which study design is the best for studying rare diseases as an outcome?

   a. Cross-sectional
   b. Case control
   c. Cohort
   d. Ecological

5. The "source population" for a case control design is:

    a. All cases in a study

    b. All controls in a study

    c. Population at midyear

    d. Population that all cases come from

6. **True or False** In epidemiology, study design is also known as "how you collect your data."

7. A study looked at the relationship between menstrual factors and breast cancer in African American women. Through a well-known national cancer registry, 304 African American women, aged 20-64, living in three Tennessee counties, and diagnosed with breast cancer between 2005 and 2008 were identified. A comparison group of 305 women was selected through random-digit dialing. Phone interviews with both groups of women were then conducted to solicit information on menstrual factors—age at menarche, time to regularity, cycle length, flow length, age at menopause—and other risk factors. What is the design of this study?

    a. Case control

    b. Cross-sectional

    c. Cohort

8. Helicobacter pylori (*H. Pylori*) infection is related to several gastroduodenal diseases, though the route of transmission remains unclear. A clinic population of 695 healthy people at the UCSD Medical Center was enrolled in a study to examine factors associated with *H. Pylori* infection. On the day of the subjects' clinic visit, *H. Pylori* status was determined, and data on other factors known or suspected to be related to infection status were collected using a questionnaire. What is the design of this study?

    a. Cohort

    b. Cross-sectional

    c. Case control

9. In 2010, investigators identified from the institute's health database a total of 11,104 older (> 65 years) nondiabetic subjects who were residents of long-term care institutions in Ontario, Canada, during 2000. These subjects were classified based on whether or not they received neuroleptic agents. Development of diabetes in these subjects between 2000 and 2010 was determined from pharmacy records and measured by newly prescribed antidiabetic drug therapy. What is the design of this study?

    a. Cross-sectional

    b. Case control

    c. Cohort

10. In choosing controls for a case control study, the most important factor to consider is:

    a. That the controls are not exposed
    b. That the controls come from the same source population as the cases
    c. That there are equal numbers of cases and controls
    d. That the controls come from the same hospital as the cases

11. Which of the following study designs is the least economical?

    a. Case control
    b. Cross-sectional
    c. Cohort

12. **For Deeper Thought** An ecological study found a strong association between the number of fast-food restaurants in a community and obesity among the children living in that community. What study design would you use to further investigate this finding?

_____

Website Resources

To look up cross-sectional data on behaviors, visit the Centers for Disease Control and Prevention at http://cdc.gov/brfss; from there, click on the "Prevalence and Trends" data tab.

Chapter 6

USING RATES AND RATIOS

Learning Objectives

Upon completion of this chapter, you should be able to:

1. Briefly discuss how rates are used to predict future disease and how rates are compared to identify determinants.
2. Describe the basic differences between ratio measures and difference measures.
3. Explain the difference between relative risk and odds ratio and how to calculate each.
4. Explain attributable risk, how to calculate it, how to use it, and give an example of its application.
5. Describe the usefulness of the confidence interval.

Key Terms

attributable risk (AR)

confidence interval
  for a measure of
  association

confidence interval for
  a rate or proportion

difference measures

direct adjustment

exposure odds ratio

incidence density ratio

indirect adjustment

measures of
  association

null value

odds ratio (OR)

outcome odds ratio

population attributable
  risk (PAR)

prevalence ratio (PR)

rate ratio

ratio measures

relative risk (RR)

risk ratio

standardized mortality
  ratio

Chapter Outline

INTRODUCTION

Remember the definition of epidemiology has two very critical words in it: *distribution* and *determinants*. As was discussed in Chapter 3, the distribution of a disease in humans is identified by measuring its occurrence, which is measured by counting cases and then developing rates and proportions from studies designed to collect the data. In this chapter, the basic methods for using these rates and proportions will be discussed and how study design affects their interpretation. One use of rates and proportions is to predict the future occurrence of a disease, whereas another use is to identify the determinants of a disease. The future of a disease may be predicted by understanding its occurrence in the past and then deciding if it will act the same way in the future. The determinants of a disease in humans, often referred to as "risk factors," are identified by measuring the disease occurrence and then comparing this occurrence between different groups of a risk factor. This chapter will discuss using rates and proportions to predict the future occurrence of a disease (*distribution*) and comparing rates and proportions to identify determinants of a disease (*determinants*).

USING RATES TO PREDICT FUTURE DISEASE

A primary purpose of measuring the rate of death or disease is to learn from its past occurrence and use this to predict the future rate of a disease. It is just like a batting average in baseball. A batting average is developed over a period of time, but it is always a measure from past occurrences and represents what the player has done up to that point. It is used to determine how well the player has hit during the season or during his career, but it is also used to help the coach determine how well the player will hit in the future. The batting average can be stratified by individual opposing pitchers to help a coach determine how the player will likely hit against that same pitcher in the future. So the batting average is a measure of past performance, but it is also used to predict future performance. Rates in epidemiology are used in the same way.

From the outset of this discussion, it is important to realize that finding the correct rate of a disease or death, as was discussed in Chapter 3, is only half the battle. The other challenge is to determine whether a disease or death will occur at the same rate in the future. In general, if conditions with respect to person, place, time, and disease remain the same, we can expect that the past rate of a disease will be the future rate of a disease. So if the infant mortality rate is 12% in Country A during 2013, we can predict that the infant mortality rate will be 12% in the same country during 2014.

However, many additional factors need to be taken into account to determine how a rate of a disease or death will behave in the future. For example, is the time period during which a rate was initially measured appropriate for determining the future rate of that disease? Suppose the rate of seasonal influenza is being measured. The seasonal nature of the disease needs to be taken into account, and it needs to be recognized that the future rate of a disease will be dependent on the season. So if the incidence rate of influenza is found to be 15% per month during the months of June to August, it would be a mistake to predict that influenza will occur at that same rate during the months of December to February. However, if we find that the incidence rate of influenza is 15% per year, it would be more likely that the rate of influenza next year would also be 15%. But even this comfort level can be threatened if the type of influenza changes, because we know that different types of influenza infect a population at different rates (see more discussion on influenza in Chapter 8, Infectious Disease).

So although the methods for developing correct rates and proportions are discussed in Chapter 3, the way to make an accurate prediction of the future rates or proportions is to understand the population, environment, time frame, and disease under study. In other words, in order to predict the future rate, you must start with the correct rate from the past and then apply knowledge about the epidemiology of the disease. To continue with the influenza example, in addition to knowing about the disease and its various types, other conditions need to be known—the immunity status of the population, the age distribution of the population, the level of vaccination in the population, the general health of the population, the travel habits of the population, the cultural habits of the community, and so forth. Only after these aspects are understood can we use the previous rate of a disease to predict the future rate.

Back to the case of influenza. A previous rate of a disease is needed to begin this prediction. For example, in 2009, a novel type of H1N1 influenza spread worldwide. In order to try and predict the rate of this type of influenza, epidemiologists looked back to rates from the last time the same type of influenza occurred in 1918. This rate was thought to be an appropriate historic rate to base predictions of the magnitude of a disease predicted for the influenza season of 2009. Although many things had changed between 1918 and 2009, which affected the predictions, epidemiologists had to begin with a known rate that had an application for the upcoming influenza season.

Using a Confidence Interval for a Rate or Proportion

The process for predicting future rates of a disease occurrence is to first make sure the past rates are accurate and then determine what factors that could influence these rates have changed. Some diseases or deaths are very consistent from year to year, but often there are changes in the populations, environment, or disease that make the future rates vary from the past ones. For this reason, investigators will often start with rates and a range that represents the rates' potential variability. For example, a familiar proportion is the percentage of people in the United States who approve of the President's job performance, which is commonly determined from polls. When reported in the news, the margin of error is also usually given. So, for example, the news anchor reports, "The President's approval rating is 52%, plus or minus 3%." This means the reality is that the President's approval rating could be as high as 55% or as low as 49%. This "interval" is commonly referred to in epidemiology as a "confidence interval."

A **confidence interval for a rate or proportion** is a range of values that represent the variability likely in any measurement of a disease or exposure occurrence. The theory is that if the same rate were calculated from many different populations or samples, the rates would vary by an amount that the interval represents. For example, if 100 separate samples are taken and a rate of a disease is calculated from each sample, the resulting rates would not be exactly the same each time. The variation in these 100 rates can be used to determine the expected range of the interval of the likely rates. One further parameter of a confidence interval (abbreviated as CI) is that investigators must decide the amount of certainty that they would like the range to represent. Most investigators choose to be 95% certain and use 95% confidence intervals (95% CI). This means that the range of all possible rates for that particular outcome from all possible samples will end up in the interval 95% of the time. The details for the calculation of a confidence interval will be presented later in this chapter.

The value of a confidence interval for a rate is that it gives an idea of the possible fluctuation of that rate in the future, if all other things remain unchanged. So when

confidence interval for a rate or proportion: a range of values that represents the variability likely in any measurement of a disease or exposure occurrence

predicting future rates, investigators measure the previous occurrence for a comparable period of time and then calculate a confidence interval for that rate. With the knowledge of the previous occurrence rate and the confidence interval, the investigator then needs to determine if there are any changes that may affect the future occurrence of the disease or exposure. If there are no changes, the expectation is that the future rate will be within the confidence interval for the previous occurrence. If there are changes in the population, environment, or disease, the future rate will need to account for those changes. Continuing the influenza example started previously, suppose the attack rate for influenza in 2008 was 18% of the U.S. population and the 95% confidence interval for the rate was 16% to 20%. If there are no changes in the population, environment, or disease, the expectation would be that the rate of influenza in 2009 would be between 16% and 20%. However, because it is known that the influenza circulating in 2009 was a different type than in previous years, this new information, plus any other changes, would need to be considered before predicting the 2009 rate.

Another important consideration for using rates to predict future disease occurrence is that it is only appropriate to make predictions using incidence rates, not prevalence rates. Remember from Chapter 3 that incidence data allows the knowledge of the entire occurrence of the disease. A very important concept is that only incidence can be interpreted as risk, and the knowledge of past risk is necessary to predict future risk. Predicting future rates is incumbent on using incidence rates.

COMPARING RATES TO IDENTIFY DETERMINANTS

Using rates and proportions to predict future rates is important to epidemiologists, but of equal importance is using rates and proportions to identify determinants of a disease or death. The concept of identifying determinants is simple and logical. If a characteristic of a population's behavior or environment influences the occurrence of a disease, it is said to be a *determinant* of that disease. For example, if disease occurrence in people who smoke cigarettes and in people who do not smoke cigarettes is measured, the occurrence in these two smoking groups can be compared to determine if smoking is related to a different level of the disease. If the disease occurrence is different in those who smoke compared to those who do not smoke, smoking is considered to be related to (or associated with) the disease. Further, if those who smoke have a higher occurrence of a disease than those who do not smoke, smoking is positively related to the disease, which increases the risk of a disease. This whole process of establishing which variables are related to (or associated with) disease is the process of identifying determinants of a disease in humans.

measures of association:
a tool that enables investigators to describe a relationship between exposure and outcome in one summary number

Although the logic of this process to compare rates of a disease among groups of a variable may seem straightforward, it can be cumbersome to explain and present. So epidemiologists have come up with a variety of tools to succinctly describe the various relationships between exposures and outcome. These tools are called **measures of association**. A measure of association enables investigators to describe a relationship between exposure and outcome in one summary number.

MEASURES OF ASSOCIATION

One of the tools that can be used to determine measures of association is comparing rates or proportions. A list of the most commonly used measures of association is listed in Table 6-1. These measures are categorized by the mathematical methods used to compare the rates and proportions. Generally, rates and proportions of outcomes from different groups are compared by subtracting one from another, or they are compared by dividing one by the other. If they are compared by subtraction, they are called **difference measures**; and if they are compared by division, they are called **ratio measures**.

As can be seen in Table 6-1, the common difference measures are the attributable risk and population attributable risk, and the common ratio measures are the risk ratio, the odds ratio, and the prevalence ratio. Each of these measures of association will be described in more detail later. In calculating one of these measures of association, it is first important to make sure the rates being used are comparable. Crude rates are not usually comparable, and it is not appropriate to calculate measures of association with them. Specific rates are more often comparable, and when they are, it is appropriate to create measures of association with them. Even better than specific rates, adjusted rates are transformed to be comparable, and calculating measures of association with adjusted rates is the best method.

difference measures: rates or proportions that are compared to each other by the mathematical method of subtraction

ratio measures: rates or proportions that are compared to each other by the mathematical method of division

TABLE 6-1 Commonly Used Measures of Association

Difference Measures

Attributable risk	Null = 0	Range −1 to 1
Population Attributable Risk	Null = 0	Range −1 to 1

Ratio Measures

Relative Risk	Null = 1	Range 0 to ∞
Odds Ratio	Null = 1	Range 0 to ∞
Prevalence Ratio	Null = 1	Range 0 to ∞
Density Ratio	Null = 1	Range 0 to ∞

*Note: "Null" refers to the value for "no relationship."

ADJUSTMENT OF RATES

In Chapter 3, adjusted rates were defined as mathematically transformed rates that provide a summary rate for an observed population after differences in specified characteristics are removed. These adjusted rates are comparable to other rates that are adjusted for the same characteristics. There are several mathematical techniques that epidemiologists use to adjust rates, and two of these basic techniques will be discussed here. It is important to understand the general steps used to perform each.

Adjustment of rates can be illustrated by an analogy in basketball. Players in the sport of basketball are at an advantage if they are tall. Although many skills and physical attributes make a good basketball player, height is a dominant attribute. Consider how height would affect accomplishments such as the number of rebounds. Taller players are at an advantage for rebounding, so it could be that players with more rebounds are simply taller. But if the intention is to compare rebounding skills, it would be necessary to eliminate the advantage that height would give some players. It is not possible to eliminate a height advantage in basketball players because all players cannot be made the same height, so it is not possible to truly determine if players with a larger number of rebounds are simply taller. The process of adjustment would be like making all players the same height in order to compare rebounding skills regardless of their height (hard to do in basketball players, but easy to do in epidemiology).

Direct Adjustment

direct adjustment: a process that eliminates the effect of extraneous variables; involves selecting a standard population and applying the rates from the populations under comparison to establish new rates that would be expected from the standard population

Direct adjustment is a process that involves selecting a standard population and then applying the rates from the populations under comparison (the *observed populations*) to establish new rates that would be expected from the standard population. This would be equivalent to choosing a single height and then making all basketball players that same height. The *standard population* is very often an actual population that is considered a good reference group, or it can be a fictitious population that is made up by combining the observed populations if we are comparing populations. An example of an actual reference population could be the population of the United States at an identified point in time, such as the U.S. population from the 2000 census. The rates from the observed populations under study would then be applied to the U.S. 2000 census. In other words, investigators would make their observed populations under study look like they have the same attributes of the U.S. 2000 population. In some cases, it makes more sense to use a standard population that is a fictitious population made up by combining the observed populations being compared. In this case, if an observed population of 5,000 people is being compared to another observed population of 5,000, the standard population would be developed by adding the two populations to become a standard population of 10,000.

The steps involved with the direct adjustment of rates are summarized in "A Closer Look" at the end of this chapter. A detailed example of these steps taken specifically in the direct adjustment for age differences is provided there. However, although the example in "A Closer Look" is about adjusting for age, the same process can be used to adjust for any attribute or variable that differs between comparison groups.

Indirect Adjustment

Like direct adjustment, **indirect adjustment** of rates is a process to mathematically transform rates to hold constant some key differences in the population so that the rates can be compared. In some cases, direct adjustment may not be possible. This may be because of the inability to determine specific rates in the observed population for categories of the variables being adjusted or because there are very few people with the outcome in the specific categories. The indirect method is basically the reverse of the direct method. In indirect adjustment, the initial steps apply the rates of the standard population to the observed population to get expected rates in each of the two observed populations. In other words, what would the expected numbers of outcome and the subsequent rates in the observed population be if the outcome was similar to the standard population? The remaining step in the use of indirect adjustment is to then create a ratio of the expected numbers of outcome to the observed numbers of outcomes in each of the populations under comparison.

indirect adjustment: a process to mathematically transform rates to hold constant some key differences in populations so that the rates can be compared

Standardized Mortality Ratio

When looking at the outcome of death, the quantity resulting from this observed versus expected ratio is known as the **standardized mortality ratio** (SMR). The formula for the SMR is:

$$\frac{\text{Observed numbers of deaths}}{\text{Expected number of deaths}} = \text{SMR}$$

This formula results in a value for each observed population being compared. Because these values are ratios, a result of 1 will indicate that the observed and expected numbers of deaths in each population are the same; a value greater than 1 will indicate that the observed number was greater than the expected number; and a value less than 1 will indicate that the observed number was less than the expected number. Then each SMR for each observed population can be compared to determine if the outcome of interest (death) is different in the observed populations after holding the variables of concern constant.

standardized mortality ratio: the ratio between the observed number of deaths as a result of a specific cause and the expected number of deaths as a result of the same cause

Many additional methods are available to epidemiologist to adjust rates. The direct and indirect methods described help make the point that rates can be different simply because of unique characteristics of populations under observation.

Only after addressing these unique characteristics, often by adjustment, can rates be compared. So in the next sections, we will describe the methods for comparing rates, but it is important to remember that before comparing rates, they must first be determined, or transformed, to be comparable.

COMPARING RATES AS RATIOS

Comparing rates is ubiquitous in epidemiology and is the cornerstone of looking for associations between exposures and outcomes (identifying determinants). *It is important to emphasize that when comparing rates, the rates must be comparable to each other.* Once there are comparable rates, the most common method for comparing them is to find the ratio between the rates of the groups or populations to be compared. As defined in Chapter 3, a ratio is a measure of the relative size between two numbers or two groups and is found by taking two different quantities and identifying how they relate to each other (by *dividing* one by the other). So a simple ratio would be, say, the ratio of men to women in a classroom. If there is the same number of men as women in a classroom (say 40 men and 40 women), it is said that there is a one to one (1:1) relationship between men and women in the classroom. Presented another way, the ratio of men to women in the classroom is 40/40 = 1. So when there is the same quantity above the fraction line as below the fraction line, the relationship is said to be 1. However, if there were 40 men but only 20 women, there are twice as many men as women, or the relationship between men and women in the classroom is 2 (40/20 = 2). Because the ratio provides a mathematical way to compare two quantities (such as rates) and results in a number that represents the relationship between the two quantities, epidemiologists can then compare rates using ratios. Refer to Table 6-1 for the types of ratio measures that will now be discussed in more detail.

Relative Risk

rate ratio: *see* relative risk

risk ratio: *see* relative risk

relative risk (RR): also known as rate ratio or risk ratio; a ratio measure of association that uses incidence rates to provide the strength and direction of the association between exposure and outcome in a population

The fundamental comparison of rates using a ratio in epidemiology is known as the **rate ratio**. If the rates being compared are incidence rates, epidemiologists call those comparisons **risk ratios** (*remember that incidence is risk*), also referred to as **relative risk (RR)**. The definition of a relative risk is a measure of association that provides the strength of association between exposure and outcome in a population. This definition has several key parts that need to be highlighted.

First, relative risk is a measure of association, which means that it has the ability to tell if two comparable groups are related to each other. The second key part of the definition of relative risk is that it provides the *strength of association*, which means that it results in a number that tells how related the comparable groups are. So a resulting relative risk of 2 indicates that the rate above the fraction line is twice as large as the rate below the fraction line. A relative risk of 3 is said to be stronger than a relative risk of 2. The third key part of the definition of relative risk is that it is between the exposure and outcome in a population. Although the terms "exposure" and "outcome" are used in the definition, the reality is that the relative risk can compare rates between any two groups. The two groups could be two populations, two geographic locations, two time periods, or two diseases, but most often relative risk is used to compare the rates of a disease in the group of people exposed to the risk factor of interest and in the group of people not exposed to the risk factor of interest. Relative risk is a very flexible tool.

The generic formula for assessing the relationship between exposure and outcome using the relative risk is:

$$\frac{\text{Incidence rate in the exposed group}}{\text{Incidence rate in the nonexposed group}} = \text{Relative risk}$$

In this form, the exposed group is identified by the hypothesis of interest to the investigator. So, for example, the exposed group could be those who smoke cigarettes, and the nonexposed group would be those who do not smoke cigarettes. The resulting relative risk will then identify the relationship between smoking cigarettes and the outcome of interest. In addition to comparing exposed and nonexposed groups, the rates above and below the fraction line can be flexible and represent any groupings that are to be compared.

Interpreting Relative Risk

The summary of the interpretation of relative risk is presented in Table 6-2. The interpretation of relative risk is the same as any ratio measure. If the rate above the fraction line is the same quantity as the rate below the fraction line, the result will be a relative risk equal to 1, which is interpreted as no relationship between the outcome being assessed among the groups of exposed and nonexposed. The implication is that if both groups have the same rate of the outcome, then being in either group is not related to a change in the outcome. Consequently, a value of 1

TABLE 6-2 Summary of Interpretation of the Relative Risk	
Relative Risk = 1	**Null value**. Same rate of outcome in both groups being compared. No relationship exists between the groups being compared in the ratio.
Relative Risk > 1	**Positive association**. Rate above the fraction line is greater than the rate below the fraction line. Subjects in the exposed group are more likely to have the outcome of interest.
Relative Risk < 1	**Negative association**. Rate above the fraction line is less than the rate below the fraction line. Subjects in the exposed group are less likely to have the outcome of interest.

for the relative risk is referred to as the **null value** because it means that there is no relationship between exposure and outcome.

The null value of relative risk is not strictly equal to exactly 1.00. Sometimes a relative risk close to 1.00 is still considered as no association between exposure and outcome. But when the result of a relative risk is different than 1, the relationship between the exposure and outcome is indicated by the strength of the association (size of the result) and the direction of the result (above or below 1). When the relative risk is above 1, the interpretation is that those in the exposed group are more likely to have the outcome than those in the nonexposed group. This is known as a *positive association* between exposure and outcome. The larger the number, the stronger the relationship between being exposed and having the outcome. The sentence that interprets a relative risk above 1 is:

> The risk that those in the exposed group will develop the outcome is XX.XX times as likely as those in the nonexposed group developing the outcome.

In this interpretation, the numeric result of the relative risk is inserted in place of the "XX.XX." Also, the actual characteristic or attribute that forms the exposure group should replace the terms "exposed" and "nonexposed." Finally, the actual outcome or disease should replace the "outcome." As an example, examine this calculated relative risk:

$$\frac{\text{Incidence rate of lung cancer in the smoking group } = 12.8\%}{\text{Incidence rate of lung cancer in the nonsmoking group } = 3.2\%} = 4.0$$

This relative risk is 4.0, which means that there is a positive relationship between smoking and lung cancer. The interpretation of this relative risk is:

> The risk that those in the smoking group will develop lung cancer is 4.0 times as likely as those in the nonsmoking group developing lung cancer.

A *negative association* is represented by a relative risk that is *less than 1*. In this case, the higher rate of outcome is below the fraction line. This finding is also an indication that the exposure is protective for the outcome. The sentence that interprets a relative risk below 1 is the same as for a relative risk above 1, except that it indicates the exposed group is less likely to develop the outcome. As an example, examine the relative risk presented here:

$$\frac{\text{Incidence rate of heart disease in the exercise group } = 2.4\%}{\text{Incidence rate of heart disease in the nonexercise group } = 8.8\%} = 0.27$$

null value: a value that indicates there is no relationship between the study factor (exposure) and the disease

This relative risk is 0.27, which means that there is a negative relationship between exercise and heart disease. Those in the exercise group have lower rates of heart disease than those in the nonexercise group. Further, from this result, there is an indication that exercise is protective against heart disease. The interpretation of this relative risk is:

> The risk that those in the exercise group will develop heart disease is 0.27 times as likely as those in the nonexercise group developing heart disease.

An important concept in the discussion of the interpretation of measures of association is that the interpretation must describe the study design. The study design used to collect the data should be reflected in the sentence used to interpret the measure of association. In the case of relative risk, the data collected must be incidence data, and incidence data only comes from *cohort studies*. Further, a cohort study compares those with exposure to those without exposure, so the sentence interpreting a relative risk will look like the cohort study design. For example, notice in the previous interpretation of relative risk, the exercise group (exposure) is compared to the nonexercise group (no exposure). This reflects the actual cohort study design. Finally, because relative risk can only come from a cohort study design, the sentence interpreting the relative risk will always be organized like a cohort study (comparing exposure to no exposure).

One further comment about relative risk resulting in a negative association is that many investigators find it difficult to present findings of relative risk less than 1 because there can be confusion about the direction of the association using the sentence as written previously. For example, it is mathematically correct to say "0.27 times as likely," but to some readers, care must be taken to notice that exercise is not "more likely." To alleviate this concern, some investigators may choose to reverse the location of each of the rates above and below the fraction line such as:

$$\frac{\text{Incidence rate of heart disease in the nonexercise group} \; = \; 8.8\%}{\text{Incidence rate of heart disease in the exercise group} \; = \; 2.4\%} = 3.67$$

This new arrangement for the relative risk still represents the same relationship between exercise and heart disease, but the investigator eliminates the possible confusion of having to interpret a relative risk less than 1. If the rates are reversed, it is critical to ensure that the correct corresponding exposure group is represented in the interpretation. Consequently, in this example, one would interpret it by saying that *nonexercisers are 3.67 times more likely to develop heart disease than exercisers* or that *exercisers are 0.27 times as likely to develop heart disease as nonexercisers*. The relationship between exercise and heart disease in both statements is the same. Finally, notice that the mathematical relationship between relative risks when the rates are reversed above and below the fraction line is that the each relative risk is the reciprocal of the other, so 0.27 = 1/3.67.

In Chapter 3, the 2 × 2 table was introduced as a way to organize data to calculate rates. An even better advantage of the 2 × 2 table is its usefulness with the calculation of relative risk. In Figure 6-1, the typical 2 × 2 table is presented to compare the number of subjects classified according exposure and outcome. Once the data are inserted in the 2 × 2 table, we can easily calculate a relative risk. The formula for relative risk using the nomenclature of the 2 × 2 table is also shown in Figure 6-1.

	Outcome	No Outcome	Total
Exposed	a	b	a+b
Not exposed	c	d	c+d
Total	a+c	b+d	a+b+c+d

Relative risk $= \dfrac{a/a+b}{c/c+d}$

© Cengage Learning 2013

FIGURE 6-1 Typical 2 × 2 Table

Odds Ratio

When incidence rates are available, comparing rates using a ratio measure of association is best done with a relative risk. However, when incidence data are not available, the most commonly used method for comparing rates as a ratio is the **odds ratio (OR).** Equally important is that an odds ratio can be used to measure associations in *any* study design. This makes the odds ratio a very widely used measure of association.

An odds ratio is a measure association that provides the strength and direction of the association between exposure and outcome in a population. This sounds very similar to the definition of a relative risk, and, in fact, the results of the odds ratio are interpreted in the same manner as the relative risk. An odds ratio equal to 1 indicates that there is no relationship between exposure and outcome in the observed populations. An odds ratio greater than 1 indicates a positive association between exposure and outcome, and an odds ratio less than 1 indicates a negative association between exposure and outcome. The formula for the odds ratio is best described by again referring to the 2 × 2 table as shown in Figure 6-1. Unlike the relative risk that uses margins of the 2 × 2 table, as well as the cells of the table, the odds ratio only uses the internal cells of a 2 × 2 table. Also unlike relative risk, the odds ratio can be calculated two different ways. Because the odds ratio does not require incidence data, the odds ratio can be either the ratio of the:

> **odds ratio (OR):** a ratio measure of association that provides the strength and direction of the association between exposure and outcome in a population

1. *Exposure* odds in those with the outcome to the exposure odds in those without outcome; or

2. *Outcome* odds in those with exposure to the outcome odds in those without exposure.

Let us consider each one of these two ways separately.

Exposure Odds Ratio

The first way that the odds ratio can be calculated is by *comparing those with the outcome to those without the outcome.* This method is based on the concept of odds, which is the probability that the event will occur divided by the probability that the event will not occur. So using this concept, the exposure odds in those with outcome and the exposure odds in those without the outcome can be calculated by the formula that uses the nomenclature in Figure 6-1.

$$\frac{a/c}{b/d}$$

This formula is known as the **exposure odds ratio**. Notice that the exposure odds in those with outcome is represented by a/c because it is the number of people in the outcome group with exposure divided by the number of people in the outcome without exposure. Likewise, the exposure odds in those without outcome are represented by b/d because it is the number of people without outcome with the exposure divided by the number of people without exposure. Solving the formula results in the traditional odd ratio formula as follows:

$$\frac{a/c}{b/d} = \frac{a}{c} \times \frac{d}{b} = \frac{ad}{bc}$$

exposure odds ratio: an odds ratio that can be calculated by comparing those with the outcome to those without the outcome using the cross-products ratio from a 2 × 2 table (ad/bc)

This final formula is also known as a "cross-products ratio" and is the standard equation for calculating an odds ratio from a 2 × 2 table.

As with the relative risk, the odds ratio interpretation must reflect the study design that produced the data. The exposure odds ratio compares those with the outcome (cases) to those without the outcome (controls), which is consistent with the *case control study design.* So when interpreting an odds ratio from a case control study, the exposure odds ratio is used.

Outcome Odds Ratio

The second way that the odds ratio can be calculated is by comparing those groups with the exposure to those without the exposure. This method is also based on the concept of odds, which is the probability that the event will occur divided by the probability that the event will not occur. Using this concept, the outcome odds in those with exposure and the outcome odds in those without the exposure is shown in the following formula, which uses the nomenclature in Figure 6-1:

$$\frac{a/b}{c/d}$$

outcome odds ratio: an odds ratio that can be calculated by comparing those with the exposure to those without the exposure using the cross-products ratio from a 2 × 2 table (ad/bc)

This formula is known as the **outcome odds ratio**. Notice that the outcome odds in those with exposure is represented by a/b because it is the number of people with exposure and with outcome divided by the number of people with exposure and without outcome. Likewise, the outcome odds in those without exposure are represented by c/d because it is the number of people with outcome and without the exposure divided by the number of people without outcome and without exposure. Solving for the formula results in the traditional odds ratio formula as follows:

$$\frac{a/b}{c/d} = \frac{a}{b} \times \frac{d}{c} = \frac{ad}{bc}$$

This final formula is also known as a cross-products ratio and is the standard equation for calculating an odds ratio from a 2 × 2 table.

In the case of outcome odds ratio, the interpretation compares the odds of outcome in the exposed group to the odds of outcome in the not exposed group. The study design that collects data in this fashion is the *cohort study design.* So in order for the interpretation of the odds ratio to match the study design, the outcome odds ratio is used to measure the association in a cohort study design. This understandably can be confusing because it would seem that if a cohort study was performed, then the chosen measure of association would be the relative risk. But remember that an odds ratio can be used in any study design, so the odds ratio must be flexible enough to reflect whatever design is used to collect the data. As a general rule, for a prospective cohort study, the relative risk is the measure of choice, but an outcome odds ratio can be used when incidence data are not available, such as in a retrospective cohort study, or because an investigator believes the odds ratio is more appropriate. Of course, if the study design is a case control study, the only option for a measure association is the exposure odds ratio.

If you found the preceding paragraphs tedious to follow, hopefully you noticed the good news. The final formula for both types of odds ratios is the same formula. The cross-products ratio can be used regardless of which type of odds ratio is needed. So with the data organized in a 2 × 2 table, calculating the odds ratio is simple and straightforward by using the cross-products ratio. However, once the odds ratio is calculated, it still must be interpreted according to one of the two methods:

Exposure odds ratio: *The odds that those with the outcome are exposed is XX.XX times as likely as those without the outcome being exposed.*

Outcome odds ratio: *The odds that those with the exposure have the outcome is XX.XX times as likely as those without exposure have the outcome.*

Odds Ratios: A Wrap Up

Although these two interpretations may seem very similar, it is very important to notice that the comparison groups differ. In the *exposure odds ratio*, those with the outcome are being compared to those without the outcome; and in the *outcome odds ratio*, those with exposure are being compared to those without exposure.

A last comment about odds ratio is that it is by far the most commonly chosen ratio measure of association. The odds ratio is a very good approximation of the relative risk in situations where the bias in a set of data is minimized and the outcome is rare. This rare outcome scenario is actually quite useful because in reality many specific diseases in humans are in fact classified as rare.

So when choosing a ratio measure of association, there is always the option to choose the odds ratio either because it provides the interpretation that the investigator is looking for, it is a close approximation of the relative risk, or the investigator is not sure which measure of association to use.

Prevalence Ratio

The **prevalence ratio (PR)** is a measure of association that provides strength and direction of the association between existing exposure and outcome in a population. The prevalence ratio can be used in a *cross-sectional study* or *any study where the outcome data is prevalence.* A prevalence ratio has the same interpretation as the relative risk and the odds ratio with respect to its null value of 1 and values greater or less than 1. The main difference is, as its name implies, the prevalence ratio compares two prevalence rates. The two rates are compared as a ratio in the following generic formula:

$$\frac{\text{Prevalence rate in the exposed group}}{\text{Prevalence rate in the nonexposed group}} = \text{Prevalence ratio}$$

This formula is the same as the relative risk, except that prevalence rates are inserted instead of the incidence rates. Also, like relative risk, the prevalence ratio is easily calculated if data are organized in a 2 × 2 table format as presented in Figure 6-1.

Although the prevalence ratios give the same numeric result as a relative risk, they are very different in the use and value for the same reasons that incidence and prevalence are very different. As with relative risk and odds ratio, once comparable rates are identified, the hypothesis and method for collection of data will determine which of these ratio measures should be used.

> **prevalence ratio:** a ratio measure of association that provides the strength and direction of the association between exposure and outcome in a population

Incidence Density Ratio

The **incidence density ratio**, a measure of association between exposure and outcome, provides strength and direction using two incidence densities. As presented in Chapter 3, an incidence density is a way to present disease occurrence using a denominator that is comprised of person time and has some advantages over using rates. Incidence densities can be compared using a ratio to determine whether either of the two groups has a greater (or weaker) density of a disease. Incidence density ratios, like relative risk, can be used as an indication of an increased (or decreased) risk of outcome.

The two densities are compared using the following generic formula:

$$\text{Incidence density ratio} = \frac{\text{Incidence density in the exposed group}}{\text{Incidence density in the not exposed group}}$$

> **incidence density ratio:** a measure of association between exposure and outcome that provides strength and direction using two incidence densities

The incidence density ratio has the same interpretation as relative risk and the odds ratio with respect to 1 and greater or less than 1 (Table 6-1).

COMPARING RATES AS DIFFERENCES

The simplest way to compare two rates would be to look at them and observe whether one is larger or smaller than the other. Determining how big (or small) the difference between the two rates is done by subtracting one rate from the other. So, for example, if the infant mortality rate (3.5% per year) in Country A is to be compared to that of Country B (2.5% per year), the rate in Country A would be subtracted from the rate in Country B. Because the infant mortality rate is higher in Country A, several conclusions can be made that may seem obvious but are important bits of information. The first conclusion is that that Country A has a higher infant mortality rate than Country B. The second conclusion is that Country B has a lower infant mortality rate than Country A. The third conclusion is that the difference in infant mortality rate between Country A and Country B is 1.0% per year. The fourth and very important conclusion is that if Country A had the same infant mortality rate as Country B, then the rate in Country A would drop from 3.5% per year to 2.5% per year. This fourth conclusion is the basis for a measure of association between the infant mortality rate in Countries A and B because the implication is that the risk of infant mortality is higher in Country A than Country B. So it can be said that Country A is associated with a higher infant mortality rate compared to Country B.

Referring to Table 6-1, the measures of association that use subtraction or differences to compare two rates are the attributable risk and population attributable risk. These concepts will be discussed in this section.

Attributable Risk

If the investigator has chosen to compare rates as a difference and if the rates being compared are incidence rates, the most common comparison is known as an attributable risk. An **attributable risk (AR)** is defined as the amount of risk in a comparison group that can be eliminated if the exposure of interest is removed from that group. This definition has several parts that are important to highlight.

The definition identifies the "amount of risk," which is that risk represented by the incidence rate. Remember that incidence rates of an outcome are also the risk of that outcome in the population; so if the rate is reduced, then the risk is also reduced. Another part of the definition is the "comparison group," which is the group or population from which the rate is calculated and is also the group or population being compared. So a comparison group could be a geographic population, a period of time, a study population, a subset of a population, or an exposure group as designated by a population. Another part of the definition is "can be eliminated," which means the amount of risk that will change. Lastly, the definition also includes the phrase "if the exposure of interest is removed," which is the key issue of the concept of attributable risk. The concept is that if the exposure is associated with the outcome, then it can be concluded that if the exposure is removed, then the outcome will be reduced or even eliminated.

Consider the example of cigarette smoking and its association with lung cancer. It stands to reason that because cigarette smoking is a cause of lung cancer, then if smokers quit, their chance of getting lung cancer would be reduced or eliminated. But remember that nonsmokers also have a risk of getting lung cancer although it is very small (it is the baseline risk that exists in the population without the risk factor). The attributable risk formula can actually calculate a number that corresponds

attributable risk: the amount of risk in a comparison group that can be eliminated if the exposure of interest is removed from that group

with the amount of lung cancer that will be prevented by getting people to quit smoking. This would be the difference between the risk in smokers and the risk in nonsmokers, or that risk attributable to smoking. Further, the attributable risk will provide the strength and direction of the association between cigarette smoking and lung cancer such that the size of the resulting number will tell how strong an association there is between cigarette smoking and lung cancer. The direction of the association will also be indicated by the calculated attributable risk. This will indicate whether there is a positive or negative association between the exposure of interest and the outcome.

The generic formula for calculating the attributable risk is:

$$\frac{\text{Incidence rate in Group 1 } - \text{ Incidence rate in Group 2}}{\text{Incidence rate in Group 1}} = \text{Attributable risk}$$

This formula is very simple, but the part that can become very complex is deciding which groups should be represented by the rates on each side of the subtraction sign. The attributable risk formula is designed to be flexible with respect to the groups and rates that it compares. The decision about what group to insert for each of the two rates is dependent on the hypothesis or goals of the data collection. For example, one example could be to insert the rate for one geographic location as Group 1 and the rate for another geographic location as Group 2. Another example could be to insert the rate for the year 2000 in the United States as Group 1 and the rate for the year 2010 in the United States as Group 2. A final example could be to insert the rate for cigarette smokers as Group 1 and the rate for nonsmokers as Group 2.

A very common use of this formula is to compare the group exposed to a potential risk factor to the group not exposed to a potential risk factor. The point is that this formula allows the comparison of any rates from two separate groups or populations. When used, this formula provides an indication of how much of the risk (rates) can be attributed to the characteristics that differ between Group 1 and Group 2. Put another way, whatever characteristic(s) are different between Group 1 and Group 2 is the unique characteristic(s) that is(are) being compared by this individual attributable risk formula.

Interpretation of Attributable Risk

A summary of the interpretation of the results from an attributable risk is presented in Table 6-3. Unlike the ratio measures of association, examining the difference between two comparable rates produces a null value that is zero. So when two rates being compared are the same and one is subtracted from the other, the result will be zero. The conclusion from an attributable risk of zero is that there is no association between exposure and outcome in the population(s) being observed. Further, if the exposure was removed there would be no change in the risk of the outcome.

However, if the attributable risk is not equal to zero, it indicates a difference in the rates between the compared groups. An attributable risk greater than zero

TABLE 6-3 Summary of Interpretation of Attributable Risk	
Attributable Risk = 0	**Null value.** Both groups being compared have the same rate of outcome. There is no relationship between the groups being compared by the difference.
Attributable Risk > 0	**Positive association.** The rate on the left side of the subtraction line is greater than the rate on the right side. Subjects being in Group 1 are more likely to have the outcome of interest.
Attributable Risk < 0	**Negative association.** The rate on the right side of the subtraction line is less than the rate on the left side. Subjects being in Group 1 are less likely to have the outcome of interest.

© Cengage Learning 2013

indicates that the rate for the group on the left side of the subtraction sign is greater than the group on the right side. Conversely, an attributable risk less than zero indicates that the rate on the left side of the subtraction sign is less than the rate on the right side. The strength of association is indicated by how far away from zero the attributable risk is. The direction of the association is indicated by whether the attributable risk is above (positive number) or below (negative number) zero.

The range for attributable risk is from 1 to -1. An attributable risk of the extreme value of 1 indicates that all of the excess risk (above the level of Group 2) of the outcome measured by the rates is the result of the unique characteristics of Group 1 (group on the left side of the subtraction sign). This also means that if the unique characteristics of Group 1 were removed, then all of the excess risk would be eliminated; or in other words, the rate would be reduced to the level seen in Group 2. An attributable risk of the other extreme value of -1 indicates a protective effect of the unique characteristics of Group 1. This means that all the decreased risk (below the level of Group 2) of the outcome measured by the rates is the result of unique characteristics of Group 1. This also means that if the unique characteristics of Group 1 were removed, then the rates in Group 1 would rise to the level of the rates in Group 2.

These extreme values of attributable risk are rare. Most of the time the finding is in the range between the extremes. This means that only a portion of the excess (or decreased) risk as a result of the unique characteristics in Group 1 can be eliminated (or increased) by removing these unique characteristics. The interpretation of the generic attributable risk formula is dependent on the direction of the result. If the result of the attributable risk is between zero and 1, the interpretation is as follows:

> Compared to Group2, the attributable risk is the amount of risk in Group 1 that can be eliminated if the unique characteristics of Group1 could be removed.

If the result of the attributable risk is between zero and -1, the interpretation is as follows:

> Compared to Group 2, the attributable risk is the amount of risk in Group 1 that would be increased if the unique characteristics of Group 1 could be removed.

Use of Attributable Risk

As previously discussed, the attributable risk formula is generally used to compare a group exposed to a risk factor to those not exposed to the risk factor. Used in this context, Group 1 would be those exposed to the risk factor, and Group 2 would be those not exposed to the risk factor. The attributable risk formula makes the most sense when used in this fashion because the unique characteristic of Group 1 compared to Group 2 is simply the exposure to the risk factor. When either of the two previous interpretations is used, the investigator is provided with an indication of the rate of outcome as a result of the exposure to the risk factor. This is a very valuable measure of association in public health because often the goal is to determine how much of a disease or outcome can be eliminated if the risk factor is removed or modified.

One other consideration for the use of the generic attributable risk formula is the choice of how to organize the comparison groups. This determines the direction of the result from the formula. The investigator can choose which group to assign to Group 1 and which group to assign to Group 2. Investigators should make this choice based on the intention of the hypothesis and the scientific sense of the intended direction. For example, in the cigarette smoking and lung cancer example, it makes sense to assign cigarette smoking as Group 1 and nonsmoking to Group 2 because the hypothesis is that smoking increases lung cancer risk. However, if the comparison is between those who exercise and those who do not and if the outcome is heart disease, an investigator will need to decide which direction makes the most sense to those interpreting the results. Is the preference to explain how exercise decreases heart disease risk, or is the preference to explain how the lack of exercise increases heart disease risk? The investigator must make this decision prior to performing the analysis, but it gives the investigator the discretion in deciding how to use the attributable risk formula.

Population Attributable Risk

Although the generic formula for the attributable risk is useful for comparing two separate groups (such as exposed and not exposed), the attributable risk can also be used to compare rates within the same populations.

Consider our continuing cigarette smoking and lung cancer example. We have been simply comparing those who smoke to those who do not smoke. However, another very important public health question would be to identify the level of lung cancer in the entire population (made up of smokers and nonsmokers) that can be eliminated by reducing cigarette smoking. For example, in the population of a county, there are smokers and nonsmokers, but the research question might be how much impact

population attributable risk (PAR): a difference measure of association, which identifies the amount of risk that can be eliminated in the entire population (exposed and nonexposed) if the risk factor is removed

a smoking cessation program might have in the entire population of the county. Although the attributable risk for this new research question uses the same format as the generic formula, the additional choice is the assignment to the two groups.

When used with an overall population in Group 1 and a subset of that population in Group 2, the attributable risk formula is referred to as a **population attributable risk (PAR)**. The modified formula of the generic attributable risk used to calculate the population attributable risk is provided here:

$$\frac{\text{Incidence rate in Total Population} - \text{Incidence rate in Subset of Population}}{\text{Incidence rate in Total Population}} = \text{Population attributable risk}$$

Interpreting Population Attributable Risk Formula

The numeric results of this population attributable risk formula is the same as the attributable risk formula, with zero being the null value, and the range being from 1 to -1. However, to interpret the population attributable risk, the characteristic(s) being compared must be identified only by the subgroup of the entire population that does NOT have the characteristic. This concept can be troubling to those using the population attributable risk for the first time because they do not see the rate (risk) of the group that has the characteristic under study.

Referring to the cigarette smoking example, the two quantities used in the population attributable risk formula are:

1. The rate of lung cancer in the entire observed population (this includes people who smoke and people who do not smoke); and

2. The rate of lung cancer in the part of the population that does NOT smoke. Notice that neither of these two quantities is the rate of lung cancer in cigarette smokers. The comparison is still between smoking and nonsmoking, but the result indicates the impact on the total population if those who smoke were able to quit smoking cigarettes.

The interpretation of the population attributable risk is dependent on the direction of the result, just like the interpretation of attributable risk. If the result of the population attributable risk is between zero and 1, the interpretation is as follows:

> The population attributable risk is the amount of risk in the entire population that can be eliminated if the characteristic of interest is removed from the population.

If the result of the population attributable risk is between zero and -1, the interpretation is as follows:

> The population attributable risk is the amount of risk in the entire population that would be increased if the characteristic of interest is removed from the population.

Like the attributable risk, the most common use of population attributable risk is to assess the impact of a risk factor on the outcome in a population. It is flexible enough to assess any measureable risk factor that is a characteristic of the population, as long as the population rates can be separated into those who have the risk factor and those who do not. Actually three rates are needed to calculate the population attributable risk, even though only two of them are used in the previous formula. The overall rate of the outcome is needed, as well as the rate for those with the characteristic of interest and the rate for those who do not have the characteristic of interest. Then the concept is that if the characteristic of interest (risk factor) is not associated with the outcome interest, then the rate of that outcome will be the same in the total population as it is in the group without the characteristic of interest, and the population attributable risk will be zero. However, if the characteristic is associated with the outcome of interest, then the rate of that outcome in the total population will be different than the rate of that outcome in the group without the characteristic of interest.

Although the range of values for either attributable risk formula is 1 to −1, notice that the results could also be presented as a percentage instead of a decimal by multiplying the result by 100. Many investigators believe that attributable risk and population attributable risk make more sense presented as a percentage. If presented as a percentage, the interpretation is then stated as the "percent of risk that can be reduced (or increased) after eliminating the characteristic of interest."

One last concept about population attributable risk: the magnitude of population attributable risk is very dependent on the proportion of exposure in the total population. If the proportion of exposure is high and if the exposure is associated with the outcome, then it can be expected that the population attributable risk will be large. On the other hand, even if the exposure is associated with the outcome, when the proportion of exposure is small, then the magnitude of the population attributable risk will be small. So population attributable risk is not very portable and should only be discussed in context of the specific population from which it was calculated.

Graphical Representation of Attributable Risk or Population Attributable Risk

Attributable risk or population attributable risk is very commonly presented as a graphic representation of the risk (rate) in the two groups being compared. To further illustrate the concept of attributable risk, examine Figure 6-2. The two vertical bars represent two comparable incidence rates of an outcome, which can also be considered the risk of that outcome in these two groups. The vertical bar on the left represents the incidence rate in Group 1, and the vertical bar on the right represents the incidence rate in Group 2. Simply by looking at the heights of the two bars, it can be seen that Group 1 has a higher rate of outcome than Group 2. This means that if these two rates are comparable, then Group 1 also has a higher risk of the outcome than Group 2. But with attributable risk, we can assign a quantity to the difference between those two bars, which then tells us how strong the relationship is between being in Group 1 and having the outcome compared to being in Group 2. The quantity identified by the bracket is the attributable risk.

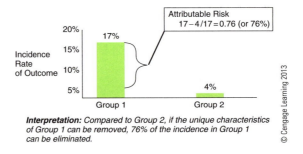

Interpretation: Compared to Group 2, if the unique characteristics of Group 1 can be removed, 76% of the incidence in Group 1 can be eliminated.

FIGURE 6-2 An Illustration of Attributable Risk

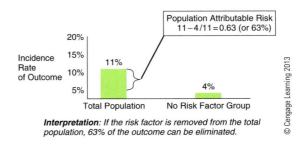

Interpretation: If the risk factor is removed from the total population, 63% of the outcome can be eliminated.

FIGURE 6-3 An Illustration of Population Attributable Risk

In Figure 6-3, an example of a population attributable risk is illustrated. The vertical bar on the left represents the incidence rate of outcome in the total population under observation. The vertical bar on the right represents the incidence rate of outcome in a subset of the population that does not have the risk factor of interest. If these two bars were the same height (which they are not), the conclusion would be that the rate in the population is no different than the rate in those without the risk factor; consequently, the risk factor does not change the risk and is not associated with the outcome. But because the vertical bar for the total population is higher than the vertical bar for those without the risk factor, we can conclude that having the risk factor does increase the rate of outcome. The strength of the association between the risk factor and the outcome in this population is represented by the difference between the two vertical bars and is identified by the bracketed area.

CONFIDENCE INTERVALS

Every measure of association calculated by comparing rates, whether it is by using ratio measures or difference measures, has "three parts." The first two parts of these measures of association, strength and direction, have already been discussed. The third part of every measure of association answers the question: Is the strength and direction of the measure of association the result of random chance? So to fully explain the association between groups being compared, it is necessary to know strength, direction, and statistical association of each comparison.

Confidence Interval for a Measure of Association

One very common tool used to establish the statistical association of a measure of association is the confidence interval. A **confidence interval for a measure of association** is a range of values that include the calculated estimate of the measure of association and represent the variability likely in the estimate. Like the confidence interval for a rate that was described earlier in this chapter, a confidence interval for a measure of association is the range of that same measure that would be seen if the same study or comparison was done in multiple samples. The ratio measures (RR, OR, and PR) and difference measures (AR and PAR) can both have confidence intervals calculated to be put around them. The generic form of a confidence interval includes three parts:

1. The estimate,

2. The predetermined level of certainty, and

3. Precision of the estimate.

The *estimate* is the actual calculated measure of association; however, if the chosen estimate is not normally distributed, some measures must be transformed before they can be used in the confidence interval calculation. All ratio measures of association must be transformed before use in a confidence interval formula, whereas the difference measures can be used without transformation. The need for transformation is that distribution of a ratio measure is skewed toward infinity on the upper end. In other words, the range of all possible results from ratio measures begins with zero on the lower end, includes the null value of 1 as the most common result, and has no limit on the upper end. In order to transform this skewed distribution to a normal distribution, it is first necessary to find the natural log of the ratio measures before calculating the confidence interval. On the other hand, it is not necessary to transform the difference measures because they are normally distributed with −1 on the lower end, the null value of zero as the most common result, and 1 on the upper end.

The *predetermined certainty level* is a decision the investigator makes before proceeding with the calculation of the confidence interval. The purpose of the certainty level is to recognize that it is not necessary (or possible) to be 100% certain, but we want to be highly certain. It is traditionally accepted to select 95% certainty for most confidence intervals, but it is possible to adjust the size of the interval by selecting different levels of certainty. A larger level of certainty will result in a wider confidence interval, and a lower level of certainty will result in a narrower confidence interval.

The final part of a confidence interval formula is the *calculation of the designated precision of the data set* under observation. From basic statistics, it is known that all calculated values come from data sets with differing variability. A data set with many diverse data points is said to have a wide variability, whereas a data set with fewer diverse data points is said to have more limited variability. The statistical measure of the variability is the standard deviation, and the standard deviation divided by the square root of the sample size gives the standard error of that data set. From a theoretical basis, the standard error of the measure of association can be calculated from the same data set and represents the precision of the measure.

confidence interval for a measure of association: a range of values that include the calculated estimate of the measure of association and represent the variability likely in the estimate

Using the criteria described for the three parts, the confidence interval can be calculated using the following formulas. The standard error formulas are presented using the nomenclature from the 2 × 2 table presented in Figure 6-1. The formula for the 95% confidence interval for a relative risk is:

$$e^{(\ln RR \pm 1.96\, *SE(\ln RR))}$$

$$SE(\ln RR) = \sqrt{\frac{b}{a(a + b)} + \frac{d}{c(c + d)}}$$

The formula for the 95% confidence interval for an odds ratio is:

$$e^{(\ln OR \pm 1.96\, *SE(\ln OR))}$$

$$SE(\ln OR) = \sqrt{\frac{1}{a} + \frac{1}{b} + \frac{1}{c} + \frac{1}{d}}$$

The formula for the 95% confidence interval for a population attributable risk is:

$$PAR \pm 1.96 \left(\sqrt{var\, (PAR)} \right)$$

$$var(PAR) = \frac{(b + d)(c)[ad(b + d) + (a + c)(c)(d)]}{(a + c)^3 (d)^3}$$

Each of these formulas is presented using the certainly level of 95%. However, the investigator can decide to be more or less certain and adjust the certainty level. To use other levels of certainty, the standard score for the chosen level of certainty would be inserted in place of the standard score of 1.96 in the formulas. To find a more comprehensive definition of the standard score, refer to any basic statistical textbook.

The practical application of the confidence interval for a measure of association is focused on the null value of the particular measure of association. Here is the logic for a ratio measure of association such as relative risk, odds ratio, or prevalence ratio. The 95% confidence interval indicates that there is 95% confidence that all possible measures for the association of interest are within this interval. So if the 95% of all possible ratio measures do not include 1 (the null value for a ratio measure), then there is a 95% confidence that our ratio is NOT 1. If our confidence interval for a ratio measure of association excludes 1, the difference between our measure and the null value is not likely the result of random chance. Stated another way, if the 95% confidence interval excludes 1, then the measure of association is sufficiently different than 1 and sufficiently large to be statistically important.

The confidence interval for the attributable risk is used in the same fashion as a ratio measure. Once the 95% confidence interval for the attributable risk or population attributable risk is calculated, we look to see if the interval includes or excludes zero (the null value for a difference measure of association). If the 95% confidence interval for the difference measure excludes zero, then the difference between the calculated measure of association and zero is not likely the result of chance. If the 95% confidence interval for the difference measure includes zero, then it is not true that the difference between our calculated measure of association and zero is not likely the result of chance.

Summary

In this chapter, we have discussed the use of rates to predict future disease or identify determinates. For epidemiologists, rates become very useful when they are compared between different populations or between groups with different characteristics such as those with a risk factor and those without a risk factor. Comparing rates is best done by calculating a measure of association. Categorized by the mathematical process to compare rates, measures of association are either ratio measures or difference measures. The most common ratio measures of association are the relative risk, the odds ratio, and the prevalence ratio. The most commonly used difference measures of association are attributable risk and population attributable risk. All measures of association have three parts: the strength of the association, the direction of the association, and whether the observed association is likely the result of random chance. The strength of association is indicated by the numeric size of the association and how different it is from the null value. The direction of the association is indicated by whether the association is above or below the null value of the measure of association. The indication of random chance for the association is most often determined by calculating a confidence interval for the measure of association.

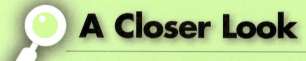

A Closer Look

Age Adjustment Using the Direct Method

The most common use of direct adjustment is to age-adjust rates. When the outcome is death or another outcome that may be related to age, it is important to adjust rates to eliminate the effect of age on the rates. This is also known as "holding age constant." If there is an attempt to compare crude rates between two populations, it may be that the only difference between the two populations is the age distribution. In that case, epidemiologists could mistakenly conclude that a difference in rates between the two populations is different because of some risk factors rather than simply the age variation. So when comparing rates between two populations, it is important to identify the age distribution of the observed populations, and if different, adjust the rates for age.

The steps for the direct adjustment method are shown in Table 6-4. Using deaths as a result of cardiovascular disease (CVD), this example will walk through those steps for an age-adjustment example. It is well known that death from CVD is related to age, so if one population is older than the other, it can be expected that the mortality rates from CVD would be higher in the older population. To compare the rates between populations, age differences would need to be eliminated to see if there are other reasons for any differences in mortality from CVD.

For this example, the information about the populations, the crude CVD mortality rates, and age distribution is presented in Table 6-5. The two populations have the same number of people but have very different crude mortality rates.

Continues

TABLE 6-4 Steps Involved with Direct Adjustment of Rates

1. Establish crude rates of the outcome of interest from observed population(s).

2. Determine the variables that are to be held constant.

3. Calculate specific rates by categories of variables in observed population(s).

4. Determine expected number of outcome in standard population.

5. Using expected numbers, calculate new specific rates.

6. Sum expected outcomes to get new adjusted rate.

© Cengage Learning 2013

TABLE 6-5 Example: Age Adjustment by the Direct Method

Outcome: Death from Cardiovascular Disease (CVD)

| **Comparing** | Population A | 5,000 people |
| | Population B | 5,000 people |

Crude CVD Mortality Rates (during 12 months)

| Population A | 74/5,000 = 14.8 per 1,000 per year |
| Population B | 29/5,000 = 5.8 per 1,000 per year |

Age Distribution

Population A	< 15 yrs	1,000 people
	15-44 yrs	1,500 people
	> 44 yrs	2,500 people
Population B	< 15 yrs	3,000 people
	15-44 yrs	1,500 people
	> 44 yrs	500 people

© Cengage Learning 2013

Step 1: Calculate the Crude Rate

The first step involved with direct adjustment of rates is to calculate the crude rate for the rate to be adjusted. This enables the investigator to see how the adjustment changes the rate. The magnitude of the change (or lack of change) will indicate the influence that the variables being held constant has on the outcome. From Table 6-5, the crude mortality rate of CVD in Population A is 14.8 per 1,000 per year, and the crude mortality rate of CVD from Population B is 5.8 per 1,000 per year. From this initial inspection, it appears that Population A has a much higher rate of mortality from CVD than Population B.

Step 2: Identify Constant Variables

Once the crude rates are calculated, the next step is to identify the variables that need to be adjusted. The criteria for determining which variables to consider for adjustment is more thoroughly discussed in Chapter 7 as part of the discussion on confounding, but very often, epidemiologists adjust rates for age, gender, occupation, etc. The idea is that to make rates comparable to either another population or the same population at another point in time, epidemiologists identify those variables that may be different and adjust for them. Because this example is about age, it is apparent that Population A has an older age distribution than Population B. So although investigators may be concerned that the crude mortality rates of CVD are higher in Population A, they need to make sure it is not just the result of the older ages of the population.

Step 3: Calculate Specific Rates

After identifying the variables to be held constant, the next step is to calculate specific rates for small categories of these variables in the observed population. So, for example, if the determination has been made to adjust for age, then the age-specific rates for subgroups of age are calculated. The size of the subgroups would be determined by the variable chosen. In the case of age, these subgroups are often in 5- or 10-year age groups, depending on the size and the distribution of the age in the observed population.

Specific rates are more comparable than crude rates, in which case this step results in rates that are comparable to other rates categorized by the same variables. But there will be many specific rates, and the goal of adjustment is to develop a single rate that can represent a population while holding the identified variable constant.

From Table 6-6, the age specific mortality rate is provided. The age-specific mortality rates are found by dividing the number of deaths in each age category by the number of people in each age category and then multiplying by 1,000. A look at the "Annual Age-Specific Rates" for each population indicates that within the more narrow age ranges, the rates are very similar; for example, in both populations, the rate for those greater than 44 years of age is 30 per 1,000 per year.

Step 4: Determine Expected Number of Outcome in Standard Population

The fourth step in direct adjustment is often referred to as applying the specific rates to the chosen standard population to get the expected number of outcome in each category for the standard population. Using the specific rates from the observed population(s) (Population A and Population B), the number of the outcome that would be expected to occur in the standard population can be estimated. The standard population for this example was determined

Continues

TABLE 6-6 Example: Age Adjustment by the Direct Method

	Age	Annual Deaths	Annual Age-Specific Rate /1,000
Population A	< 15 yrs (1,000)	3	3
	15-44 yrs (1,500)	12	8
	> 44 yrs (2,500)	75	30
Population B	< 15 yrs (3,000)	9	3
	15-44 yrs (1,500)	12	8
	> 44 yrs (500)	15	30

© Cengage Learning 2013

by combining the two observed populations into a larger population as seen in Table 6-7. Using the two observed populations and this new standard population, the number of expected outcomes can be obtained for each age group. So if the age-specific rate of the outcome is 3 per 1,000 per year in < 15 year olds in Population A, and there are 4,000 people aged < 15 years old in the standard population, 12 people would be expected to have the outcome in that age group in the standard population (Table 6-8). This same step is repeated for each subgroup of the chosen variables. This then provides the number of expected deaths by age group for each population as shown in Table 6-8. The number of expected deaths is then totaled to get the expected number of CVD deaths for each population. Of course, it is important to have the information to be able to separate both the observed population(s) of interest and the standard population into the same subgroups. One of the limitations of direct adjustment occurs if the information about the subgroup categories is not available for all populations.

TABLE 6-7 Example: Age Adjustment by the Direct Method

Standard Population (10,000 people)

Age	Number of People
< 15 yrs	4,000
15-44 yrs	3,000
> 44 yrs	3,000

© Cengage Learning 2013

TABLE 6-8 Example: Age Adjustment by the Direct Method

Standard Population (10,000 people)

Age	Number of People
< 15 yrs	4,000
15-44 yrs	3,000
> 44 yrs	3,000

Observed	Age	Annual Age-Specific Rate/1000	Expected Number of Deaths
Population A	< 15 yrs	3	4,000 * 3/1,000 = 12
	15-44 yrs	8	3,000 * 8/1,000 = 24
	> 44 yrs	30	3,000 * 30/1,000 = <u>90</u>
			TOTAL 126
Population B	< 15 yrs	3	4 000 * 3/1,000 = 12
	15-44 yrs	8	3,000 * 8/1,000 = 24
	> 44 yrs	30	3,000 * 30/1,000 = <u>90</u>
			TOTAL 126

© Cengage Learning 2013

Step 5: Calculate Expected Specific Rates

Once the expected numbers of outcome in the standard population are obtained using the rates from the observed population, new expected specific rates for the observed population can be calculated using the distribution of the variables from the standard population. This is the stage where specific rates have removed the variability of the variables that we intend to adjust. Using the basketball player analogy, now all the players are the same height. For example, when adjusting for age, the new specific rates are now using the age distribution of the standard population, not the age distribution of the original observed population. The purpose of this step in direct adjustment is mainly to be able to observe expected specific rates to better understand the outcome of interest. You will see in step 6 that these specific rates from the standard population are not directly used in the calculation of the adjusted rates.

Continues

Step 6: Combine Expected Outcomes for New Adjusted Rate

The last step of direct adjustment is to combine the new expected numbers of the outcome from each subgroup into a total expected number of the outcome for the standard population, while using the specific rates from the observed population(s). This step is done as many times as there are observed populations. So this step is done once if there is just one observed population that needs adjusting. However, if there are several observed populations, then this step will be done as many times as the number of observed populations. Remember, the adjusted rate will be for the observed population, so if there is more than one observed population, there will be more than one adjusted rate.

In this step, sum the expected number of outcome from each subgroup into one total expected number that will be the numerator for the new adjusted rate (Table 6-8). So in Population A, there is expected to be a total of 126 people with CVD; and in Population B, there is expected to be a total of 126 people with CVD after using the numbers of people in each age category from the standard population. The denominator for the new overall adjusted rate will be the total number of people in the standard population. Using this numerator and denominator will provide an adjusted rate that has standardized the distribution of the variables that we were concerned about. For an age-adjusted rate, we use the rates from the observed population, but make the distribution of age look like the standard population, rather than the distribution of age from the observed population. So if there is more than one observed population or the same observed population over a long period of time, we can keep calculating age-adjusted rates so that any differences in age in the observed population are held constant or eliminated.

Table 6-9 presents the new age-adjusted rate for each of the two observed populations. It is interesting to note that the crude rates indicated that Population A was at higher risk for CVD death than Population B. Although it is true that the crude rate was higher in Population A, when the effect of age distribution was eliminated (held age constant), the rates are actually the same in both populations. In other words, if the age distribution of Population A was the same as Population B, there would be no expected difference in CVD mortality rates either.

TABLE 6-9 Example: Age Adjustment by the Direct Method

	Crude CVD Death Rate/1,000	Age-adjusted CVD Death Rate/1,000
Population A	14.8 per year	126/10,000 = 12.6 per year
Population B	5.8 per year	126/10,000 = 12.6 per year

© Cengage Learning 2013

Review Questions

Using the table below, answer the next question:

	LUNG CANCER	NO LUNG CANCER	TOTAL
Smoker	127	3,400	3,527
Nonsmoker	45	3,100	3,145
Total	172	6,500	6,672

© Cengage Learning 2013

1. What is the odds ratio for the relationship between NOT smoking and lung cancer in the above table?

   a. 0.388
   b. 1.00
   c. 2.57
   d. 1.5

2. Using the table above, what is the odds ratio for the relationship between smoking and lung cancer?

   a. 0.388
   b. 1.00
   c. 2.57
   d. 1.5

3. **True or False** Using odds ratio measures requires access to incidence data.

4. Match the terms in column A with the definitions in column B.

Column A	Column B
Attributable risk	Estimates the amount of risk that can be eliminated as a result of removing an exposure
Relative risk	Provides strength and direction of an association between outcome and exposure using incidence data
Prevalence ratio	Provides strength and direction of an association between outcome and exposure using prevalence data
Confidence interval	A range of values that represent the variability likely in any measurement of a disease or exposure
Standardized mortality ratio	A ratio between the observed and expected number of deaths as a result of a specific cause

5. If the confidence interval for a measure of association includes the value of 1.0, then the measure is said to be:

    a. Statistically significant
    b. Not statistically significant
    c. A strong measure
    d. None of the above

6. When attempting to determine if the death rate in Country A is different than would be expected and the standardized mortality ratio is below 1.0, then the most likely interpretation is:

    a. There is no difference in mortality between the two groups.
    b. The mortality rate in Country A is higher than expected.
    c. The mortality rate in Country A is lower than expected.
    d. None of the above

7. You reported that from a group of people with lung cancer, 87 smoked and 24 did not smoke. This quantity is known as a(an):

    a. Rate
    b. Ratio
    c. Proportion
    d. Odds ratio

8. Subtracting the incidence rate of heart attack among those with normal blood pressure from the incidence rate of heart attack among those with high blood pressure is known as a(an):

    a. Attributable risk
    b. Relative risk
    c. Population attributable risk
    d. Attack rate

9. Smokers are 4.25 times more likely to develop lung cancer than nonsmokers. The measure of association used to establish this finding is a(an):

    a. Attributable risk
    b. Relative risk
    c. Population attributable risk
    d. Attack rate

10. In measuring an association using a ratio measure, which of the following indicates no relationship between exposure and outcome?

    a. 1
    b. > 1
    c. < 1

11. What term describes the absolute difference between the rates of a disease in the entire population and the rates of a disease among the nonexposed?

    _____

12. What term describes the risk of a disease in the exposed group divided by the risk of a disease in the nonexposed group?

    _____

13. **True or False** A relative risk of 4.0 for smoking and lung cancer is considered a positive association.

14. **True or False** The null (or no risk) value for an attributable risk is 0.

    The following table presents the number of diabetes-related deaths by age in 2005, in two California counties.

Age	RIVERSIDE COUNTY		IMPERIAL COUNTY	
	Deaths	**Population**	**Deaths**	**Population**
35-44	16	406,405	1	17,779
45-54	21	283,238	2	16,229
55-64	57	187,973	6	16,478
65-74	131	185,482	10	16,986
75-84	144	112,547	9	7,788
TOTAL	**369**	**1,175,645**	**28**	**75,260**

© Cengage Learning 2013

15. **For Deeper Thought** When comparing the rates of diabetes mortality between Riverside and Imperial Counties, you realize that Riverside County has a higher proportion of young adults than Imperial County. These different age structures lead you to suspect that the crude rates calculated earlier may not be accurate. You decide to perform an age-adjustment on your data. What is the age-adjusted rate of diabetes mortality in Riverside and Imperial Counties?

    a. Riverside, 3.18 per 10,000 per year; Imperial, 3.14 per 10,000 per year
    b. Riverside, 3.14 per 10,000 per year; Imperial, 3.72 per 10,000 per year
    c. Riverside, 3.38 per 10,000; Imperial, 52.3 per 10,000
    d. Riverside, 2.95 per 10,000; Imperial, 0.22 per 10,000

Website Resources

For more information and hands-on experience about adjusting rates, visit the tutorials found at: http://seer .cancer.gov

Chapter 7

ACCURACY

Learning Objectives

Upon completion of this chapter, you should be able to:

1. Describe at least one issue related to data accuracy.
2. List at least three types of bias that can affect epidemiologic studies.
3. Explain the distinction between different types of validity.
4. Give one example of how to measure reliability.
5. Understand the use of sensitivity and specificity when evaluating screening tests.

Key Terms

accuracy	external validity	random sampling
adjustment	information bias	reliability
bias	internal validity	sample size
confounding	inter-rater reliability	selection bias
construct validity	nondifferential bias	statistically significant
controlling	power of a study	stratification
convenience sampling	precision	test-retest reliability
differential bias	*p*-value	validity

Chapter Outline

INTRODUCTION

accuracy: the degree to which a measurement or an estimate based on measurements represents the true value of the attribute that is being measured

validity: the degree to which a study accurately reflects or assesses the specific concept that the researcher is attempting to measure

One key assumption when using, evaluating, or interpreting health data or health studies is that the data elements used are **accurate**, meaning, how closely the measured values represent the true values. Another assumption has to do with **validity**, or the degree to which a study accurately reflects or assesses the specific concept that the researcher is attempting to measure. The confidence we have in the data or the study results is based on the belief that the data are correct and a true reflection of reality. The rules necessary to foster this confidence will be discussed in detail in this chapter.

Things that may interfere with the accuracy of the data or studies include:

1. Random errors; and

2. The lack of validity of the data or procedures.

Most of us understand the concept of random errors or simply making a mistake, and we recognize the need to minimize mistakes in epidemiology. But a more difficult concept in accuracy is the lack of validity, which is also an error, but an error caused by flawed processes, tools, or systems used in gathering subjects, collecting data, analyzing data, or interpreting results. In epidemiology, the term most often used to describe this lack of validity is **bias**.

A further threat to the accurate interpretation of a health study is when misleading or distorted results occur as a result of extraneous factors or characteristics. These extraneous factors or characteristics that cause distortion in study findings are known as "confounders," and the distortion itself is known as **confounding**. The types and sources of random error, bias, and confounding that are often present when collecting or interpreting epidemiological data are discussed in this chapter. This chapter also deals with related matters concerning how to determine if the results of a study are important from a statistical viewpoint, as well as from a clinical viewpoint.

bias: any systematic error in the design, conduct, or analysis of a study that results in a mistaken estimate of an exposure's effect on the risk of disease

confounding: the confusion or distortion of measures of association between exposure and outcome as a result of third (or more) variable(s)

WHY ACCURACY IS IMPORTANT

From the earliest use of epidemiologic data, accuracy has been important. In the 1600s, John Graunt began the Bills of Mortality by keeping counts of the causes of death in London. Although simply counting the number of deaths from specific causes sounds easy, it can be quite inaccurate. Inaccuracy can result from simply miscounting, keeping incorrect records, or from the coroner being incorrect in the determination of death. One can only imagine how John Graunt must have worried about the accuracy of these statistics as he was trying to convince the London government how important it was to have accurate data for this new concept.

Now in modern times, it is much more complicated and even more important to be accurate. Consider the collection and use of mortality data from death certificates in a health department. Although computerized records are easier to count, there are multiple steps required to enter data into the computer systems, each step a potential for error. Further, death certificates have options to enter multiple causes of death. Many causes may not be apparent to the medical examiner, or the true cause may have a stigma associated and consequently not readily listed. For example, a study of suicide using death certificate data may not be able to identify all true cases of suicide. Listing suicide as the cause of death on a death certificate is potentially an uncomfortable label for the cause of death, and another cause may be listed out of respect for the deceased. The result can be an underestimate of the rate of suicides. In addition, the ability to identify risk factors for suicide from the same study may be hindered because some study subjects may be misclassified with respect to their suicide status, which could result in true risk factors appearing to be unrelated to suicide.

Accuracy is also important to ensure that associations seen in epidemiologic studies are not spurious. One of the most common reasons for misleading associations is confounding. An example of confounding can be seen in an often cited study published by MacMahon in 1981. In that study, an association was reported between coffee drinking and cancer of the pancreas. If true, these results could suggest many things—from individual behavior change to economic impact to legal liability and to warnings about coffee drinking. But consider that coffee drinking and cigarette smoking are closely associated because smokers often drink coffee. Further, cigarette smoking is a known risk factor for pancreatic cancer. So how can we be sure that it is coffee drinking that is the potential cause of pancreatic cancer, or if the reported association is simply because coffee drinking is related to cigarette smoking? Further studies since the MacMahon study have shown that cigarette smoking *was* confounding the relationship between coffee drinking and pancreatic cancer.

Much of the health information available to the general public, government policy makers, and health care providers comes from epidemiologic studies that involve data collection, analysis, and interpretation. Because these studies are used to guide personal behavior, health policy, and even your individual health care, it is important that the data and conclusions be as accurate as possible. The relationship between results of a study and the actual truth is never absolute. For example, when a study identifies an association between a risk factor and a disease, the study-derived association is only an estimate of the actual association. It is always hoped that the study estimate of the association is close to the actual association, but there is always some deviation that can be the result of random chance or validity of the study. This is a major reason that epidemiology requires repeated looks at data and studies to ensure that any one finding is not an outlier from what other data and studies have shown. Repeated and consistent findings from multiple studies help provide confidence that the results reflect the actual truth.

Finally, accuracy is important because it is always in need of improvement. In order to improve accuracy, its two major components need to be understood: validity, the degree to which the study measures what the researchers plan to measure, and **reliability**, the consistency of the study instruments to measure the same thing at different times. Inaccuracy can occur as a result of problems with validity or reliability or both. A good analogy can be seen in baseball when a pitch is called a "ball" instead of a "strike." When a pitcher misses throwing a strike, it is either because he cannot reliably hit what he is throwing at, or because he does not know the rules that determine the strike zone, or both. A pitcher can be very talented and able to hit the exact spot that he is aiming at, but unless he knows the rules, he is likely to miss the strike zone. Conversely, a pitcher can know the exact location of the strike zone, but not be very talented, such that he unintentionally misses the strike zone. So in order to throw strikes, the pitcher much be talented (reliable) and know the rules (valid). If he misses, the pitcher must determine which part of accuracy he needs to improve.

> **reliability:** the consistency of a procedure or a set of measurements to give the same results under different conditions

VALIDITY

Validity is often defined in terms of what it is, and what it is not. Validity can be defined as the degree to which data elements or health studies reflect or assess the specific concept that the researcher is attempting to measure. Validity can also be defined as the absence of bias in data elements or health studies. Both of these definitions reflect a similar concept but represent a different perspective of validity. Data elements are said to be valid if the information is determined to reflect reality. For example, if the researcher reports there were 55 males in a study, and it can be confirmed that there are in fact 55 subjects who were truly male, and the remaining subjects were female, then that data element is said to be valid with respect to gender.

Data elements are also said to be valid if there is no bias in the collection of the data. For example, a behavior very often studied in public health is cigarette smoking, but smoking status is not simply "yes or no." Many investigators have studied the best methods to ascertain accurate smoking status. When methods are used for the first time, the investigator will need to take the steps to confirm if the collected data elements are correct. If the methods result in incorrect information about the cigarette smoking status of the subjects in the study, those methods are said to be biased. However, once a method is found that provides a valid assessment of cigarette smoking status, the investigator may publish the degree of validity of this method. As others use the same method, additional confirmation of the validity may also be published. Then for future research, using methods that have been shown to be unbiased is considered a good strategy to collect valid data.

One additional perspective is that the degree of validity is often dependent on a number of different biases. Consequently, one particular bias may be minimized, but the data or conclusions may still not be valid. But in general, the degree of validity and bias go in opposite directions. An increase in biased methods results in a decrease in validity, whereas the minimization of bias results in increased validity.

Validity has several components. One component of validity is **construct validity**, meaning that a measurement (questionnaire item or several items, for example) correctly identifies the trait that it was designed to measure. For studies where you are looking for cause and effect, another component is **internal validity**, meaning that what you believe to be a cause and effect based on the observations in your study truly is the real relationship. Another component of validity is **external validity**: the extent to which the (internally valid) results of a study can be generalized beyond the study sample or for different people, places, or times.

> **construct validity:** the degree to which a measurement (questionnaire item, for example) correctly identifies the trait that it was designed to measure
>
> **internal validity:** the degree to which what you did in the study *caused* the effect you observed
>
> **external validity:** the extent to which the (internally valid) results of a study can be generalized beyond the study sample or for different people, places, or times

Construct Validity

Any time epidemiologists collect data from human subjects, they are concerned about construct validity. No matter how simple the information, it still must be collected and organized before it can be analyzed. Any initial data collection from subjects is accomplished through a variety of methods such as interview, questionnaire, laboratory test, medical examination, or record review. These methods are generically known as "constructs," and the degree to which these constructs correctly collect and record the true information from each subject is construct validity.

The importance of ensuring good construct validity cannot be understated. From the earliest planning of any study or data collection, the appropriate methods and measurement tools need to be considered. Data can frequently be collected through a variety of methods, and the decision about which to choose should include the construct validity of each method. For example, consider the case of collecting and recording a subject's age. It can be collected by directly asking the subject, including a question about age on a questionnaire, asking for birth date on a questionnaire, or recording birth date directly from a driver's license. Even in collecting very straight-forward data, such as age, each of these methods has variable construct validity that should be considered when deciding which method to use.

In more complicated data collection, technical expertise, field experience, and knowledge of the literature are required to determine construct validity. Consider the situation of a study assessing alcohol use as a variable. Alcohol use has physiological and psychological effects on the body, which contribute to a number of health out-comes, and these effects are the true variable being measured. Further, these effects differ by person. There are many options for methods available to assess the alcohol use of a group of subjects. Many of these methods include asking subjects for the amount of drinking, types of drinks, and frequency of drinking. Although it is a threat to construct validity that subjects may provide misleading information to these questions, even with truthful responses from subjects, the research tools must enable the investigators to classify each subject according to a valid alcohol use category.

For example, a commonly used category of alcohol use is "heavy alcohol use," defined as five or more alcohol drinks in a two-hour period at least once a week. So first the investigator must obtain true information from the subjects, and then the investigator must make sure that the data elements are handled correctly. Finally, the investigator must make correct classifications of each subject in this category of alcohol use (or not). But even this classification is just an estimate of the ultimate effects that heavy alcohol use has on the body. So, consider all of the levels at which construct validity can suffer:

- Misleading information from the subject;

- Incorrect classification of category;

- Variability within category;

- Variability of the category on different individuals; and

- Variability of the actual alcohol effects on the body.

Internal Validity

Internal validity is most often discussed with studies that are investigating cause and effect. These studies of cause and effect can be observational or experimental, but the ability to draw conclusions from either type of study is dependent on good internal validity. In the absence of random error, good internal validity depends on true mea-surement of information, correct classification and use of that information, and control of confounding (see discussion of confounding later in this chapter). To continue the example of alcohol use discussed previously, if subjects in a study are incorrectly clas-sified with respect to heavy alcohol use, then the internal validity of that study suffers, and any conclusions about the effects of heavy alcohol use from that study are suspect.

External Validity

Epidemiologists use many terms to describe external validity including "generalizability" and "representativeness." External validity is the extent to which the (internally valid) results of a study can be generalized beyond the study sample or for different people, places, or times. In other words, do the results of the study apply to groups of people beyond the study subjects themselves?

For example, in most studies performed among 15–20-year-old males, the results would not be considered externally valid to 60–65-year-old females. The degree of external validity depends on the perspective of those who are using the results of a study. If the study results will only be applied to the subjects themselves, then that study is considered to have very good external validity. However, if the study results will be applied to a group of people very different from the study subjects themselves, then the study will likely not be considered to have good external validity.

The underlying concern about external validity is that the epidemiology (distribution and determinants) of health and disease often varies in populations that are diverse or different from each other. These health differences may only depend on very basic population attributes, such as age, or on more complicated factors such as culture, socioeconomic status, geography, or genetics.

Finally, the diversity or differences in the study population from the preferred external population may result from the intentional goals of the investigators or to errors in the selection and enrollment of the subjects. Many studies are performed very well with very little error, but the external validity is limited.

For example, a well-performed study in young male military members may be externally valid to the young male population of the military. But this same study may have poor external validity to other populations. However, if the same study is expected to be externally valid to the young male military population, but is performed poorly, the external validity will suffer. For example, the study may fail to enroll all of the selected subjects as a result of poor procedures. The resulting population may be a group of subjects who are not similar to the young male military population, and subsequently have poor external validity.

UNDERSTANDING BIAS

Bias in epidemiology is defined as any systematic error in the design, conduct, analysis, or reporting of a study that results in a mistaken estimate of an exposure's effect on the risk of disease. This definition of bias has several key concepts that need to be highlighted.

Bias is *systematic*, which means that it is not random and that it can be expected to occur whenever the procedure is performed. Bias is also an *error*, which means that we want to avoid it. Bias occurs in the *design, conduct, analysis, or reporting*, which means that it can occur in all aspects of epidemiologic studies. Finally, bias results in a *mistaken estimate of an exposure's effect on the risk of disease*, which means that when it occurs, we draw a wrong conclusion from our study (an example of poor internal validity).

All of these things are threats to good epidemiology and obviously need to be avoided or at least minimized. Although is it often impossible to totally eliminate bias in the performance of a study, it is a high priority to minimize it to every extent possible.

Another perspective on bias is that it can also be defined as an inclination, predisposition, partiality, or prejudice that well-meaning, but inexperienced, investigators can inflict on the performance of a study. For example, consider a study that includes interviewing women about their experiences during childbirth. By definition, the subjects are all women who have had children, but it is conceivable that the choice for individuals to do the interviewing could have an influence on the type of information provided by the subjects. Could it be expected that the subjects would provide the same information if the interviewer was also a woman who has had children versus an interviewer who was a 50-year-old man who has never been married and has no children? Further, if there are any judgments left to the interviewer about any of the information provided by the subjects, it could be expected that the background of the interviewer may influence the information recorded for a subject.

To minimize bias, the only person who should have influence over the information provided by the subject should be the subject. Or if that is not possible, the influence over any information should be done in a consistent manner for all subjects.

Differential and Nondifferential Bias

Bias can occur in one of two types, **differential** and **nondifferential**. Although nondifferential bias suggests that the errors are consistent, the most concerning of these two types is differential bias, or systematic errors that do not affect all subjects equally. Differential bias causes the most damage to internal validity. For example, in a study comparing sick people to healthy controls, bias is most damaging to internal validity when the systematic errors occur differentially between cases and controls. Consider a study investigating the relationship between smoking cigarettes in cases of lung cancer compared to controls without lung cancer. If the information about cigarette smoking is underestimated in cases, but is correct in the control group, the conclusion from the study will be distorted simply because of the bias. However, if there are consistent errors (nondifferential bias) in classifying smoking status, then the results may be weakened, rather than distorted, because the errors occur throughout the study population.

Differential bias must be avoided to every extent possible. The most troubling result is the unpredictability of the distortion that can occur from this type of bias. In some cases, the differential bias could result in spurious associations, and in other cases, the differential bias can result in a weakened association. In many cases, the investigator cannot ascertain which direction the bias is occurring. On the other hand, nondifferential bias is more predictable, so arguably less damaging than differential bias.

In the case of nondifferential bias, the expectation is that the result will be a weakening of the association between exposure and outcome. Nondifferential bias is a result of the systematic errors occurring consistently and equally throughout the entire study population. This applies to methods used to enroll subjects, as well as to

differential bias: systematic errors resulting in bias, which affect the comparison groups of a study differently

nondifferential bias: systematic errors resulting in bias, which affect all subjects and comparison groups of a study the same

gather information from subjects. Although it is counterintuitive to recognize that more error is better, the reality is that if flawed methods are used in the performance of a study, it is better for the flawed methods to affect the entire study rather than specific groups or categories of subjects. So although it is of course preferable to have no flawed methods, nondifferential bias will result in a distortion in a single and predictable direction, a weakening of the association.

The expected weakened association resulting from nondifferential bias can be described as washing out the relationship. To illustrate the concept, a study comparing physical activity and cardiovascular disease (CVD) is displayed in Figure 7-1. The study looked at 10 subjects who exercise (people running) and 10 sedentary

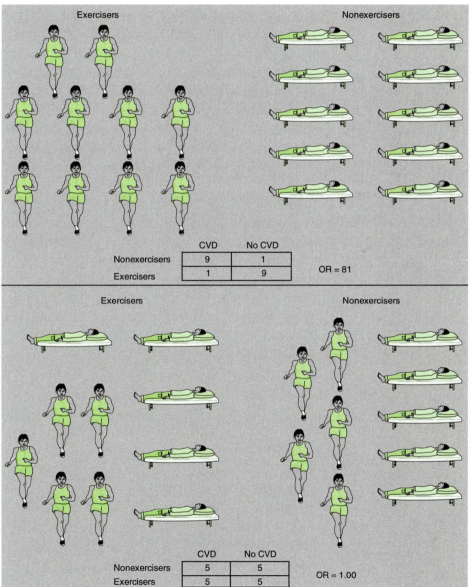

	CVD	No CVD	
Nonexercisers	9	1	OR = 81
Exercisers	1	9	

	CVD	No CVD	
Nonexercisers	5	5	OR = 1.00
Exercisers	5	5	

© Cengage Learning 2013

FIGURE 7-1 Study of the Relationship between Cardiovascular Disease and Exercise

subjects (people lying on the couch). These 20 subjects were followed to see who developed CVD. Those who developed CVD are identified with a box around the subjects. The upper half of Figure 7-1 displays the true findings of the study, and it is clear that being sedentary was very highly associated with CVD.

However, consider the conclusion that would be seen from a study that misclassified the exercise/sedentary status. In the lower half of Figure 7-1, notice that some subjects who exercised were misclassified as sedentary, and some subjects who were sedentary were misclassified as exercisers. Because the misclassification affected both comparison groups, it is considered nondifferential misclassification. Also notice that although the CVD status was not misclassified, some of those subjects with CVD will now be mistakenly arranged into the wrong comparison group so the resulting conclusion appears to indicate that there is no relationship between exercise/sedentary status and CVD.

Bias can occur in all aspects of the performance of a data collection or a study. Some references have labeled well over 150 specific types of biases that can occur in epidemiologic studies (*Encyclopedia of Biostatistics*). Some of the most common and well-known types and sources of bias are shown in Table 7-1. The majority of all biases can be categorized into two large groups: (1) selection bias and (2) information bias. Further, selection bias can be differential or nondifferential, and information bias can also be differential or nondifferential.

TABLE 7-1 Types and Sources of Bias		
Bias	**How It Occurs**	**Effect on Results**
Biases Associated with the Study Sample		
Selection	Occurs when the study sample is drawn such that certain segments of the population are not eligible for selection	Differential and may overestimate or underestimate the true effect
Volunteer or Self-Selection or Convenience	Occurs when the study subjects are volunteers and may not represent the target population	Differential and may over- or underestimate the true effect
Loss to Follow-up	Occurs when subjects enrolled in a study are successfully tracked throughout the entire follow-up period	May be differential or nondifferential and may over- or underestimate the true effect
Nonresponse	Occurs when a sample is selected scientifically, but not all respondents choose to participate and the resulting sample may not be representative of the target population	May be differential or nondifferential and may over- or underestimate the true effect

Healthy Worker Effect	Occurs when individuals healthy enough to be working are selected with the intent to represent the entire population	Differential and may over- or underestimate the true effect
Survival	Occurs when the disease is associated with mortality and those who die early are not available to be studied	Differential and may over- or underestimate the true effect

Biases Associated with the Data

Information Bias	Occurs when data concerning exposure or disease is misclassified or measured incorrectly	May be differential or nondifferential, depending on the circumstances and may over- or underestimate the true effect
Response Fatigue	Occurs when a questionnaire is not completed or completed incorrectly because of its length or repetitiveness	Probably nondifferential, unless fatigue is associated with the disease
Recall	Occurs when subjects remember past exposures differently, especially when recall varies by disease status	Differential if the disease status affects recall of related exposures; could overestimate the true effect
Interviewer	Occurs when interviewers actively extract information more directly from those who have the disease than from those who do not	Differential and can overestimate the true effect
Ascertainment	Occurs when certain groups are more likely to be diagnosed with a disease than other groups in the same target population	Can be differential or nondifferential and could over- or underestimate the true effect

© Cengage Learning 2013

Selection Bias

selection bias: a large category of systemic errors in the performance of epidemiology studies that affect the characteristics of the group of subjects selected for enrollment in a study

Selection bias occurs when the methods used to select and enroll subjects are flawed and cause a distortion in characteristics of the study groups. The distortion from selection bias has an adverse effect on the external validity of the data set and internal validity of the study. Typically, studies with multiple selection biases have limited external validity, but selection bias can also result in limited internal validity. Conversely, studies with good external validity tend to have minimal

Historical Note 7-1

William Ogle

William Ogle (1827-1912) observed two problems in 1885 when he studied death rates in different industries. The first was "the considerable standard of muscular strength and vigour to be maintained" in order to keep on performing many tasks in the industry. If the individual's health or strength fell below this standard, he was compelled to move to a more suitable activity or even retire. The second problem was that "some occupations may repel, while others attract, the unfit at the age of starting work and, conversely, some occupations may be of necessity recruited from men of supernormal physical conditions." These observations explained why people who worked were usually healthier than the general population and led to the description of the "healthy worker effect." (Vineis & McMichael, 1998)

selection bias. For example, if a phone survey was conducted to assess use of clinical services by subjects with low income, many of the target population may be missed because they do not have a phone. Furthermore, their access to services may be very different from the people who were surveyed (and who had a telephone). Interpretations made from this study may be biased because of the way the subjects were selected or sampled.

A particularly troubling example of selection bias in studies that follow people over a period of time is known as *loss to follow-up bias*. Loss to follow-up bias occurs when subjects who are enrolled in a study are not successfully tracked throughout the entire follow-up period and subsequently lost from the study population. Loss to follow-up bias is most troubling when it occurs differentially. For example, if the loss to follow-up in a study occurs more frequently among women than among men, the differential loss to follow-up between men and women results in a study group that is different from the originally collected group. This difference could result in misleading conclusions (poor internal validity) or damage to the external validity.

There are various ways to decide who will be included in the study, but only two of them will be discussed. The most common method of collecting subjects for small studies is called **convenience sampling**, a method by which volunteers are approached and asked to participate. This type of sampling is often conducted in shopping malls or other places where people might congregate. Of course, those who volunteer to participate may not represent the general population because (1) they are frequenting the place where the study data are collected and (2) their volunteer status may make them less similar to others who do not volunteer. This type of sampling may impair the external validity of the study.

convenience sampling: a method by which volunteers are approached and asked to participate

A more formal method of selecting a sample involves **random sampling**, a systematic method of approaching individuals to participate in the study. In this situation, the random aspect involves a statistical method that allows every person in the target population to have an equal opportunity to participate. Studies based on random sampling are more likely to represent the target population and to reduce study biases as a result of sampling.

> **random sampling:**
> a systematic method of approaching individuals to participate in the study

Information Bias

Information bias occurs when the methods used to collect data (information) from enrolled subjects are flawed and result in incorrect data being recorded for subjects. Further, when the flawed information results in misclassification of a subject, a distortion in findings and conclusions from the study can be expected. Typically, studies with one or many information biases have poor internal validity and/ or construct validity. Conversely, studies with good internal validity and construct validity tend to have minimal information bias.

> **information bias:** a large category of systemic errors in the performance of epidemiology studies that result in reduced validity of the information gathered from study subjects

A classic example of information bias is asking subjects to report something that they will have a hard time remembering. Referred to as "recall bias," this type of bias is common in many studies such as those using dietary information. Do you remember what you had for lunch last Tuesday? Other examples of information bias were presented in Table 7-1.

Aligning Bias with Validity

Although it may be desirable for discussion purposes to simply align concerns about selection bias with external validity and concerns about information bias with internal validity, the practical reality is that it is not that simple. Generally, information bias is aligned with internal validity, but in some cases, collecting inaccurate information can result in misleading information during the enrollment of subjects; this can lead to problems with external validity. But although information bias is mostly associated with internal validity, selection bias is often a concern for both internal validity and external validity. As discussed previously, it makes intuitive sense that problems with the selection of the study subjects can affect external validity, but very often selection bias can distort the relationship between the study factors and the outcome of interest.

Consider an example comparing the cell phone use while driving between subjects in fatal automobile accidents to nonfatal automobile accidents. In order to get informed consent and personal information from the fatal accident group, investigators must approach living relatives as surrogates for the deceased drivers. To get the same information from the comparison group, the investigators would approach the subjects themselves. This could cause a differing probability of enrollment between, and within, the comparison groups resulting in a selection bias. The results could be that the subjects in the different groups may represent different attributes solely because of the methods of enrollment, which could further result in a misleading interpretation of the relationship between cell phone use and fatal accidents: poor internal validity. This is an example of *differential selection bias*. But, as with differential information bias, it is impossible to predict which direction the distortion will occur, resulting in the true association being underestimated or overestimated.

CONFOUNDING

The general dictionary definition of the word confound is to "baffle or frustrate." In older language usage, it also can mean "bring to ruin or destroy." Who can forget a line made famous by the movie *Mary Poppins*: "Confound it, Banks!" In epidemiology, the term confounding is not any less ominous.

Confounding is defined as the confusion or distortion of measures of association between exposure and outcome as a result of third (or more) variable(s). Several parts of the definition of confounding are important to highlight. Confounding causes *confusion or distortion*, which means it is something to avoid or control. Confounding confuses or distorts measures of association, which means that the results of a study are numerically wrong such that a study may find that smoking is related to a decrease in lung cancer when in fact it is related to an increase in lung cancer. Confounding is *a result of a third (or more) variable(s)*, which means that the distortion is caused by the actual influence of variables other than the hypothesized exposure of interest or the outcome of interest.

As discussed in Chapter 2, variables in a study are identified as exposure and outcome by the hypothesis of each study, and different study investigators often choose different variables for their hypotheses. Further, there are often many other variables collected in a study, in addition to those designated as exposure and outcome. These additional variables are the ones that can qualify as a "third (or more) variable(s)."

Confounding Criteria

The variable(s) that cause confounding are known as "confounders." Although confounders are not the exposure of interest or the outcome of interest, they may be any other variables collected in the study, or worse, they can be variables that are not collected in the study. The criteria for a variable being a confounder are listed in Table 7-2. From this table, it is important to realize that the label of confounder is applied only with respect to the specified exposure and outcome relationship. So in some studies a particular variable will be a confounder, but the same variable may not be a confounder in another study with a different hypothesis.

The first two criteria in Table 7-2 are different and the distinction is very important. The first criterion requires that the potential confounder be a risk factor for the hypothesized outcome, but the outcome does not change the effect of the risk factor. For example, cigarette smoking has been shown to increase the risk of lung

TABLE 7-2 Criteria for Confounding

The following three criteria must all be met for a variable to be considered a confounder of the association between the hypothesized exposure and outcome:

1. Confounder must be a risk factor for the outcome.

2. Confounder must be associated with the exposure in the study population.

3. Confounder cannot be an intermediate step in the causal pathway between exposure and outcome.

© Cengage Learning 2013

cancer and has been referred to by many as a cause of lung cancer. However, the opposite cannot be said to be true. Lung cancer is not a risk factor for smoking.

The second criterion in Table 7-2 requires that the potential confounder is associated with the exposure of interest. This criterion applies to the potential confounder's relationship to the exposure of interest, but not to those variables that are risk factors for the exposure. An example is drinking coffee and smoking cigarettes. Coffee drinkers are often smokers, and smokers are often coffee drinkers, but neither drinking coffee nor smoking cigarettes causes the other to occur. So these two variables are said to be associated, but not risk factors for each other.

The third criterion in Table 7-2 requires that the potential confounder is not simply an intermediate step in the casual pathway from exposure to outcome. As discussed in Chapter 2, variables can be a direct cause or indirect cause of an outcome. Variables that are direct causes can alter the outcome simply by the change in that variable. However, variables that are indirect causes need to alter other attributes in order to alter the outcome, and consequently, there are intermediate steps between a change in the exposure and an alteration of the outcome. An example of this would be the situation where a driver who has been drinking alcohol causes an automobile accident that causes a broken leg. The direct cause of the broken leg is the automobile accident, whereas the indirect cause (intermediate step) is alcohol use.

To graphically display the relationship of a confounder to the exposure and outcome, the Confounding Triangle in Figure 7-2 is commonly used. The Confounding Triangle illustrates that the purpose of the study is to identify the association between the exposure of interest and outcome. But the association of interest can be affected by a potential confounder if that confounder is a risk factor for the

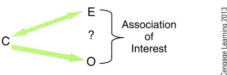

E = exposure; O = outcome; C = possible confounder   © Cengage Learning 2013

FIGURE 7-2 Confounding Triangle

outcome (single pointed arrow) and is associated with the exposure of interest (double pointed arrow).

Two Methods to Identify Confounding

There are two typical methods to identify variables that are confounders: (1) literature based and (2) data based. Investigators often choose between these two methods to search for confounders, but it is wise to use both methods simultaneously.

Literature-Based Confounding

The use of previously published confounders for a proposed specified hypothesis is a very sound starting point and should be utilized during the development of research proposals. If previous studies have shown that the criteria for confounding was met, and if previous authors have controlled confounding in their methods, those confounding variables should also be included in future studies with similar hypotheses and populations. Identifying confounders through literature-based methods can also be done by looking at research that used potential confounders in the role of the exposure of interest. In these studies, an investigator can determine if criteria for confounding have been met. For example, if the decision is made to determine if cigarette smoking is a confounder of the relationship between diet and CVD, previous studies on smoking and diet, as well as other studies on smoking and CVD, could be reviewed to determine whether smoking is associated with diet and is a risk factor for CVD.

Data-Based Confounding

The assessment of data-based confounding is often used to confirm literature-based confounding but also can be the sole reason that variables are chosen to be addressed as confounders. However, the method of data-based confounding assessment is dependent on the predetermination to collect information on the potential confounding variables from subjects. So it is often best to perform a literature-based assessment of confounding prior to determining which information will be collected from the subjects. In data-based confounding assessment, investigators will use the actual data collected for their study to see if potential confounders will meet the criteria for confounding. Once all their data have been collected, organized, and edited, they can analyze the relationships between potential confounders and the exposure and those between the potential confounders and the outcome of the study. Based on the findings of these preliminary analyses, data-based confounders can be identified.

controlling: mathematical transformation of rates or measures of association to account for external variables; also known as "minimizing confounding," "holding confounders constant," and "eliminating the effect of confounding"

Another data-based method for assessing confounding is to actually test the findings from the study several times to see whether the confounding variable(s) cause a distortion in the findings. This involves an iterative process performed by testing the study hypothesis without considering the effect of the confounder, then testing the hypothesis again while considering the effect of the confounder. This process is known as **controlling** for confounding in the analysis of the data. Other terms used for controlling confounding are "minimizing confounding," "holding confounders constant," and "eliminating the effect of confounding." Many techniques are available that control for confounding, but the purpose is to obtain study results as if the confounding did not occur. If investigators perform their analysis without controlling for confounding, then they perform the same analysis while controlling for confounding; the investigators will be able to ascertain whether there is any distort in results as a result of the confounding. If there is distortion and if the variable meets the other criteria for confounding, that variable is a data-based confounder for that specific hypothesis.

CONTROLLING FOR CONFOUNDING TECHNIQUES

Epidemiologists spend a large part of their time learning and using the wide variety of techniques used to control for confounding. Some of these techniques are performed in the early stages of the planning and implementation of a data collection or research study. Others of these techniques are statistical tools used during the analysis of collected data. The list of techniques used to control for confounding in the early stages of planning and implementing data collection or research study includes:

1. Conducting literature reviews to identify confounding variables from other studies;

2. Deciding to collect data on these known confounding variables;

3. Restricting data collection to limited groups of the confounders;

4. Randomizing subject enrollment;

5. Randomizing subjects to intervention groups in an experimental trial; and

6. Collecting data such that comparison groups are matched on confounding variables.

Detailed discussion of each of these techniques is beyond the scope of this text, but each technique takes planning and upfront work before starting data collection. The first two techniques simply identify the need to know which literature-based confounders are important for the chosen hypothesis. As discussed previously, a review of the literature is an important step in identifying confounders. The worst-case scenario in the controlling of confounding would be for the investigators to not realize that particular variables are confounders and, consequently, not plan to collect data about them from subjects. For example, an investigator who does not realize that cigarette smoking is a confounder for the relationship between coffee drinking and pancreatic cancer may not collect data on cigarette smoking or may not decide to include cigarette smoking in the processes to control for confounding. This would not allow the investigator to observe the distortion that this confounder would cause. Although it seems simple to identify confounding variables and collect data about them, it is one of the most important steps in controlling for confounding, without which the other techniques are not possible.

Another technique for controlling confounding variables in the early stages of a study is to restrict enrollment of subjects to narrow categories of a known confounder. If the technique is implemented correctly, it ensures that all subjects have the same value for the confounders, and it holds the confounders constant. An example of this restriction would be in the case where gender is a confounder to conduct the study among men only (or women only).

The other three techniques for controlling for confounding in the early stages of a study cannot be covered with adequate depth in this introductory text. Briefly, randomizing of either selection of subjects or assignment of subjects to intervention groups are both techniques that use scientific randomization to attempt to keep the variation of the confounding variables within the subject groups constant. This hopefully is accomplished because every subject, regardless of confounder category, has an equal chance of being in any one of the groups. Lastly, matching is a traditional method in epidemiology, which, although complicated to design and implement, is very easy for nonresearchers to understand how the confounders are controlled. In essence, the idea behind matching is that the investigator intentionally enrolls subjects such that the variation of confounders in the comparison groups is the same. To continue with the gender example, in a situation where gender is considered a confounder of the hypothesis, and the study is designed to compare those with the outcome to those without the outcome, the decision to match on gender would mean that the comparison groups (outcome versus nonoutcome) are selected and enrolled so that each comparison group has an equal number of men and women.

CONTROLLING CONFOUNDING: STATISTICAL TECHNIQUES

stratification: separating and analyzing data according to categories of a variable or characteristic

adjustment: mathematical transformation of rates or measures of association to account for external variables

In addition to controlling for confounding in the early stages of planning or implementing a study, another method involves controlling for confounding through statistical techniques used during the analysis of data. The process of controlling confounding in the analysis of data is performed in two steps: (1) **stratification** and (2) **adjustment**. A great deal of planning and experience, as well as statistical expertise, needs to go into both stratification and adjustment. One or both of these steps can be used in the analysis of data, but both individually will provide control of confounding.

Stratification

Stratification is the process of separating data in the sample into several subsamples (strata) according to specified criteria such as age groups, socioeconomic status, and so on, when these variables are identified as confounders. This is a very straightforward but powerful tool for both assessing confounding, as well as for eliminating the distortion as a result of confounding. Once the strata are formed, the subjects within each stratum have similar values for the confounders. Data can then be reanalyzed within each stratum, and the results of this reanalysis will be unaffected by the confounders for which the stratification was performed.

Examples of stratification are provided in Tables 7-3 and 7-4. In Table 7-3, the data from a study investigating the relationship between salt in the diet and high blood pressure is presented among the 200 subjects in the study. Because the total study population is 200 subjects, the analysis of the entire study data set is referred to as the crude analysis. A crude relative risk is calculated as 1.67, implying that salt in the diet may be related with an increase in blood pressure. However, the investigators know that the age of subjects is a confounder for the relationship between salt in the diet and blood pressure. So fortunately the investigators also collected information about the age of each subject. The subjects' ages were categorized into "old" and "young" (this is an oversimplification for the purposes of this example).

In Table 7-4, the data from the 200 subjects in this study were stratified by age, which resulted in 130 subjects being classified as young and 70 subjects being classified as old. The data are now reanalyzed within each age-specific stratum. The relative risk among the young subjects is 1.00, and the relative risk among the old subjects is also 1.00.

These two relative risks are referred to as "stratum-specific relative risks," and each one is performed among subjects with similar ages. The result is to look at the relationship between salt in the diet and blood pressure while holding age constant or, in other words, while eliminating the effect of age on the hypothesis. The investigators can now look at the crude (without controlling for age) relationship between salt and blood pressure and compare it to the age-specific stratum (controlling for age) relationship between salt and blood pressure. This comparison will identify whether there is a distortion as a result of age in the diet and blood pressure relationship. The conclusion between Tables 7-3 and 7-4 is that there appears to be a moderate relationship (RR = 1.67) between salt intake and high blood pressure; but once the investigators eliminated the effect of age, that relationship appears to disappear (RR = 1.0 in both age-specific strata). So the conclusion is that age does distort the relationship between salt intake and blood pressure and is therefore a confounder.

TABLE 7-3 Crude Results from a Study of Dietary Salt Intake and Hypertension in 200 Subjects

	High Blood Pressure	**Normal Blood Pressure**	
Use Salt in Diet	30	70	100
No Salt in Diet	18	82	100
	48	152	200

Relative risk $= \dfrac{30/100}{18/100} = 1.67$

TABLE 7-4 Results from a Study of Dietary Salt Intake and Hypertension in 200 Subjects Stratified by Age Group

Age group: YOUNG

	High Blood Pressure	Normal Blood Pressure	
Use Salt in Diet	5	45	50
No Salt in Diet	8	72	80
	13	117	200

Relative risk $= \dfrac{5/50}{8/80} = 1.00$

Age group: OLD

	High Blood Pressure	Normal Blood Pressure	
Use Salt in Diet	25	25	50
No Salt in Diet	10	10	20
	35	35	70

Relative risk $= \dfrac{25/50}{10/20} = 1.00$

Further, the distortion caused by the confounder made the relationship between salt intake and blood pressure appear to exist, but it likely was simply the result of the relationship of age with both salt intake and blood pressure.

Adjustment

Although stratification in the process to control for confounding is valuable and should always be attempted, it is very easy to imagine how cumbersome it can become when there are multiple confounders or multiple categories of a single confounder. Further, it does not leave the investigator an overall measure to report because the crude measure is no longer considered valid and there may be many stratum-specific measures. The solution is to take a remaining step and calculate a single measure that summarizes the relationship while also controlling for confounding. This single measure is known as a *summary measure*, and the mathematic processes used to calculate summary measures are known as *adjustment*. The discussion of statistical adjustment in epidemiology is a very broad and, of course, a very mathematical discussion. Statistical adjustment for confounding in epidemiology can include very straightforward techniques that can be calculated by hand, as well as very complicated regression techniques that require matrix algebra and computers to perform.

Although there will be no attempt to describe the mathematics of statistical adjustment of confounding in this text, it is important to understand the general concept and to identify the key methods used in epidemiology. The reason to adjust rates is to eliminate the difference as a result of external variables on the magnitude and comparability of the rates. This is the same concept behind adjusting measures of association. (See Chapter 6, Using Rates and Ratios, for a discussion of adjusting rates.)

Methods for adjusting measures of association to control for confounding in epidemiology are generally categorized in two groups—those used to control for a few variables or those used to control for many variables simultaneously. The statistical procedures to control for a few variables generally involve performing stratification first, then using various formulas to calculate a single measure that can be interpreted as the measure of association between exposure and outcome while controlling for the confounders.

The most traditional epidemiologic method to calculate this single measure was developed by Mantel and Haenszel (1959). They developed formulas that have led to the calculation of summary measures of association such as summary odds ratios, summary relative risks, and summary density ratios. The property of each of these is that they combine the multiple stratum-specific measures into one new estimate that is calculated as the weighted average of the stratum specific measures. Once the summary measure is calculated, it is the single measure of association that can be reported as the findings that are now controlled for the confounders. Continuing the example in Tables 7-3 and 7-4, the crude measure of association between salt intake and high blood pressure was RR = 1.67. Then the data were stratified by age and the stratum-specific associations were both RR = 1.00. A summary relative risk can then be calculated according to the Mantel and Haenszel process, which would give a measure of RR = 1.00. The conclusion from this calculation is that after controlling for age, there is no relationship between salt intake and high blood pressure. Using this same general idea, it is possible to control for multiple confounders using mathematical adjustment techniques that provide one summary measure.

PRECISION

A second component that affects the accuracy of data or a study is **precision**. Unlike validity, precision is not a systematic problem, but instead involves collecting incorrect data as a result of random errors. These random errors can occur for a wide variety of reasons, but many can be prevented by being careful and detail-oriented. Because reliability is defined as the consistency of a procedure or a set of measurements to give

precision: how close a measurement is to its true value

the same results under different conditions, some reasons for precision errors may be poor reliability of a procedure, measurement, or staff member.

Another precision issue involves evaluating if the results are **statistically significant**, meaning that the results observed were unlikely to be the result of chance. Statistical significance takes on a perspective with an opposite view of reliability. Statistical significance assesses how often random errors occur in data, and then determines when any data point is different from another NOT as a result of random chance. And finally, precision is easier to achieve when there is a large, unbiased sample of people to study.

statistically significant: the results observed were unlikely to be the result of chance

Reliability

Recall the baseball pitcher example used at the beginning of this chapter. A reliable pitcher can hit the same spot every time. It is usually a result of practice and skill. When a reliable pitcher misses the intended spot, it is often infrequent and random. A reliable data collection tool has minimal random error and is able to be repeated correctly in many different scenarios.

The best way to improve reliability of data measurement tools, like a pitcher in baseball, is to utilize measurement tools many times prior to the data collection or study implementation. In epidemiology, this can be done by reviewing the literature to see what others have successfully used to measure the same information. It can also be done by training staff and piloting measurement tools.

One way to assess whether a measure is reliable and will give the same result every time it is used is to test it by administering the measure to the same people at two different times. This kind of reliability is called **test-retest reliability** and can assess the consistency of a measure across time. Of course, this test assumes that there will be no change in the construct being measured. For example, if a questionnaire is used twice with the person, it could differ the second time because the subject changed his or her mind. So it is best used for things that are stable over time. Generally, test-retest reliability will be higher when a short amount of time has passed between tests.

Another type of reliability is **inter-rater reliability**, or the degree to which independent raters score the same information in the same way. This is very important, if several data collectors are used, and takes effort on the researcher's part to make sure that they are trained to collect the information in the same way. Further, often one data collector is identified as the gold standard. This data collector can be used to repeat measures on subjects previously assessed by other data collectors to increase inter-rater reliability and overall reliability.

test-retest reliability: can assess the consistency of a measure across time by administering it to the same people at different times

inter-rater reliability: the degree to which independent raters score the same information in the same way

The adage that "practice makes perfect" is the key to reliability in the precision of data and study results. Although no investigator intends to make random errors in his or her research, it is the experienced investigator who knows that reliable tools and process will minimize random errors. But even with reliable tools and procedures, investigators still need to work on ensuring random errors do not occur because of mundane problems such as sloppy data entry or handwriting, filing problems, losing records, or typos in manuscripts.

Statistical Significance

A related use of the concept of precision is a wide variety of statistical tests that are used to determine whether a deviation from the expected findings of a study is the result of random chance. In other words, the concept of precision is concerned with any deviations from the expected truth that are random, but the opposite perspective is the question: How far from the expected truth does a finding need to be before it is too far to be random? When a finding is too far from the expected truth to be random, the finding is considered to be statistically significantly different, or often just referred to as "statistically significant."

Note that not all statistically significant findings are, in fact, important. There is a distinction between mathematically assessing the likelihood that a result is the result of chance and whether the finding is meaningful in the real world.

The logic behind statistical significance is that there is a true value for everything that is measured, and the goal of accuracy is to get to that true value. So anytime there are differences, the goal is to try to fix the errors. But what if the hypothesis involves determining if something is in fact supposed to be different? For example, say the infant mortality rate was measured in two distinct populations and the result is two different rates. The reason for the two different rates could be the result of: (1) an error was made in one or both of the rates or (2) they truly are different. To address the first reason, statistical tests can be used to determine if the difference in rates is likely the result of errors. Then if these tests confirm there was not an error, it can be concluded that the rates are truly different.

To illustrate significance testing using our baseball pitcher example in Figure 7-3 the pitcher is asked to aim at the same spot for 100 pitches. If he is reliable (precise), he will hit very close to the same spot every time, and the few that he misses will only miss by a small amount, so the pattern will be very tightly packed together. However, another pitcher might be less reliable, and the pitches that he misses will

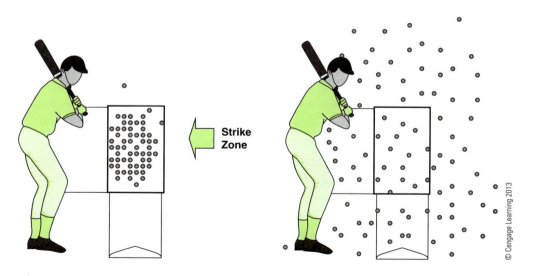

FIGURE 7-3 Precision of Pitching from Two Different Pitchers

be more frequent and farther from the same spot for a more scattered pattern. For each pitcher, those pitches that stay within the pattern will simply be labeled as random error in missing the target. But as the pitches get closer to the outside of the pattern of each of the pitchers, the location of these outside pitches becomes less and less likely. Further, there is a distance from the target that is so far outside the pattern that an observer would begin to wonder if the pitcher is now throwing at another target. Statistical significance testing can tell the observer that based on the first 100 pitches, what is the likelihood that a pitch will land beyond any specified distance from the target? Hitting farther and farther from the target becomes less and less likely. Also, notice that the distance that seems less and less likely will be different based on the precision of the two pitchers.

From this example, it can be seen that the underlying precision of a data set is both a problem to be improved and an attribute that can be used to help make scientific decisions. Once the precision of a data set is determined, investigators testing hypotheses with that data set can use statistical significance testing to help accept or reject a hypothesis that is based on an observed change either between data sets or between different categories within the same data set.

P-Values

Regardless of the statistcal significance test used, all of them calculate a *p*-value to determine the probability that the difference is the result of random error. The **p-value** is the probability of obtaining a test statistic at least as extreme as the one that was actually observed, assuming that the null hypothesis is true.

The *p*-value can range from 0 to 1, where numbers closer to zero are less likely to have occurred by chance. Typically, a *p-value of 0.05 or lower* is considered to be statistically significant or unlikely to have occurred by chance. However, the investigator can predetermine a cut point to use for considering statistical significance; this predetermined cut point is referred to as an "alpha (α) level." Again, the typically accepted alpha level is 0.05, which means that a *p*-value of less than 0.05 is considered statistically significant.

Using Statistical Significance

The primary use of statistical significance is to determine whether two measures with different values are different from each other simply because of random chance or not. It is a method to assist with decision making. Statistical significance is used to test a scientific hypothesis, assuming that study bias is minimal. A hypothesis is a statement about an anticipated relationship between risk factors and outcomes. An example of a simple hypothesis is stating that cigarette smoking is a risk factor for lung cancer. If a researcher wants to test this hypothesis, it would be necessary to develop and implement a study to investigate it. It is standard in statistical testing to state the research hypothesis as if there is no relationship between the study factors and the outcome. For the smoking and lung cancer example, a null hypothesis is that "cigarette smoking is not related to lung cancer." We can use statistical significance testing to determine whether the null hypothesis is likely, which means that cigarette smoking is not a risk factor for lung cancer. But if the significance

p-value: the probability of obtaining a test statistic at least as extreme as the one that was actually observed, assuming that the null hypothesis is true

testing finds that the null hypothesis is not likely, then there is evidence that cigarette smoking may, in fact, be related to lung cancer.

The steps to testing a hypothesis are to first develop and state a null hypothesis. Then develop, design, and implement a study to test the null hypothesis. Perform the study with as little bias as possible. Once the study has resulted in good clean data, the data can be used to perform statistical procedures to begin the testing. The statistical procedures will result in *p*-values, and these *p*-values will be used to see if the null hypothesis is likely. If the null hypothesis is likely, then the null hypothesis is accepted, and the evidence leans toward no relationship between the study factors and the outcome. However, if the null hypothesis is unlikely, then the null hypothesis is rejected, and the evidence leans toward a relationship between the study factors and the outcome. It is important to reemphasize that statistical significance testing is not the only information used to make a decision, but it does contribute to the decision.

Sample Size

The good news about precision errors is that they can be minimized by the size of the sample to collect for a study. In order to improve the precision of a data set, a larger sample can be collected. The large **sample size** makes any one random error less of a proportion of the overall data set. So although it would be better to have no random errors, one way to keep the effects of these to a minimum would be to dilute them. For example, consider the situation of a thimble full of a toxic material dumped into water. If you were forced to take a drink of that water afterward, would you prefer that the toxic thimble be dumped in to glass of water or a swimming pool of water before you drink it? Unfortunately, in the case of nonrandom errors (differential errors), a larger sample size does not dilute the effect and may magnify the problem.

Although there is no set number that identifies an appropriately large sample size, there are formulas that can be used to estimate the needed sample. In the case of only having access to a fixed sample size, there are also formulas for the **power of a study**, which is the probability of finding a positive result if one is present given that sample size. In general, the larger the sample size, the less error introduced by variations in the population and the easier it is to be confident in the results of the study.

sample size: number of subjects who participate in a study

power of a study: the probability of finding a positive result, if one is present

Summary

This chapter provided some important tools and concepts that epidemiologists use to ensure that data are collected accurately. These included the types of validity and a discussion of the effects that different types of bias might have on the results. Also discussed were ways to recognize confounding and how to control this type of bias through stratification or adjustment. To put these concepts into context, the role of precision, including its components of reliability, statistical significance, and *p*-values, sampling techniques, and sample size, were also introduced.

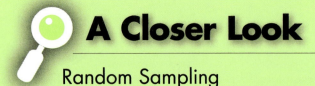

A Closer Look

Random Sampling

The whole point of selecting a sample of the population is to get general data about the entire (source) population without having to gather information from every person. For example, if there are 10,000 people in the population, an accurate characterization of this group could be obtained by getting surveys from 1,000 people. However, if the source population distribution is 60% men and 40% women and the survey distribution is 30% men and 70% women (as often happens with surveys), the results will not accurately represent the source population.

This example using men and women is easy to understand, but consider that there could be many other differences between the source population and the surveyed population. To protect against selection bias, the sampling method of choice is random sampling, rather than convenience sampling. However, many people mistake random sampling for convenience sampling (because the people included are chosen for the survey "at random"). However, "random" in the statistical sense means that everyone in the source population has an equal chance to be included in the survey. There are several ways to do this. The easiest to understand (but the hardest to implement) is to make a list of all 10,000 people and assign them a number from 1 to 10,000. Then using a random number generator (computer programs or apps are available to do this), keep drawing numbers until there are 1,000 in the survey sample. Or, use the random number to start the process and then select every tenth number after that until you have 1,000 subjects. This method helps to remove bias in selecting potential subjects, but it is not usually possible to use this approach.

Another random sampling approach is to stratify the population first (by neighborhood or income or other characteristic) and then use a random number for a starting point within each stratum and select the number needed to complete the survey sample by taking every tenth person. This is often done with telephone sampling where the phone numbers are stratified by the first three digits and a random number generator selects subsequent numbers. These are just a few of the techniques that can be used to conduct random sampling. The field of sampling is diverse and includes many options, depending on the goals of the study.

Review Questions

1. What are the two "parts" of accuracy?

   i. _____

   ii. _____

2. The type of validity that correctly measures variables of a study population is known as:

   a. Internal
   b. External
   c. Reliability
   d. Interaction

3. **True or False** In general, as study biases decrease, validity increases.

4. **True or False** Another term for convenience sampling is "random sampling," because they have the same meaning.

5. **True or False** Nondifferential bias is less damaging to a study than differential bias.

6. **True or False** The finding from the study suggesting that coffee drinking was associated with pancreatic cancer is an example of confounding.

7. **True or False** A p-value close to zero is probably a mistake.

8. If a strong finding goes away after adjustment, this is an example of:

   a. Nondifferential measurement of the exposure
   b. High test-retest reliability
   c. Confounding
   d. Stratification
   e. None of the above

9. Which one of the following is NOT an information bias?

   a. Volunteer bias
   b. Interviewer bias
   c. Reporting bias
   d. Response fatigue bias

10. Match the characteristics in the left column with the appropriate letter from the list in the right column. (Letters from right column may be used more than once.)

____ Lack of cause/effect bias in a study	a. construct validity
____ Measures what it is intended to measure	b. external validity
____ Enables generalization to similar populations	c. internal validity
____ Causes confusion or distortion	d. reliability
____ Consistency in measurement	e. confounding
____ Controls for confounding variables	f. precision
	g. adjustment

11. Which are important elements in evaluating whether a study is relatively free of bias? (Circle all that apply.)

   a. Large sample size
   b. Convenience sampling
   c. Low internal validity
   d. Nondifferential assessment of disease state
   e. Control of confounders

12. **For Deeper Thought** A study found a strong and statistically significant association of smoking and being involved in an automobile accident. Because people who smoke often drink alcohol, what are some strategies to determine if the smoking and automobile accident finding was confounded by alcohol use?

Website Resources

For more information on health statistics: http://www.cdc.gov/nchs

For more information and history on sampling, visit Wikipedia: http://en.wikipedia.org

References

Encyclopedia of Biostatistics. John Wiley and Sons, Inc., 1999–2010. Online ISBN: 9780470011812. doi: 10.1002/0470011815.

MacMahon, B., Yen, S., Trichopoulos, D., Warren, K., & Nardi, G. (1981). Coffee and cancer of the pancreas. *New England Journal of Medicine, 304*(11):630–633.

Mantel, N., & Haenszel, W. (1959) Statistical aspects of the analysis of data from retrospective studies of disease. *Journal of the National Cancer Institute, 22,* 719–748.

Vineis, P., & McMichael, A. J. (1998). Bias and confounding in molecular epidemiology studies: Special considerations. *Carcinogenesis, 19*(12) 2063–2067.

PART II

APPLICATIONS IN EPIDEMIOLOGY

In Part I, the basic concepts and tools of epidemiology were presented. Although the presentation of these tools is an important first step, the tools become more apparent when they are shown in use with specific diseases. The application of epidemiologic tools is one of the unique strengths of this text. Each of the chapters in Part II first describes the basic physiology and symptoms of the major diseases and conditions studied in epidemiology. The application of the basic tools of epidemiology is then described for each disease and condition. The diseases and conditions chosen for each chapter are the infectious diseases and chronic diseases that are traditionally studied in epidemiology, plus some added presentations of reproductive epidemiology and epidemiology in developing countries. In addition, a chapter on outbreak investigations as another fundamental application of epidemiologic tools is also included to give students the concepts used in this very important function of epidemiology and public health.

Chapter 8

INFECTIOUS DISEASES

Learning Objectives

Upon completion of this chapter, you should be able to:

1. Name three methods used to classify infectious diseases and give two examples of each.
2. List the six modes of transmission and give an example of a disease that is transmitted for each mode.
3. Name an infection of the central nervous system, respiratory system, gastro-intestinal system, and a sexually transmitted infection and basically describe key characteristics of each (infectious agent, incubation period, disease caused, and unique features, if any).
4. List the five goals of infectious disease control.
5. List the three major methods of transmission of the HIV virus and provide an example of each method.

Key Terms

Acquired Immunodeficiency Syndrome (AIDS)

active carrier

antiretroviral therapy (ART)

CD4 T cells

carrier

convalescent carrier

diarrhea

encephalitis

enterocolitis/colitis

fomite

food borne intoxication

gastritis

gastroenteritis

Gram stain

healthy or passive carrier

horizontal transmission

human immunodeficiency virus (HIV)

index case
latent TB infection
meningitis
mother-to-child
transmission (MTCT)

opportunistic infections
pathogenicity
per-act risk
primary case
reservoir

seroconversion
vector
vertical transmission
virulence
zoonoses

Chapter Outline

INTRODUCTION

This is where the field of epidemiology got its start, studying infectious diseases! Epidemiology is the historical cornerstone of the study of infectious diseases for clinicians, as well as for public health professionals and researchers. The term *epidemiology* itself is indicative of its history in the study of infectious diseases. The name originates from the study of epidemics throughout history. Finally, infectious diseases have had the largest impact on the history of health in humans.

Fewer than 100 years have passed since infectious diseases caused the most death and suffering around the world. In developed countries, chronic diseases have now surpassed infectious diseases as the most common causes of death and disability, but the study of the epidemiology of infectious disease is still the most fundamental part of the study of the distribution and determinants of disease in humans.

Infectious disease epidemiology is the study of circumstances under which both infection and disease occur in a population and the factors that influence their frequency, spread, and distribution. Infectious diseases are generally short-lived and, with treatment, can often be quickly cured. There is, however, with some agents, the potential for widespread infection that crosses community, state, country, and continental lines. In all epidemics, morbidity and mortality are costly from a public health standpoint.

In infectious disease epidemiology, a *case may also be a source* of disease. So when discussing infectious diseases, one has to recognize that the distribution and determinants of disease include new cases transmitted from a person who already has the infection. For example, the risk of becoming infected with chickenpox is dependent on being exposed to another person who currently has chickenpox. Furthermore, a *case may be a source of disease without being recognized as a case* of disease at the time. Many infectious diseases, such as chickenpox, can be transmitted to others by a person who is not yet clinically ill. Also, *people may be immune, either because of immunization or previous disease, and therefore, not get the infection even if adequately exposed.* So although a person may be exposed to others with chickenpox, he or she may not get ill if she or he has already had the disease or has had the vaccine. When studying infectious disease epidemiology, *there may be a need for urgency* such as when an outbreak of disease has occurred like the 2009 influenza pandemic. Finally, *infectious diseases very often have clear opportunities for prevention measures* that have a good scientific basis. Prevent exposure to the etiologic agent or make one resistant to an infectious agent (e.g., with vaccination) and the disease is prevented.

Most recently the epidemiology of infectious disease has been dramatically changed by the recognition that control of infectious disease and emerging disease is now a global priority. Infectious diseases are no longer confined to local populations and communities because of the global "travel" of these diseases. A susceptible person exposed to an infected person in an endemic country without an organized immunization program can then get on an airplane back to the United States prior to the onset of any symptoms. After that person's arrival, symptoms develop and diagnosis occurs, but not before others are put at risk for disease and complications of the infection. For example, measles is still considered endemic in many parts of the world. In fact, 87% of the 692 cases of measles in 6–23-month-old infants in the United States from 2001–2010 were imported from other countries. Another well-documented example of global "travel" of disease are cases of malaria occurring from infected mosquitoes that have "stowed away" on airplanes while still on the ground in malaria endemic areas, biting passengers and transmitting malaria in the air. Most of the recent outbreaks of vaccine preventable infections in the

United States, which are usually controlled by immunization programs, arrived in this country via a susceptible person returning from a foreign country where this person was infected.

The purpose of this chapter is to provide the fundamental concepts in the epidemiology of infectious disease, as well as some fundamental concepts of microbiology and the diseases themselves. Although the epidemiology of the large categories of infectious disease will briefly be identified here, this chapter is not intended to be a definitive text of microbiology for the diseases presented.

THE SCOPE OF THE PROBLEM

human immunodeficiency virus (HIV): RNA virus that infects human immune cells and destroys them

Acquired Immunodeficiency Syndrome (AIDS): the most severe stage of HIV infection

Infectious diseases are the leading cause of death worldwide; influenza and pneumonia are the eighth leading cause of death in the United States. Everyone will have multiple infectious diseases in his or her lifetime. This may be anything from the common cold to something as severe as **human immunodeficiency virus (HIV)** infection or **Acquired Immunodeficiency Syndrome (AIDS)**, the most severe stage of HIV infection. Infectious diseases are responsible for 98% of worldwide deaths in children under 15 years old and 50% of deaths in persons 15–59 years old. The probability of death as a result of infectious disease in sub-Saharan Africa is 22%, but only 1.1% in developed countries, such as the United States.

Prevalence

Most infections are time limited either by their natural course or by the medications like antibiotics used to treat them. This makes prevalence data non-existent for most of the infectious diseases. Some of the longer-lasting infections like tuberculosis or HIV/AIDS can have prevalence data. Because these data are disease-specific, it will not be discussed here. Further, as discussed in Chapter 3, prevalence equals incidence times duration. Because infectious diseases are usually short in duration (either because of recovery or death), epidemiologists generally do not see a difference between the prevalence and incidence of infectious disease.

Incidence

In the United States, state health department workers collaborate with the Centers for Disease Control and Prevention (CDC) specialists in Atlanta, Georgia, on a periodic basis to determine which infectious diseases will require reporting to the public health departments (see Chapter 4). A report at the local level protects the public health by identifying cases, following up on treatment, and instituting necessary control measures. Public health workers track contacts and investigate outbreaks. During the year, CDC collects and compiles data from the states on certain reportable diseases, and these statistics are published annually in the *Summary of Notifiable Disease—United States*. The last report was published in 2011 for data

TABLE 8-1 New Cases of Reportable Infectious Diseases, United States, 2009

Infection	Total No. New Cases, 2009
HIV infection	36,870
Giardia	19,399
Gonorrhea	301,174
Salmonella	49,192
Syphilis	44,828

Based on: CDC, *Summary of Notifiable Disease–United States, 2009;* http://www.cdc.gov/mmwr/PDF/wk/mm5853.pdf

obtained in 2009. See Table 8-1 for the data for a few of the infections that are discussed later in this chapter.

Similarly, the World Health Organization collects data from countries across the world and compiles and reports on infectious diseases. The latest compiled data available as of November 2011 is from 2004, but data on a couple of the specific diseases are available from 2009. Information on the number of new cases of the top five infectious diseases is presented in Table 8-2 with the 2004 data, unless otherwise noted.

TABLE 8-2 New Cases of Infectious Diseases, Worldwide, 2004

Infection	Total No. New Cases, 2004
Diarrheal Disease	4,620,419,000
Lower Respiratory Infection	446,814,000
Malaria (2009)	225,000,000
Measles	27,118,000
Pertussis	18,387,000
HIV/AIDS (2009)	2,600,000
Tuberculosis (2009)	9,400,000

Based on: WHO, Disease and Injury Regional Estimates for 2004 and World Health Statistics 2011 Report; http://www.who.int/healthinfo/global_burden_disease/estimates_regional/en/index.html; http://www.who.int/gho/publications/world_health_statistics/EN_WHS2011_Part1.pdf

Death Rates

The most dramatic and concerning result of any disease is death. The discussion of death from infectious disease in the United States is highlighted by the trend in the last 100 years that shows the rate of death from infectious diseases has been declining. In Figure 8-1, the overall crude death rate from all infectious diseases in the United States is shown from 1900 to 1996. There is a clear decline in the death rate during this time period, beginning with a rate of 800 deaths per 100,000 persons per year in 1900 and ending with a rate of 30 per 100,000 persons per year in 1996. Many technologic and public health accomplishments have contributed to this decline in death from infectious disease. Dramatic declines can be seen when health departments were established in the beginning of the 1900s. Although infections still occurred, deaths from those infections were substantially reduced. The widespread use of penicillin in the early 1940s prevented the deaths of many people who previously would have died from their infectious disease.

As can be seen in Figure 8-2, a concurrent shift in the leading causes of death can also be seen in the United States since the beginning of the twentieth century.

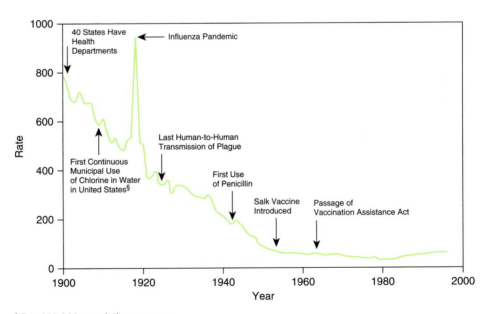

* Per 100,000 population per year.

+ Adapted from Armstrong, G. L., Conn, L. A., & Pinner, R. W. (1999). Trends in infectious disease mortality in the United States during the 20th century. *Journal of the American Medical Association, 281,* 61-66.

§ American Water Works Association. (1973). *Water Chlorination Principles and Practices: AWWA Manual M20.* Denver, CO: American Water Works Association.

FIGURE 8-1 Crude Death Rate* for Infectious Diseases—United States, 1900–1996+

Courtesy of Centers for Disease Control and Prevention: http://www.cdc.gov/mmwr/preview/mmwrhtml/mm4829a1.htm)

In 1900, the top three leading causes of death (as a percentage of all deaths) in the United States were infectious diseases. Almost 100 years later, deaths caused by infectious diseases have dramatically dropped such that only two infectious diseases are in the top 10 leading causes of death. This drop in deaths caused by infectious disease has paved the way for the emergence of chronic disease to become the most frequent killer of the U.S. population in 1997, led by heart disease, cancer, and stroke (as discussed in later chapters). In 2008, in the United States, pneumonia

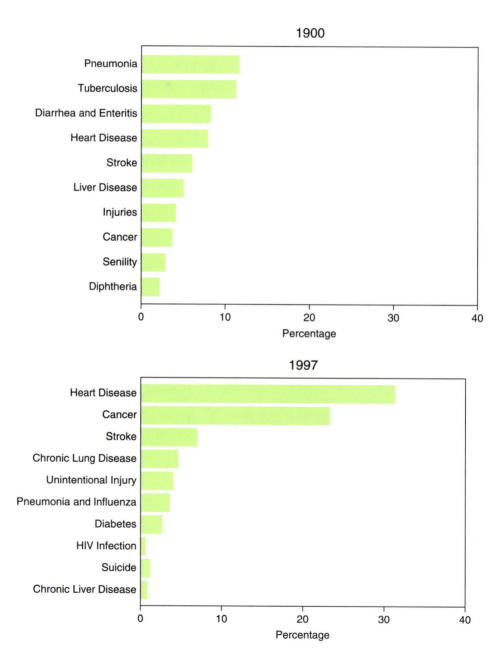

FIGURE 8-2 The 10 Leading Causes of Death as a Percentage of All Deaths—United States, 1900 and 1997
Courtesy of Centers for Disease Control and Prevention: http://www.cdc.gov/mmwr/preview/mmwrhtml/mm4829a1.htm)

TABLE 8-3 Leading Causes of Infectious Disease Deaths Worldwide, 2004

Lower respiratory infections (4.2 million)

HIV/AIDS (2.0 million)

Diarrheal diseases (2.2 million)

Tuberculosis (1.5 million)

Malaria (0.9 million)

Based on: World Health Report, 2004 data; http://www.who.int/health-info/global_burden_disease/estimates_regional/en/index.html

and influenza were the eighth leading cause of death (down from sixth in 1997) and septicemia was the tenth. HIV infections are no longer among the top 10 causes of death in the United States.

In 2004 (latest data available as of November 2011), WHO reported that infectious diseases were responsible for 30.6% of all deaths worldwide, with over 9.5 million deaths each year from infectious diseases, mostly in developing countries. The United Nations considers infectious diseases important enough that the sixth Millennium Development Goal is "to combat HIV/AIDS, malaria and other diseases" with a target date of 2015. See Table 8-3 for the leading causes of death worldwide from infectious diseases.

Financial Costs

The total economic costs of infectious diseases are difficult to pinpoint. There are costs for outpatient visits and medications for simple infections, which are direct costs. The cost as a result of lost employment when someone is ill or has to stay home to care for a loved one with an infection accounts for indirect costs. Hospitalizations to treat complications for infections, like dehydration resulting from severe diarrhea or/and vomiting or for intravenous antibiotics for more serious infections, add to direct costs. About 5–10% of all hospitalizations are for infectious diseases, and that number peaks to almost 15% in the winter months. About 34% of these hospitalizations are for lower respiratory tract infections, and 10% each are for kidney/urine, cellulitis/skin infections, and septicemia. There are costs for hospital-acquired infections and costs to treat infections that occur as complications of surgeries or procedures. In addition, investigating infectious outbreaks lead to high economic costs to public health agencies. This includes the costs for the public health workers who track and investigate these outbreaks and for the medical treatment.

BASICS OF INFECTIOUS DISEASE

To understand the epidemiology of infectious disease and the investigation of outbreaks (discussed further in Chapter 9), it is important to understand some basic concepts about infectious diseases—the stages of transmission, how organisms are transmitted, the organisms that cause infectious diseases and how they are classified, and how the epidemiologic triangle that was discussed in Chapter 2 applies specifically to infectious diseases.

Transmission of Infectious Diseases

Knowledge of the transmission of infectious diseases includes understanding the process of transmission from exposure to disease, the modes of transmission (horizontal vs. vertical), and the specific mechanisms of how the agents are transmitted.

Stages of Transmission

The key to understanding how diseases are spread is the concept of "stages" of transmission. The three stages of transmission include: (1) exposure, (2) infection, and (3) clinical disease (see Figure 8-3). The occurrence of one stage does not necessarily mean that the next stage will occur, but understanding these stages is fundamental to the epidemiology and prevention of infectious disease. For example, consider chickenpox. A person who has had the disease in the past or has been vaccinated may be exposed but will not become infected. An unimmunized person who has never had chickenpox before would be almost certain to become infected. An important fact is *that there is a difference between infection and disease*. While very often being infected with the etiologic agent will result in disease, it is not certain, and there can be a varying period of time between infection and disease.

Measuring disease occurrence depends on the stage of disease in individuals. Remember from Chapter 2 that once a disease occurs, it can be preclinical, subclinical, and clinical. The distinction between these types is especially important in infectious diseases. People with any of the three types have been exposed and infected with the etiologic agent, but only the person with clinical disease has the signs and symptoms that make the disease apparent. However, the infected person with preclinical or subclinical disease is usually able to transmit the disease to others.

Once the infectious disease manifests itself, there are three possible outcomes. Most commonly, the infection resolves with or even without treatment. Death from the infection is less common in the United States but more common worldwide. In addition to these two outcomes, an infected person can become a carrier of the disease. A **carrier** is person who has been exposed and infected by the etiologic agent and who is capable of transmitting the disease to others for a prolonged period of time. Carriers can transmit disease to others in a variety of ways. An **active carrier** is an infected individual capable

carrier: person who has been exposed and infected by the etiologic agent and who is capable of transmitting the disease to others for a prolonged period of time

active carrier: an infected individual capable of transmitting disease during and after clinical disease

EXPOSURE ⟶ INFECTION ⟶ CLINICAL DISEASE

FIGURE 8-3 Three Stages of Transmission
© Cengage Learning 2013

convalescent carrier: a person who can transmit the etiologic agent while recovering from the disease

healthy or passive carrier: an infected person who never gets clinically ill but who can transmit the etiologic agent to others

of transmitting disease during and after clinical disease. Active carriers are most concerning once they are no longer clinically ill. A carrier can also be a **convalescent carrier** and can transmit the etiologic agent while recovering from disease. But the most concerning carrier is known as a **healthy or passive carrier**. An infected person who never gets clinically ill, the healthy or passive carrier can transmit the etiologic agent to others. The most famous healthy carrier was known as Typhoid Mary (see Historical Note 8-1).

Historical Note 8·1

Typhoid Mary

Mary Mallon was born in Ireland in 1869. She immigrated to New York with her aunt and uncle when she was about 15 years old and took up employment as a cook. In 1906, she was working for the Warren family who had rented a summer home on Long Island. An outbreak of typhoid fever occurred and several members of the family, two maids, and a gardener became ill. The owners of the home knew that if they did not find the source of the infection, they would have difficulty renting the home again so they hired George Soper, a civil engineer with experience in typhoid fever, to investigate. He examined the food and water and decided that a human carrier probably transmitted the disease.

The cook, Mary Mallon, had disappeared so he tracked down her previous employment history only to find out that during her work at her previous seven jobs, 22 persons had become ill with typhoid fever and one had died. When she refused his request for stool, blood, and urine specimens for testing (she was healthy and could not understand how she could be responsible for the outbreaks!), he turned the case over to the New York City Department of Health. When Mary was finally found, she refused treatment because of her belief that she was healthy. She was placed in quarantine on North Brother Island for three years as she was considered a threat to the public. In 1910, she was released by a judge who ordered her not to work as a food handler. She agreed because she was anxious to be released. She tried working several other jobs but returned to cooking because of better pay. But in 1915, another outbreak occurred in a hospital in New York; and 25 persons became ill; two of them died. This infection was traced to the cook, Mrs. Brown, who was actually Mary Mallon using a different name for employment. Mary was found and placed in custody in quarantine again on North Brother Island, which is where she died in 1938. Mary was the first healthy carrier of an organism that could cause disease in others that was identified by the public health department.

Modes of Horizontal and Vertical Transmission

A basic concept of disease transmission is to understand that there are two modes: horizontal and vertical. **Horizontal transmission** is transmission of disease from person to person and may be directly from one person to another or indirectly from one person through an intermediate item to another person. An example would be any of the respiratory infections such as the common cold, as well as gastrointestinal infections and sexually transmitted infections. **Vertical transmission** is transmission of disease from mother to child during pregnancy or delivery. An example is the acquisition of Group B streptococcus infection by a newborn exposed to the agent during labor or passage through an infected birth canal. Most diseases are transmitted horizontally only—such as pneumonia, food borne infections, cholera, syphilis, and malaria. Some diseases may be transmitted horizontally or vertically—such as HIV, hepatitis B, and syphilis.

Horizontal Mechanisms of Transmission

To fully understand the concept of horizontal transmission, know that infectious diseases can be organized by the mechanisms of transmission. Table 8-4 shows the six mechanisms that account for most all infectious disease transmission. Some infectious agents can be transmitted by more than one mechanism.

The *first* mechanism of horizontal transmission includes **vectors** (insects) as an intermediate step between an infected individual and a susceptible person. The microbiological organism may require the metabolism of the insect for its own life cycle or may simply use the insect as a mode of transportation to a new host. Malaria is a major worldwide disease transmitted by the *Anopheles* mosquito and is discussed later in this chapter.

The *second* mechanism is food or water borne transmission of disease. This is the major mechanism that accounts for acute gastrointestinal infection outbreaks. There are more than 200 diseases transmitted in this nature where the agent is shed by the infected individuals and then carried by food or water to susceptible individuals. See Tables 8-8 and 8-9 for examples of diseases transmitted by food or water. A few of the more common agents are also discussed in more detail later in this chapter.

The *third* mechanism of horizontal transmission, as listed in Table 8-4, is direct person to person contact. Diseases are passed in this mechanism through contact with contaminated skin (e.g., hands), saliva, and respiratory secretions. These diseases are primarily the respiratory infections, as well as some of the gastrointestinal diseases. Other diseases such as chickenpox and meningitis may also be transmitted in this way. Some diseases may be transmitted from animals to humans. These diseases are called **zoonoses**.

A *fourth* mechanism of horizontal transmission includes inanimate objects (**fomites**) as an intermediate step between an infected individual and a susceptible individual. This mechanism succeeds because the agent is able to survive for a period of time on an object, contaminate it, and then come into contact with a susceptible individual. The fomite can be kitchen equipment, tissues used during a cold, and money exchanged. Agents that are transmitted in this manner

---

horizontal transmission: transmission of disease from person to person; may be directly from one person to another or indirectly from one person through an intermediate item to another person

vertical transmission: transmission of disease from mother to child during pregnancy or delivery

vector: an organism (usually an insect) that transmits or carries an infectious agent from its reservoir to its host

zoonoses: infectious diseases that are transmitted from animals to humans

fomite: an inanimate object that may serve as an intermediary for transmission of an infectious disease between an infected person and a susceptible host

TABLE 8-4 Horizontal Mechanisms of Infectious Disease Transmission

Vectors	Malaria, yellow fever, dengue fever, Lyme disease, plague, leishmaniasis, West Nile virus
Food/Water	Cholera, typhoid fever, salmonellosis, *E. coli* infection, botulism, *Giardia*, *Staphylococcal* food poisoning, shigellosis
Direct Contact	Common colds, influenza, chickenpox, Epstein Barr virus (mononucleosis), meningitis, herpes simplex virus-1, tuberculosis
Fomites	Common colds, influenza, rotavirus, adenovirus, anthrax
Feces/urine	Cholera, salmonellosis, *E. coli* infection, most food-borne diseases, Hantavirus
Sexual Contact	HIV/AIDS, chlamydia, herpes, syphilis, gonorrhea, human papillomavirus, and pubic lice (crabs)

need to be hearty organisms that are able to survive outside of the body without dependence on living cells or tissues. This mechanism is often concerning to the general public, but it is generally difficult for diseases to be transmitted through fomites.

Horizontal transmission of disease can also be accomplished through the shedding of the infectious agent in the feces or urine of infected individuals, the *fifth* mechanism. The feces or urine then contaminates a water supply or is not sufficiently cleaned from hands or equipment. Diseases transmitted in this mechanism include many of the gastrointestinal diseases such as cholera, salmonellosis, and *E. coli* infection.

The *sixth* mechanism for horizontal transmission includes those infections transmitted through sexual contact. Sexually transmitted infections include a broad variety of diseases that are spread by intimate contact with exposed genital sores or with the exchange of bodily fluids during sexual activity.

Case Concepts: Incubation Period, Primary versus Index Case

Case concepts, case definition, and case severity were presented in Chapter 3. These case concepts are very important to the measurement of infectious diseases. In addition to those concepts provided previously, several additional concepts are important when considering infectious diseases.

Incubation Period

One important concept in discussing infectious disease is the incubation period. As seen in Figure 8-3, infectious diseases begin with exposure, followed by infection, followed by clinical symptoms. The incubation period (similar to the latency period as discussed in Chapter 2) is the time between infection and appearance of clinical disease. When infection occurs, usually quickly after exposure, the amount of time until clinical signs and symptoms appear can vary greatly and is dependent on the disease and the individual. Most infectious diseases have a known incubation period "window," which can typically range from as little as 1–2 hours, as in the case of *Staphylococcal* food poisoning, to as long as a month or more. In the case of leprosy, the incubation period can be as long as 5 years!

If the infectious agent causing symptoms is known, this window can help to look backwards in time to determine when exposure and infection occurred. This may enable investigators to identify the original source of infection (e.g., exposure to certain foods in the case of food borne illnesses). Conversely, if the infectious agent is not known, but the time from exposure to clinical symptoms is known, this window can help investigators identify the infectious agent, which will help with treatment of the infections, as well as with control and prevention activities. The incubation period can also be used to enable investigators to estimate when the exposure occurred once the infectious agent and date of symptom onset are known, which will help with further control and prevention activities. The incubation period is also very important for two other reasons:

1. During this period when an infected person has not yet developed symptoms, *infection may be transmitted* to other susceptible hosts.

2. During this time, there may be many persons who have been infected but have not yet developed symptoms and, therefore, *cases will miss being counted*, leading to inaccurate and confusing data.

Primary versus Index Case

The primary case versus the index case, a second concept in infectious disease epidemiology, is particularly important when a rapid increase in cases occurs, such as in an outbreak. The **primary case** is the *first case of a specific infectious disease that occurs* in a population. The primary case is very specific to the infectious agent. For example, during the influenza season, there is frequently more than one subtype of influenza virus that circulates in the population. The primary case would be different for each of the subtypes of the virus. In some cases, the primary case in a population is not known. Then the *first case of a disease in a population that is identified* is known as the **index case**. Frequently, the primary case and the index case are the same, but in some situations, investigators may not be able to ascertain the primary case and may only be able to identify the index case. In fact, it is not always necessary to identify both cases. If the primary case is not certain, labeling the first case identified as an index case allows flexibility in the investigation of the outbreak. Later if more cases are identified that have occurred before an index case, the earliest case identified becomes the index case.

primary case: the first case of a specific infectious disease in a population

index case: the first case of a disease that is identified in a population

Basic Microbiology

From a public health standpoint, understanding the type of organism that is causing an outbreak or epidemic helps to anticipate signs and symptoms to use in surveillance, medications to use for treatment or prevention, and potential preventive control measures to initiate. The most common types of infectious agents (bacteria, viruses, and parasites) are described in this chapter.

Bacteria

Bacteria are single celled organisms that may cause disease themselves or through the toxins they produce. Bacteria are classified by their shapes—rods (bacilli), round (cocci), or spiral (spirilla)—as well as whether they take up **Gram stain**—either positive or negative. The shape and staining of bacteria give clues as to which bacteria may be responsible for a certain infection and therefore can guide treatment. Figure 8-4A illustrates cocci or round bacteria, and Figure 8-4B demonstrates bacilli, or rods, bacteria. For example, a pneumonia caused by Gram-positive cocci in pairs and chains is most likely Streptococcus pneumonia and therefore may be treated with penicillin. Bacterial infections are generally treated with antibiotics.

Gram stain: stain used in a microbiology lab to help classify bacteria according to the property of whether the bacteria take up the stain (Gram-positive) or not (Gram-negative)

Viruses

Viruses are infectious agents that use the metabolic processes of their host cells to reproduce and carry on their functions. They consist of genetic material, either DNA or RNA, and a protein capsule. The viral agent can coexist with the host cell, and infection is present but no disease is active. Later, some factor such as stress, a nutritional deficiency, or another infection, occurs and activates the virus to take over the cell processes

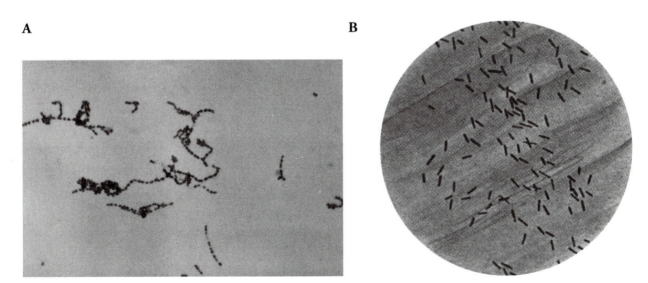

A   **B**

FIGURE 8-4 Types of Bacteria. (A) Gram-Positive Cocci (B) Gram-Negative Rods (Bacilli)
Courtesy of Centers for Disease Control and Prevention Public Health Image Library (PHIL): http://phil.cdc.gov/Phil/details.asp

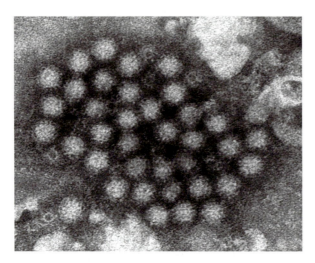

FIGURE 8-5 Electron Microscopy of the Norovirus
Courtesy of Centers for Disease Control and Prevention Public Health Image Library (PHIL): http://phil.cdc.gov/Phil/details.asp

causing cell death and spread of infection, thereby causing disease. An example is the varicella-zoster virus that causes chickenpox usually during childhood. The virus then resides in the nerve roots, coexisting there, to reactivate in later years and cause shingles infection. There are antiviral agents, but most of the more common viral infections will resolve on their own with supportive symptomatic care. Viral infections are NOT cured with antibiotics. See Figure 8-5 for an electron microscopy photo of a common virus.

Parasites

Parasites may be single-celled or multicelled organisms that are dependent on their host for their existence. They may release toxins and enzymes that destroy their hosts' cells or disrupt their function. Common examples are worms (helminthes) like the tapeworm, protozoa (single-celled organisms) like Giardia, or the Plasmodium species that cause malaria. There are specific drugs to treat parasitic agents. Figure 8-6 shows a common protozoan parasite.

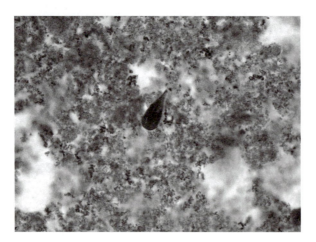

FIGURE 8-6 Giardia Protozoan
Courtesy of Centers for Disease Control and Prevention Public Health Image Library (PHIL): http://phil.cdc.gov/Phil/details.asp—CDC/DPDx/Melanie Moser

Classifications of Infectious Diseases: Clinical, Type, and Natural Habitat

reservoir: the natural host in which an organism grows and multiplies without causing disease to the host; serves as a source of infection for a susceptible individual

Infectious diseases may be classified in several ways, and the method used is usually based on the reason needed. Table 8-5 shows the classification by clinical picture. This is generally done according to the organ system that is the site of primary infection and source of symptoms. Table 8-6 shows the classification according to the type of infectious agent. It would not be uncommon to use both the clinical picture and the infectious agent to categorize the infections. A third way to classify infectious diseases, as shown in Table 8-7, is according to their natural habitat or where they reside before they attack their intended host, also known as the **reservoir** of the agent.

TABLE 8-5 Classification of Infectious Diseases (According to Clinical Picture)

Clinical Picture	Infection
Central Nervous System Infections	Meningitis
	Encephalitis
Respiratory Infections	Sinusitis
	Upper Respiratory
	Lower Respiratory
Gastrointestinal Infections	Vomiting
	Diarrhea
Sexually Transmitted Infections	Gonorrhea
	Syphilis
	Herpes Simplex

© Cengage Learning 2013

TABLE 8-6 Classification of Infectious Diseases (According to Infectious Agent)

Infectious Agent	Characteristics
Bacterial	Gram-negative
	Gram-positive
Viral	DNA virus
	RNA virus
Parasitic	Protozoa
	Helminths
	Trematodes
	Cestodes

© Cengage Learning 2013

TABLE 8-7 Classification of Infectious Diseases (According to the Reservoir)

Reservoir	Examples
Human	Neisseria gonorrhea
	Hepatitis B & C
Animal (Zoonoses)	Yersinia pestis (plague)
	Rabies
Soil	Clostridium tetani (tetanus)
	Clostridium botulinum (botulism)
Water	Pseudomonas aeruginosa
	Legionella

© Cengage Learning 2013

The Epidemiologic Triangle of Infectious Disease

Acquiring an infectious disease is more complicated than simply being exposed to an infecting organism. For example, some diseases can be caused by exposure to a single organism, whereas most diseases will only be caused if there is exposure to a high volume of organisms. Some organisms must maintain exposure over a period of time. Some organisms will only cause disease if the exposed individual is susceptible (not immune) to infection and illness. Some organisms require an optimal environment in order to be successfully transmitted. The optimal environment for transmission might be poor sanitation or a high-density population. All of the conditions must be right for an infectious disease to be transmitted and cause illness.

The traditional model of disease in humans, known as the epidemiology triangle, was introduced in Chapter 2. The epidemiology triangle graphically demonstrates the relationship between the infectious agent, environment, and individual/host as a function of time and is presented in Figure 2-2. The sides of the triangle each indicate that these three are necessarily interrelated in order for successful transmission of infection and subsequent clinical disease to occur. More importantly, this model indicates that in order to prevent disease, all that is necessary is to "break" just one of the legs of the triangle, and then the model will not be successful.

Individual/Host

In the epidemiology triangle, the *individual/host* on one vertex of the triangle is the person "at risk" for infection and disease. There are a variety of ways to protect the individual, such as hand washing, isolation, immunization, or respirator masks.

If the individual is sufficiently protected, even exposure to the agent will not result in infection and/or illness. The individual can also be a reservoir of disease, which also can affect the transmission of disease. If humans are the only reservoir of disease and if the individuals with the illness are kept away from susceptible individuals, transmission can be impeded.

Agent

On another vertex of the triangle is the *agent*, which is the etiologic cause of the disease. The characteristics of the infectious agent vary widely, and these characteristics determine how effective an agent is at causing infection and disease. Two common characteristics of infectious agents that describe the ability to cause disease are pathogenicity and virulence. **Pathogenicity** is the ability of an agent to cause disease. For example, some organisms live normally in the human body and do not cause illness, but if other organisms were to enter the same location, disease would occur. Those that make us sick are called pathogenic. **Virulence** is the degree of pathogenicity that is characteristic of a particular organism or agent. Some organisms that make us sick can do so easily or with very few organisms (highly virulent). Other organisms have a more difficult time making us sick or require many more organisms to do so. The pathogenicity and virulence of an agent will influence the model of disease and the epidemiology triangle.

pathogenicity: the ability of an agent to cause disease

virulence: the degree of pathogenicity possessed by an infectious agent

Environment

The third vertex of the epidemiology triangle is the *environment*. The surroundings, both internal and external to the individual, play a role in the effectiveness of infectious disease transmission. Most pathogenic organisms do not survive well outside of the human host or the natural reservoir of the disease. But an environment such as poor sanitation or overcrowded living conditions can be helpful (which is bad) to the successful transmission of a disease.

Time

The last concept of the epidemiology triangle is *time*. Time is part of the model as it pertains to the incubation period of the disease, the length of duration of the disease, the survival time of the infected individual, and the time that the host remains infectious to others.

The utility of the epidemiology triangle as it relates to infectious diseases is only apparent after understanding all of the components of the model. Preventing transmission of a given disease can be as simple as interrupting one aspect of the triangle, or it may take several different interruptions.

TYPES OF INFECTIONS

The standard text used by epidemiologists and public health care workers in the field is *Control of Communicable Diseases Manual*, edited by David L. Heymann and currently in its 19th edition (2008). It is a small paperback manual designed to be carried in the investigator's pocket. However, because of the immense expansion of knowledge in the field of infectious diseases, this book is too thick to fit in most pockets, but the information is available online and accessible from mobile devices. An understanding of the clinical picture is important when assessing how to proceed during an outbreak investigation. This section is not a substitute for more complete texts on infectious diseases, but it gives basic information about some infectious diseases and is set up primarily by clinical picture. For each clinical picture, at least one example is given. These were chosen based on how frequently they occurred, how important they are to public health, or those with unique features.

Central Nervous System Infections

Central nervous system infections include infections that involve the brain (encephalitis), the meninges (the lining of the spine and brain), or both. They can be caused by a variety of agents, including bacteria, viruses, and protozoa.

Meningitis

Meningitis is an inflammation of the meninges, the membranes that line the brain and spinal cord. See Figure 8-7 for a picture of infected meninges surrounding the brain. Viruses, bacteria, or parasites can cause meningitis although viruses are the most common cause. Bacterial meningitis, the second most common form of meningitis, will be discussed in Chapter 10 (Vaccine Preventable Diseases).

Viral or "aseptic" meningitis is most often caused by enteroviruses. These are spread through contact with infected feces, through contact with respiratory droplets directly, or via fomites. Coxsackie virus, herpes simplex virus, varicella-zoster virus (chickenpox), measles virus, and the influenza virus all may cause viral meningitis. The incubation period is generally 3–7 days. Symptoms of fever, headache, and stiff neck with sensitivity to light may appear suddenly on their own or follow cold or stomach flu symptoms. One is contagious from the onset of symptoms

meningitis: inflammation of the meninges, the membranes that line the brain and spinal cord

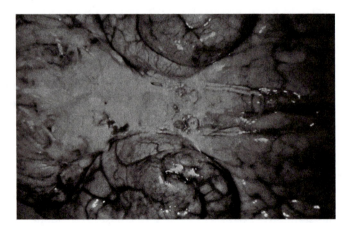

FIGURE 8-7 Purulent Discharge Seen Surrounding Part of the Brain in Meningitis
Courtesy of Centers for Disease Control and Prevention Public Health Image Library (PHIL): http://phil.cdc.gov/Phil/details.asp

until symptoms go away. There is no specific treatment and symptoms usually resolve in 7–10 days, usually without aftereffects. Meningitis caused by viruses is much different from bacterial disease and is rarely fatal in persons with normal immune systems.

Encephalitis

Encephalitis is the inflammation and swelling of the brain and is generally caused by a viral infection. It is most severe in young infants and the elderly. Transmission can be by infected mosquitoes (West Nile virus), by person to person spread through respiratory droplets (measles or chickenpox), by contaminated food or drink (*Listeria*), or by animal bites (rabies virus). Herpes simplex virus is the most common virus responsible for severe encephalitis in all ages. Because the viral etiology varies, so does the incubation period. Symptoms may follow cold or stomach flu symptoms and can include a change in the level of consciousness, unsteady gait, headache, confusion, vomiting, light sensitivity, seizures, and fever. Some antiviral agents are available to treat certain specific viral brain infections. Recovery varies from full resolution without aftereffects to persistent brain damage.

encephalitis: inflammation and swelling of the brain

Respiratory Infections

Respiratory infections can occur anywhere along the respiratory tract and include rhinitis (inflammation of the nose), sinusitis, otitis (ear infection), laryngitis, pharyngitis (sore throat), tracheitis, bronchitis, and pneumonia. The most common symptom is cough, whether the infection is in the upper (above the vocal cords) or lower (below the vocal cords) respiratory tract. Other symptoms may include runny nose, congestion, fever, sore throat, and/or ear pain.

Most respiratory infections are transmitted by respiratory droplets either directly or on hands or other fomites. These types of infections are major problems in any crowded conditions like schools, daycare facilities, nursing homes, or military barracks. Routine preventive and control measures include respiratory droplet control—that is, minimizing contact with infected droplets. Although most of us were taught to "cover your mouth with your hand" when you cough, it is now known that hands are the major source of spreading respiratory infections. The newer recommendations are that a person should cough into the fold of an elbow. This is because the elbow is much less likely to come into contact with another susceptible person's body and thus minimizes spread. Another major control measure is frequent hand washing by those who are ill and those who come into contact with persons ill with respiratory infections.

Viruses cause the same spectrum of respiratory diseases that bacteria do but are usually self-limited, less severe, and require no treatment. Viral respiratory diseases include the common cold, ear infections, pharyngitis, croup, pneumonia, and bronchiolitis (infection of the smaller airways of the lungs). Antibiotics treat bacterial infections and have *no effect* on viral infections. Overuse or misuse of antibiotics lead to resistance by the organisms they are supposed to kill.

Common Cold

The common cold is an upper respiratory infection caused by over 200 different viruses, the most common of which is the highly contagious rhinovirus. Children average 3–8 colds per year and are the usual sources for adults' infections. The incubation period is usually 48 hours but may range from 12 hours to 5 days. One is contagious from 12 hours before symptoms appear to the fifth day of symptoms. Symptoms are runny nose, congestion, cough, and sneezing. Spread is by direct respiratory droplet contact and by contact with contaminated hands and fomites. The course is self-limited, lasting 7–10 days, although the cough may last for up to 4 weeks. There have been no reported deaths from the common cold. Antibiotics that treat bacterial diseases are not effective against viruses and, therefore, not indicated in the treatment of the common cold. The major public health impact of the common cold is that it is the leading cause of work and school absenteeism.

Pneumonia

Together with influenza, pneumonia accounts for the eighth leading cause of death in the United States and has been among the top 10 causes of death in the United States since at least the early 1900s. Because there are various organisms that cause pneumonia, the disease can vary from mild to severe. The most common bacterial organism causing this infection is *Streptococcus pneumonia*, and the most common viral etiology is influenza or respiratory syncytial virus (in infants). *Mycoplasm pneunomiae* is a small bacterium that causes atypical pneumonia or what is commonly known as "walking pneumonia," which is common in school-aged children and younger adults. Those at highest risk for lung infections include the young (≤ 5 years old), the elderly (≥ 65 years old), smokers of any age, and those with underlying medical conditions (HIV/AIDS, diabetes, asthma). It is commonly seen when there are crowed living conditions like homeless shelters or military barracks.

Tuberculosis (TB)

According to the Centers for Disease Control and Prevention, one-third of the world's population is infected with *Mycobacterium tuberculosis*, and each year 9 million more people become infected. *Mycobacterium tuberculosis* is an acid-fast (a different stain is used because the organism is resistant to Gram stain) bacillus that primarily causes lung infections but can also infect other organs such as the brain or bones of the spine. See Figure 8-8.

Not everyone who becomes infected with the organism becomes sick with tuberculosis. Some people who become infected have the organisms kept in check by their immune system and have no symptoms of disease. They will however test positive for infection but are not contagious at this stage. These people are said to have **latent TB infections**, and they are treated to prevent later emergence of disease. The incubation period for those who do develop disease is 2–10 weeks.

People who do develop the disease when infected with the organism have cough, which is frequently bloody, and constitutional symptoms such as poor

latent TB infection: when infectious organisms are kept in check by the immune system and no symptoms of disease are present

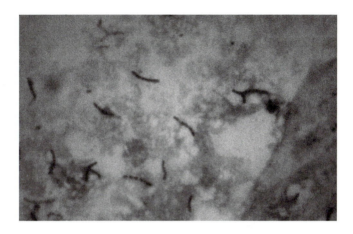

FIGURE 8-8A Tuberculosis—Mycobacterium Tuberculosis
Courtesy of Centers for Disease Control and Prevention Public Health Image Library (PHIL): http://phil.cdc.gov/Phil/details.asp

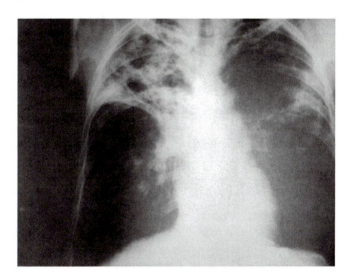

FIGURE 8-8B Chest X-ray Showing Advanced TB
Courtesy of Centers for Disease Control and Prevention Public Health Image Library (PHIL): http://phil.cdc.gov/Phil/details.asp

appetite, fatigue, and weight loss. The disease is spread through respiratory droplets from coughing or sneezing or even with droplets spread with speech. People with immune deficiencies like HIV infection or AIDS are at particular risk for this disease.

There are two major issues with TB worldwide. The first is that HIV infection weakens the immune system and allows for severe TB disease, which is the leading cause of death in HIV positive patients. Both infections, TB and HIV, are most prevalent in the sub-Saharan Africa region, and HIV is the most important factor in the rising TB rates there. The other significant public health issue is the emergence of multi-drug resistant tuberculosis (MDR-TB) strains. This has come about because of partial or inconsistent treatment of tuberculosis. Although still treatable, MDR-TB requires longer treatment by second line medications.

Gastrointestinal Infections

Gastrointestinal (GI) infections are among the most common infectious diseases worldwide and are a frequent cause of outbreaks. They can be caused by bacteria, viruses, or protozoa. (See Table 8-8.) Transmission is through contaminated food or water, person to person spread via the fecal-oral route, or contact with infected animals.

Symptoms most often include fever, abdominal cramping, and may predominate with upper GI symptoms like emesis (vomiting) or lower GI symptoms like **diarrhea** (passage of three or more loose or liquid stools per day), or both. Terms used to describe these infections include **gastritis** (infections targeting the stomach and causing vomiting), **enterocolitis** or **colitis** (infections affecting the intestines/colon and causing diarrhea), and **gastroenteritis** (infections that affect the stomach and intestines and cause both vomiting and diarrhea), also known as the "stomach flu" (which is not really the "flu" as in influenza). The predominating symptoms may indicate the causative agent. Whether diarrhea is bloody or not also gives important clues as to the responsible infectious agent.

Because persistent vomiting and diarrhea associated with gastrointestinal infections can lead to significant body fluid losses, especially in infants and children, these infections may be life-threatening. Diarrhea is the second leading cause of death in children under 5 years old worldwide and, in 2004, was the third leading cause of death in low-income countries worldwide. It is a major cause of childhood

diarrhea: passage of three or more loose or liquid stools per day

gastritis: infections targeting the stomach and causing vomiting

enterocolitis/colitis: infections affecting the intestines/colon and causing diarrhea

gastroenteritis: infections that affect the stomach and intestines and cause both vomiting and diarrhea; also known as the stomach flu

TABLE 8-8 Common Causes of Gastrointestinal Infections	
Causative Agent	**Examples**
Bacterial	*E. coli*
	Staph aureus
	Salmonella
	Cholera
Viral	Norovirus
	Rotavirus
Protozoan	*Giardia*
	Amobea

TABLE 8-9 Top GI Pathogens in the United States

Top 5 Pathogens Causing Food Borne Infections	Top 5 Pathogens Causing Food Borne Infections Requiring Hospitalization	Top 5 Pathogens Causing Food Borne Infections and Resulting in Death
Norovirus (58%)	*Salmonella*, nontyphoidal (35%)	*Salmonella*, nontyphoidal (28%)
Salmonella, non-typhoidal (11%)	Norovirus (26%)	*Toxoplasma gondii* (24%)
Clostridium perfringens (10%)	*Campylobacter* spp. (15%)	*Listeria monocytogenes* (19%)
Campylobacter spp. (9%)	*Toxoplasma gondii* (8%)	Norovirus (11%)
Staphylococcus aureus (3%)	*E. coli* 0157 (4%)	*Campylobacter* spp. (6%)

Based on: Centers for Disease Control and Prevention; Food Safety at CDC; http://www.cdc.gov/foodsafety/facts.html

malnutrition worldwide. In the United States, the Centers for Disease Control and Prevention predicts that 1 in 6 Americans will become infected, 128,000 will require hospitalization, and 3,000 will die from food borne illnesses each year. See Table 8-9 for a summary.

Escherichia coli (E. coli)

E. coli is a Gram-negative bacillus with several strains that cause a variety of conditions such as traveler's diarrhea and severe diarrhea in developing countries. Enterohemorrhagic *E. coli* 0157:H7 is a major source of food borne epidemics in the United States, frequently associated with contaminated ground beef. It is a toxin-producing bacteria first recognized in 1982 in the United States during an outbreak of hemorrhagic colitis (bloody diarrhea).

See Table 8-10 for examples of *E. coli* outbreaks in the United States over the past several years to see the variety of foods involved. *E. coli* may be spread via contaminated food or water, directly person to person, or through contact with infected animals. The incubation period is 3–4 days, and an infected adult is contagious for 1 week; but infected children are infectious for about 3 weeks. The disease this organism causes ranges from mild, nonbloody diarrhea to severe bloody diarrhea and may lead to a major complication called "hemolytic-uremic syndrome."

TABLE 8-10 *E. coli* Outbreak Sources in the United States, 2007–2011	
2011:	Bologna
	Hazelnuts
2010:	Cheese
	Romaine lettuce
	Beef
2009:	Prepackaged cookie dough
	Beef
2008:	Beef
2007:	Frozen pizza
	Ground beef patties

Based on: Centers for Disease Control and Prevention; *E. coli* Outbreaks; http://www.cdc.gov/ecoli/

Staphylococcus aureus

Staph aureus is a Gram-positive coccus that produces enterotoxins, which cause what is commonly referred to as "food poisoning." It is the most common cause of acute **food borne intoxication** worldwide. Because it is the toxins in the contaminated foods, rather than the infecting organisms, that produce the disease, it is not transmitted person to person. Food handlers with skin infections are a major source of spread. If foods they have infected are inadequately heated or refrigerated or left out at room temperature for several hours before being eaten, toxins are produced. These toxins are heat tolerant and are not destroyed by cooking. The disease occurs with the rapid onset of severe nausea, abdominal cramps, and vomiting about 2–4 hours after exposure and may or may not be associated with diarrhea for 1–2 days. About 25% of healthy people will become chronic carriers and harbor the organism on the skin and in the nose. They are another potential source of disease spread.

food borne intoxication: toxins in the contaminated foods, rather than the infecting organisms, produce the disease

Salmonella

Salmonella is the second leading cause of gastrointestinal infections in the United States and a major cause of food borne illness throughout the world with millions of cases reported annually. In the United States, it causes more hospitalizations and deaths from gastrointestinal disease than any other organism. Table 8-11 lists several of the recent U.S. outbreaks occurring over the past several years. The one that obtained the most recent notoriety was the *Salmonella enteritidis* outbreak from contaminated egg shells associated with two egg suppliers in the Midwest that sickened

TABLE 8-11 *Salmonella* Outbreak Sources in the United States, 2010–2011

2011:	Turkish pine nuts—*Salmonella enteriditis*
	Ground turkey—*Salmonella* Heidelberg
	Fresh imported papayas—*Salmonella* Agona
	African dwarf frogs—*Salmonella typhimurium*
	Alfalfa sprouts—*Salmonella enteritidis*
	Chicks and ducklings—*Salmonella* Altona and Johannesburg
	Turkey burgers—*Salmonella* Hadar
	Cantaloupe—*Salmonella* Panama
2010:	Alfalfa sprouts—*Salmonella* I and *Salmonella* Newport
	Shell eggs—*Salmonella enteritidis*
	Cheesy chicken rice frozen entrée—*Salmonella* Chester
	Red and black Peppers/Italian-style meats—*Salmonella* Montevideo
	Water frogs—*Salmonella typhimurium*

Based on: Centers for Disease Control and Prevention; *Salmonella* Outbreaks; http://www.cdc.gov/salmonella/outbreaks.html

almost 2,000 persons in a multistate epidemic occurring from May to November, 2010. The incubation period is 12–36 hours. Clinical symptoms include a sudden onset of headache, pain, diarrhea, nausea, and fever, with or without vomiting. Most often these symptoms resolve spontaneously without treatment, but the young and elderly are at risk for severe disease. The period of contagion varies from several days to several weeks. In about 10% of cases, the infection goes on to cause extra-intestinal focal infections or even widespread infections because it can enter the blood.

Salmonella is a Gram-negative bacillus with over 2,500 serotypes and is divided into two major groupings—*Salmonella* nontyphoidal and *Salmonella typhi*. Although most infections are caused by ingesting infected foods of animal origin (meat, poultry, eggs, milk) or vegetables contaminated with infected feces, *Salmonella* is also well known to be associated with handling infected pet reptiles, particularly small turtles (see Figure 8-9). Currently there are about 74,000 cases per year related to spread by reptiles. In 1975, the Food and Drug Association (FDA) banned the sale of turtles that were less than 4 inches in length that had previously been popular pets for small children because of the increased risk of salmonellosis in younger children. It is anticipated that this ban has prevented about 100,000 cases of clinical salmonellosis per year since that time.

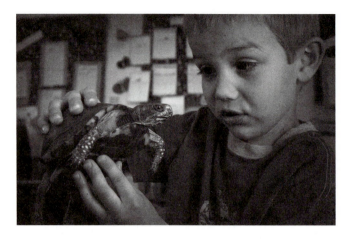

FIGURE 8-9 Pet Turtles Can Spread Salmonella Infections
Courtesy of the Centers for Disease Control and Prevention Public Health Image Library (PHIL): http://phil.cdc.gov/Phil/details.asp

Norovirus

Norovirus is a group of small RNA viruses, previously known as "Norwalk virus," and is the leading cause of food borne infections in the United States, with more than 50% of the 21 million cases of gastroenteritis each year being caused by norovirus. The infection is frequently called viral gastroenteritis or "stomach flu." The most common symptoms are vomiting, diarrhea, and abdominal pain that occur 24–48 hours after exposure. Norovirus is highly contagious with as few as 10 viral particles required for infection. It spreads rapidly in confined spaces so outbreaks are common, particularly on cruise ships (21%), daycare centers/schools (13%), and nursing homes (35.5%), according to data from the CDC from 1994–2006. About 31% of outbreaks occurred from restaurant or catered meals. During outbreaks several modes of transmission may be responsible for the propagation of the disease. For example, the index case may have been infected by contaminated food in a restaurant and then spread the disease person to person or by fomites to household contacts. Once infected, a person remains infectious for up to 48 hours after the diarrhea stops.

Giardia intestinalis

Giardiasis is a diarrheal infection caused by a protozoan found in soil, in food, or on surfaces. It is frequently spread person to person by the fecal-oral route, but the infection may also be spread by water contaminated from fecal matter of infected animals (rivers or lakes, swimming pools) or humans (including diapers). *Giardia* has also been known to be transmitted through sexual contact in which there is contact with infected feces (e.g., oral-anal). This parasite lives in the intestines of its host and passes its cysts in the host's stools. *Giardia* can survive for weeks to months outside the body. Humans swallowing as few as 10 cysts in infected food or water may become ill within 7–10 days and once infected may shed up to 1–10 billion cysts per day. The infection is capable of being transmitted for as long as cysts are being shed, which may be months. Globally, *Giardia* infects nearly 2% of adults and 6–8% of children in developed countries and about 33% of people in developing countries. In the United States, it is the most common parasite to cause gastrointestinal infections. The symptoms of the infection are primarily intestinal and include diarrhea or greasy stools, gas, and abdominal cramps. Worldwide asymptomatic carriage rates range from 16–86%.

Sexually Transmitted Infections (STIs)

Previously called "venereal diseases" and then "sexually transmitted diseases," this group of infections is now more appropriately referred to as *sexually transmitted infections*. After years of decreasing incidence, several of these infections are now making a reemergence, chiefly among young adults.

Syphilis

Adolf Hitler, Mussolini, Al Capone, Napoleon Bonaparte, and Leo Tolstoy—all are reported to have had syphilis.

Syphilis is caused by a spirochete bacterium, *Treponema pallidum*. Transmitted during oral, anal, or genital sex when there is contact with the syphilitic ulcer, syphilis occurs in three stages. The primary chancre seen in Figure 8-10 is a painless ulcer that occurs at the site of initial invasion and appears about three weeks after infection. Especially in women, this first stage may go completely unnoticed. The secondary infectious stage involves a rash of the skin and mucous membranes. After years of latency, tertiary disease involves the brain, heart, bone, and skin. Syphilis can cause fetal death in up to 40% of pregnancies if a pregnant woman is infected early in pregnancy and can cause fetal infection in up to 80% of pregnancies if primary disease occurs anytime within the four years preceding pregnancy. If left untreated, the disease allows for easier transmission of HIV during sexual contact.

Historical Note 8-2

Early History of Syphilis

The first written records of an outbreak of syphilis in Europe occurred in 1494-1495 in Naples, Italy, during a French invasion. Because syphilis was spread by returning French troops, it was initially known as the "French disease." It is only in 1530 that an Italian poet and physician, Girolamo Fracastoro, first used the term "syphilis." In his epic poem, Fracastoro created a protagonist, a shepherd, named Syphilis. Apollo sent this classical disease to Syphilis to punish him for defiance. Over the ages, the disease has also been known as "Lues," "Cupid's disease," and the "Great Pox."

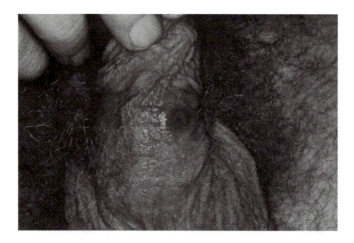

FIGURE 8-10 Chancre of Syphilis
Courtesy of the Centers for Disease Control and Prevention Public Health Image Library (PHIL): http://phil.cdc.gov/Phil/details.asp

Gonorrhea

Gonorrhea is caused by *Neisseria gonococcus*, a Gram-negative diplococci and is the second most commonly reportable disease in the United States. Transmission is through sexual contact: anal, genital, or oral. The incubation period is 1–14 days. The disease is different in males and females in regards to course, severity, and ease of recognition. Males develop a purulent discharge from the urethra as seen in Figure 8-11 and have pain with urination. Females are often asymptomatic, but there may be vaginal discharge, cervicitis, or pelvic inflammatory

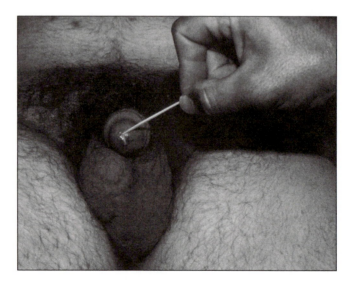

FIGURE 8-11 Discharge of Gonorrhea
Courtesy of the Centers for Disease Control and Prevention Public Health Image Library (PHIL): http://phil.cdc.gov/Phil/details.asp

disease. Complications in women include infertility. Pharyngeal and anorectal infections are common with oral and anal sexual contact. Eye infections can occur in neonates born to infected women. Untreated infected persons will be contagious for months, but within hours of adequate antibiotic treatment, they are no longer contagious.

Genital Herpes

Genital herpes is most often caused by herpes simplex virus type 2 (HSV-2). Although the herpes simplex virus type 1 can also cause the disease, it is more often the cause of the common cold sore or fever blister. Transmission is during sexual contact and is more commonly passed from men to women than from women to men. Most infected persons show no symptoms or only mild symptoms once infected. Transmission may occur when there is active lesion present or when there is no obvious lesion. The lesion of small grouped vesicles may or may not be apparent at the initial infection and can take up to four weeks to heal completely (see Figure 8-12). Once healed, the lesions tend to recur during times of stress or illness when the immune system is compromised. There is no absolute cure at this time for genital herpes, but there are medications that may shorten outbreaks.

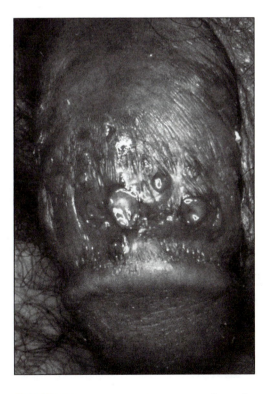

FIGURE 8-12 Cluster of Fluid-Filled Lesions of Genital Herpes
Courtesy of the Centers for Disease Control and Prevention Public Health Image Library (PHIL): http://phil.cdc.gov/Phil/details.asp

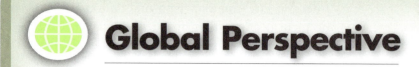

Global Perspective

Malaria

Malaria kills a child every 45 seconds. This is such an important problem that four Nobel prizes have been awarded based on work associated with malaria. The United Nations has recognized this infection (along with tuberculosis and HIV/AIDS) as worthy of worldwide effort to decrease its rising incidence and mortality. This serious infection that causes an acute, but preventable, febrile illness is caused by the parasite, *Plasmodium*. Worldwide there are four species of this parasite that cause the disease, but there are two that are the most common: *Plasmodium falciparum* (the most deadly) and *Plasmodium vivax*.

Transmission to humans is through the bite of the *Anopheles* mosquito (see Figure 8-13). In Africa, this mosquito has adapted to be the most effective vector of malaria for several reasons: (1) it has a long life span that allows the *Plasmodium* to complete its life cycle, (2) it bites primarily at night, and (3) it prefers humans over other animals. Because of these reasons, over 85% of malaria deaths occur in Africa, where it is the second leading cause of death from infectious diseases (HIV is the first). In the United States, about 1,500 cases of malaria are reported annually. Most of these are related to immigrants traveling back to the endemic country of origin without taking the appropriate medicine to prevent infection. There have been only a handful of cases over the years that have been transmitted through blood transfusions.

The incubation period for malaria is 10-15 days. Initial symptoms are fever, chills, and flu-like symptoms. *P. falciparum* can progress to severe disease and death soon after if it is left untreated. In endemic areas, presentations

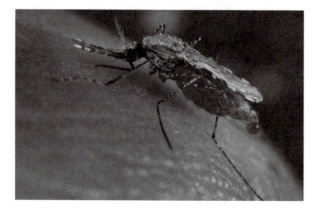

FIGURE 8-13 *Anopheles* Mosquito
Courtesy of the Centers for Disease Control and Prevention

such as anemia, respiratory symptoms, or cerebral malaria may occur. In some cases, the parasite may seed in the liver and cause relapses for its host. There are medications available that, if taken before exposure, will prevent malaria. These medicines are generally recommended for all persons travelling to endemic areas. For persons living in endemic areas, the primary method of prevention is vector (mosquito) control. This is generally accomplished by the use of insecticide-treated mosquito nets and indoor spraying with residual insecticides.

Check It Out

For information on other infectious diseases (particularly in the United States), go to: http://www.cdc.gov/. Click on "Diseases and Conditions" for an alphabetized list of the diseases discussed.

For information on other infectious diseases (particularly worldwide), go to: http://www.who.int/en/. Click on "Health Topics" for an alphabetized list of the diseases discussed.

INFECTIOUS DISEASE CONTROL

Control of the spread of infectious diseases can be at the global, national, state, or local public level. Maintaining an adequate public health infrastructure is the foundation of preventing transmission of disease. Sanitary measures such as the availability of clean, safe drinking water and the proper handling of sewage are key measures that are used. In the United States, county and state level programs monitor and survey certain high-risk workers such as food handlers and health care workers. County, state, and federal level programs maintain surveillance programs for certain diseases, and when the diseases are detected, these agencies manage the investigation and control measures to prevent epidemic spread.

Public health intervention in the control of communicable diseases also includes education programs for the public. This can include instruction for proper food preparation and storage, thorough cooking of meat, washing of fruits and vegetables, exclusion of food handlers with skin infections, and proper hand washing to prevent the spread of gastrointestinal diseases. Surveillance of cattle and food processing plants and chlorinating public pools is also done to prevent disease.

When gastrointestinal disease is already present, precautions such as hand washing and the proper handling of stools become important. In the case of norovirus epidemics where disease is transmitted on fomites, cleaning and disinfecting surfaces and washing clothes are all necessary as well. The transmission of respiratory illnesses can be prevented primarily at the personal level by proper hand washing, minimizing the spread of respiratory droplets by coughing into the elbow (not covering the mouth with the hand as your mother taught you!), and minimizing the spread of respiratory droplets transmission on fomites such as tissues and money. In the cases of mosquito borne infections, vector control is paramount. As discussed in the section on malaria, this can be done with pesticide impregnated mosquito nets and indoor spraying with residual insecticides. As will be discussed in a later chapter, vaccines play an important role in the prevention of many infectious diseases.

Five Goals to Control Infectious Disease

On a broader level, there are five goals for the control of infectious disease:

- Control of the disease,
- Elimination of the disease,
- Elimination of an infection,
- Eradication of an infection, and
- Extinction of an infection.

The first goal is basic *control of the disease*, which consists of reduction of the disease incidence, prevalence, morbidity, and mortality to a locally acceptable level. Ongoing intervention efforts are required. Examples include the use of nets and insecticides to control malaria and the screening of high-risk persons and treatment of latent disease in the case of tuberculosis.

Second, the *elimination of disease* involves reducing the incidence of a disease in a specified geographical area to zero. This too, requires ongoing intervention efforts. Improved personal and environmental hygiene is used in an attempt to prevent the spread of trachoma, an eye infection caused by *Chlamydia trachomatis* that is the leading cause of blindness worldwide.

A third goal of infectious disease control is the *elimination of an infection*, which is the reduction of the incidence of infection by a specific agent in a specified area to zero. Onchocerciasis, an infection caused by a parasitic worm and transmitted by blackflies, is controlled by spraying breeding sites with insecticides.

Eradication of an infection is the fourth goal and implies the permanent reduction of the worldwide incidence of an infection caused by a specific agent so that intervention measures are no longer required. The only disease that has achieved worldwide eradication at this time is smallpox, but measles and polio are targeted by WHO and may meet this goal in the foreseeable future.

The fifth and final goal of infectious disease control is *extinction of an infection*, which occurs when the specific infectious agent no longer exists in nature or in the laboratory. It was once thought that smallpox would be the first disease to become extinct, but the increased interest in this disease as a potential biological warfare agent makes it unlikely in the near future. Stockpiles of the virus are kept in only two laboratories worldwide—one in Russia and one in the CDC in Atlanta, Georgia.

THE FUTURE OF INFECTIOUS DISEASES

One of the most important emerging problems with the control of infectious diseases has to do with antibiotic-resistant bacterial infections. In this situation, a microorganism is able to survive exposure to an antibiotic. Genes that confer resistance then can be transferred between bacteria. Thus, a gene for antibiotic resistance that had evolved via natural selection may be shared. This can occur when stress, such as exposure to antibiotics, selects the antibiotic-resistant trait. If a bacterium carries several resistance genes, it is called "multidrug resistant" or, informally, a "superbug" or "super bacterium." The increasing prevalence of antibiotic-resistant bacterial infections seen in clinical practice stems from antibiotic use both within human medicine and veterinary medicine. Any use of antibiotics can increase selective pressure in a population of bacteria to allow the resistant bacteria to thrive and the susceptible bacteria to die. As resistance toward antibiotics becomes more common, a greater need for alternative treatments arises. However, despite a push for new antibiotic therapies, there has been a continued decline in the number of newly approved drugs. Antibiotic resistance therefore poses a significant problem.

Summary

The field of epidemiology began with the study of infectious diseases. This field is different than the epidemiology of chronic disease in several ways. An infectious disease can be a minor, brief, self-limiting condition or a more serious disease that is spread globally causing severe morbidity or mortality. There are various types of organisms that cause infections—bacteria, viruses, parasites—and each has its own unique characteristics that may help with investigating outbreaks, determining control measures, and deciding on treatment modalities. These diseases can be classified according to the causative agent, the clinical picture, or the natural reservoir of the organism.

Transmission of infections to susceptible hosts can be achieved in several ways, and knowing how a disease is spread is important in breaking the chain of infection. Understanding the traditional model of disease involving the individual, agent, and environment and the factors that impact each of these also aids in breaking the spread of disease. These techniques are important whether the disease is endemic, epidemic, or even pandemic.

Several of the more common infections in various categories and their characteristics were discussed. The advantages of understanding the various individual diseases and their modes of transmission are that public health control methods can be instituted for that particular infection to prevent its spread. There are also broader goals of infectious disease control that are used at the global level. The emerging problem of resistant infections was also discussed.

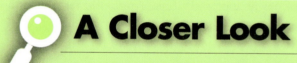

A Closer Look

Human Immunodeficiency Virus

Infection with the HIV and its most severe stage, AIDS, has been responsible for over 27 million deaths since its discovery in 1981. The source of infection in humans has been found to be similar to a virus that infected chimpanzees in West Africa. It most likely mutated into its human form after being transmitted to hunters who ate the meat of the chimpanzees. The Millennium Development Goals were adopted by the United Nations in 2000 as a global action plan to target worldwide poverty, hunger, and disease. Part of the Sixth Millennium Development Goal was to halt and begin to reverse the spread of HIV/AIDS by 2015 and to achieve universal access to treatment to all those who need it by 2010. By the end of 2009, however, about 10 million people who needed treatment still had no access to medical treatment.

Epidemiology of HIV

In 2009, there were 33.3 million people worldwide living with HIV infection (see Figure 8-14). Over two-thirds of the infected persons lived in sub-Saharan Africa. The prevalence of HIV/AIDS is increasing as the success of treatment becomes more widespread and effective. New cases still outpace the increase of those cases receiving appropriate treatment: for every two infected persons beginning treatment, five new cases are diagnosed. Worldwide each day,

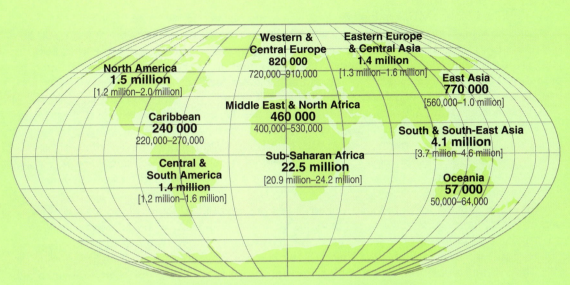

North America
1.5 million
[1.2 million–2.0 million]

Western &
Central Europe
820 000
720,000–910,000

Eastern Europe
& Central Asia
1.4 million
[1.3 million–1.6 million]

East Asia
770 000
[560,000–1.0 million]

Caribbean
240 000
220,000–270,000

Middle East & North Africa
460 000
400,000–530,000

South & South-East Asia
4.1 million
[3.7 million–4.6 million]

Central &
South America
1.4 million
[1.2 million–1.6 million]

Sub-Saharan Africa
22.5 million
[20.9 million–24.2 million]

Oceania
57 000
50,000–64,000

Total: 33.3 million [31.4 million–35.3 million]

FIGURE 8-14 Adults and Children Estimated to Be Living with HIV, 2009
Source: UNAIDS 2010 AIDS Epidemic Update (November, 2010); http://www.unaids.org/en/dataanalysis/epidemiology/epidemiologyslides

over 7,400 persons develop new infections, and 5,500 persons with the infection will die of a related illness. The total number of new infections per year has dropped from its peak in 1996 of 3.5 million new cases per year to 2.6 million new cases per year in 2009. In addition, the total number of deaths per year has dropped from 2.2 million in 2002 to 1.8 million in 2009. Although new cases are decreasing or at least stabilizing in many of the areas of the world, they are still increasing in Central Asia and Eastern Europe.

Since the epidemic began, there have been about 617,025 deaths as a result of AIDS in the United States. There are currently more than one million persons living with HIV/AIDS. In 2008, there were 56,300 new cases, primarily among men having sex with other men (MSM), as well as among African-American men and women. An estimated 17,343 deaths occurred as a result of HIV/AIDS that same year. Almost one-third of those infected with HIV in the United States are not aware of their HIV status.

Perinatal HIV infection and subsequent AIDS in women and children are part of the global HIV/AIDS epidemic. Over 90% of the 370,000 new infections in children that occurred in 2009 worldwide were transmitted vertically through **mother-to-child transmission (MTCT)**, but this represented a 24% decrease in incidence since 2004. Worldwide there are 2.5 million children living with HIV/AIDS, with 2.2 million of those children living in sub-Saharan Africa. Slightly less than 52% of the 32.8 million people living with HIV/AIDS are women, most of them living in sub-Saharan Africa. South Africa is one of the few countries in sub-Saharan Africa where child and maternal mortality from AIDS is increasing. It is the major cause of maternal mortality and accounts for 35% of childhood mortality. The other area of the world where MTCT HIV infection is increasing is in Eastern Europe/Central Asia.

mother-to-child transmission (MTCT): transmission of HIV infection from an infected mother to her child during pregnancy, labor, delivery, or breastfeeding

Continues

In the United States, MTCT of the HIV infection is the most common route of infection in children and now accounts for almost all cases in children. There are currently fewer than 200 HIV infected infants born each year in this country. For the most recent data available from 2008, the CDC used data from 37 states and 5 U.S. dependent areas. For this group, there were an estimated 182 new diagnoses of HIV infection in children less than 13 years old and 10,332 new cases (25% of all new diagnoses) in women. Of the new infections in children, 141 (77%) were transmitted perinatally. At the end of 2007, in the 37 states with surveillance, there were 2,919 infected children less than13 years old (0.5% of total infected persons). In 2008 in the entire United States, there were 41 new cases of AIDS in children less than 13 years old and 9,567 new cases (27% of all new cases) in women. At the end of 2007, there were 908 children less than 13years old living with AIDS. There were 6 deaths in children with AIDS less than 13years old in 2007.

Most of the infected children in the United States belong to minority races/ethnicities. At the end of 2005, there were about 6,051 persons alive with HIV/AIDS who had been infected perinatally; and of these, 66% were black and 20% were Hispanic. Women account for 25% of new cases of HIV infection in the United States and for 27% of those currently living with HIV. The incidence of HIV infection in black women is almost 15 times that of white women and nearly 4 times that of Hispanic women.

The Disease

The HIV virus is a RNA virus of the family retrovirus that infects specific immune cells (CD4 cells), and impairs their function. **CD4 T cells** are also known as "T-helper cells" and are a type of white blood cell that fights infection. The HIV virus attacks these cells, uses them to replicate, and later destroys them. Over time, with progressive deterioration of the immune system, the inability to fight off infection occurs. HIV is the virus that can cause AIDS and is known to have two types: HIV-1 and HIV-2. HIV-1 is the most common type worldwide. HIV-2 causes similar disease to HIV-1 but occurs primarily in West Africa.

HIV disease occurs as a continuum: After an incubation period of a few weeks, some infected persons will have a mild flu-like illness, but many newly infected persons will have no symptoms at all. Within 2 weeks to 3 months after the infection occurs, **seroconversion** develops. Seroconversion is the point where an HIV test becomes positive. This is usually followed by an asymptomatic period that can last 5–10 years. If left untreated, as the HIV virus destroys the function of the immune system, then **opportunistic infections**, infections that occur when the immune system is weakened, begin to develop. AIDS, the most severe stage of the disease, occurs at the final end of the spectrum, which may be 10–15 years after the initial infection. AIDS is characterized by decreased immune capability, decreased CD4 levels (<200), an increased viral load, and the presence of opportunistic infections. Tuberculosis is the most common life-threatening opportunistic infection that occurs in patients with AIDS.

CD4 T cells: T-helper cells; specific immune cells that are infected and destroyed by HIV

seroconversion: occurs when the laboratory test for HIV becomes positive

opportunistic infections: infections that occur when the immune system is weakened

There are three major methods of transmission for the HIV virus: blood inoculation, sexual contact, and MTCT. *Blood inoculation* can occur in the medical setting through transfusion of HIV-infected blood and blood products, needle sticks that can occur in health care workers caring for HIV positive patients, or in developing countries, reuse of unsterilized, contaminated injection supplies. Other possibilities of blood inoculations include needle sharing among IV drug users and HIV contaminated instruments that pierce the skin (e.g., ears, tattoos). *Sexual contact* can spread the virus through the exchange of semen, vaginal fluids, or blood between men, women, or homosexual contacts. This would include genital sex, anal sex, and oral sex. *Mother-to-child* (MTCT) or *perinatal HIV* is defined as an HIV-infected mother who transmits the infection to her baby during pregnancy, labor, and delivery (through contact with infected maternal blood), or by breastfeeding (through contact with infected maternal breast milk). *HIV is not spread through saliva, tears, or sweat.*

When discussing the risk for transmitting HIV infections to unborn children, one must understand the risk factors to infections in the women themselves. Heterosexual contact accounts for 84% of infections in women in the United States, whereas injected drug use accounts for only 15%.

Once a woman is infected, the main risk factor for MTCT transmission is her lack of awareness of HIV status during pregnancy. Approximately 25% of infected persons do not know their status, and this is true with pregnant women as well. Current recommendations for pregnant women include universal screening of pregnant women, but this assumes an infected woman presents for timely prenatal care. The fact is, however, that the practice of universal screening is not consistent across the United States, and this becomes an additional risk factor for MTCT transmission.

The **per-act risk** is the risk of acquiring the infection during an individual episode of exposure to the agent. The transmission method that has the highest "per-act" risk may not be the method that accounts for the majority of disease. For example, although the per-act risk of acquiring HIV infection is the highest with blood transfusions, this method of acquisition has become rare because of the routine screening of blood donors.

Sexual activity is the mechanism of transmission of HIV infection that accounts for the majority of cases of HIV worldwide because it occurs so much more frequently, but the risk of acquiring infection during a single sexual act with an HIV-infected person is less than the per-act risk of transfusions or needle sharing. The per-act risk of needle sharing during IV drug use is the next highest after transfusion of infected blood and is consistent with the higher risk associated with the contact with infected blood. Sexual contact, which accounts for the majority of new cases worldwide, has a per-act risk that is highest among the receptive anal intercourse group. This is followed by receptive penile-vaginal intercourse, insertive anal intercourse, insertive penile-vaginal intercourse, receptive oral intercourse, and lastly, insertive oral intercourse.

Current Treatments and Prevention of Future Infections

Treatment of HIV infection is usually done with a combination of medications and is referred to as **antiretroviral therapy (ART)**. ART has been responsible for the change in life expectancy after infection with HIV, for the decrease in infections that progress onward to full AIDS, and for the increased prevalence of the disease. The Millennium Development Goal of universal access to treatment has not yet been achieved, but at the end of 2009, about 5.2 million infected persons in the poorer nations were receiving treatment. Major reasons for the increased number of those receiving ART include the decreased cost of the drugs, as well as improved infrastructure and the financial commitment of the global community.

Treatment of the infected mother with antiretroviral medication was shown in 1994 to significantly reduce the transmission to the fetus and newborn. In 1999, the Institute of Medicine, with support from the American Congress of Obstetricians and Gynecologists and American Academy of Pediatrics, recommended universal screening

per-act risk: risk of acquiring the infection during an individual episode of exposure to the agent

antiretroviral therapy (ART): combination of medications used to combat HIV infection

Continues

of pregnant women to identify those with infection early for preventive treatment. Treatment works by decreasing the viral load of the mother, as well as providing pre- and post-exposure prophylaxis to the infant.

In the United States, the transmission rate in nontreated, HIV-infected mothers to their newborns is 25%. With proper management, this rate can be reduced to less than 2%. Medical treatment consists ideally of antiretroviral medications given to the woman during pregnancy and labor and to the newborn within the first hours of birth for up to six weeks. Even if treatment is not instituted during the pregnancy, treatment during labor for the mother and to the infant within 1–2 days of birth will still significantly decrease transmission of the infection to the infant to less than 10%. Once the amniotic sac surrounding the baby breaks, the risk of transmission of the HIV virus is increased because of increased exposure to maternal blood and body fluids. Therefore, an additional preventive measure to decrease the risk of transmission during delivery is to schedule a Cesarean section prior to the due date.

The HIV infection can also be transmitted via breast milk, and for this reason in the United States, the recommendation is for HIV-positive mothers to avoid breastfeeding. This is not a reasonable prevention in much of the developing world because breastfeeding is the primary source of infant feeding and formula is not economically possible, safe, acceptable, or available. In these countries, breastfeeding accounts for about 40% of all infant infections, and prevention of its transmission is primarily through the use of antiretroviral agents.

Prevention programs focusing on harm reduction may vary by global region based on the predominant transmission mechanism of the area. Figure 8-15 highlights sources of HIV infections by geographic regions. For example, IV drug use is the primary transmission method in Eastern Europe, and prevention targets there would be different than in Latin America/Caribbean where men having sex with men (MSM) is the major way the disease

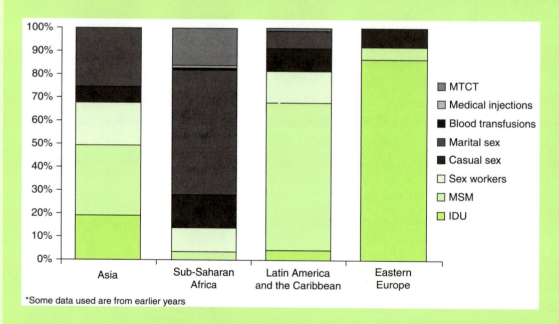

FIGURE 8-15 Source of New HIV Infections by Region
Source: Global HIV Prevention Working Group (June 2007); Bringing HIV Prevention to Scale: An Urgent Global Priority; http://www.malecircumcision.org/advocacy/documents/PWG_HIV_prevention_report_web.pdf

is transmitted or in sub-Saharan Africa where heterosexual sex is the most common mode of transmission. Prevention modalities used in Africa that have worked give a basis for intervention programs. Because sexual transmission is a major source of spread in Africa, multiple methods aimed at prevention have been used, including education of those at highest risk about behavior changes. The focused behaviors include abstinence, reduction in the numbers of partners, and use of condoms. Other methods of prevention that have proven successful include instruction on condom use, treatment of other sexually transmitted infections, and counseling of those who test positive regarding prevention of disease spread. Routine testing of those at risk for earlier diagnosis and prevention of spread has been found to lead to better prevention.

Barriers to full prevention of perinatal HIV in the United States include absent or delayed prenatal care (especially in higher risk women), acute infection late in pregnancy, acute infection in breastfeeding women, noncompliance in adhering to medication regimens, and lack of full implementation of universal screening for HIV in pregnant women. These issues are currently being addressed.

In the United States, the current recommendations are for universal testing in certain circumstances, such as pregnancy, but allowing patients to opt-out of testing for personal reasons. This reduces the stigma previously associated with testing only in high-risk patients after full counseling, called the "opt-in practice." Male circumcision in the adult population, although not 100% protective, has been found to decrease the risk of the spread of the HIV virus and is now a part of prevention programs in Africa.

Worldwide, prevention arms that target the spread via blood borne transmission have included the testing of donated blood and blood products, supply of clean needles and injection supplies to IV drug abusers, education programs aimed at IV drug abusers, and infection control. Increasing the availability and use of antiretroviral therapy to pregnant women has had the most positive impact on the prevention of the perinatal spread of HIV infection. According to the WHO, in 2008, 45% of pregnant women received ART, up from 10% in 2004. Delivery of the newborn via cesarean section decreases the risk of exposure to infected maternal blood.

In the United States and other developed countries, alternatives to breastfeeding are available in the form of commercial infant formulas and can be used to prevent the spread of HIV through infected breast milk. In developing countries where alternatives are not readily available, breastfeeding continues with treatment of the mothers with ART. A vaccine effective against the HIV virus is currently being researched and is a future hope for complete global protection.

Review Questions

1. Match the following terms in Column A with their corresponding terms in Column B.

Column A	Column B
___ Infection that can be spread by reptile pets like turtles and lizards	a. Common cold
___ Many outbreaks occur with ground beef	b. *Salmonella*
___ Causes food "intoxication"—e.g., enterotoxin causes disease, not bacteria itself	c. Tuberculosis
___ The etiology of many cruise ship outbreaks of food borne illness	d. *Giardia*
___ Has become a major problem with patients with HIV infections or AIDS and because of multidrug resistance	e. *Staph aureus*
___ Sexually transmitted disease that presents with a purulent discharge	f. *E. coli* 0157
___ Viral respiratory disease that is not cured with antibiotics	g. Gonorrhea
___ Infection of the lining of the brain and spinal cord	h. Norovirus
___ Sexually transmitted disease that mainly causes skin lesions	i. Meningitis
___ Protozoa that causes diarrhea	j. Syphilis

2. Which of the following is NOT a method of classification of infectious diseases?
   a. By clinical picture
   b. By reservoir
   c. By incubation period
   d. By infectious agent

3. **True or False** Because persons with latent tuberculosis have no clinical evidence of disease, they do not need treatment.

4. **True or False** The majority of people worldwide who are infected by HIV are not aware of their HIV status.

5. HIV can be transmitted through a number of routes. Which of the following has the highest estimated per-act risk of transmission?
   a. Needle sharing
   b. Receptive anal intercourse
   c. Receptive vaginal intercourse
   d. Blood transfusion

6. The prevalence of HIV infection worldwide is approximately 33 million. However, in 2007, the prevalence only increased by a proportionally low amount. This is the result of:

    a. A very low death rate compared to incidence
    b. Successfully curing people with HIV infection
    c. A very high death rate compared to incidence
    d. A very low incidence of infection

7. List three examples of modes of transmission and a disease associated with each.

    1. _____   _____
    2. _____   _____
    3. _____   _____

8. Put the following five goals of infectious disease control in order of achievement (with the easiest first): elimination of infection, control of the disease, eradication of an infection, extinction of an infection, elimination of the disease.

    _____,   _____,
    _____,   _____,
    _____,

9. The most common agent causing food borne infections in the United States is _____, whereas the most common agent causing deaths from food borne infections in the United States is _____.

10. **True or False** Transmission of malaria occurs via the bite of the *vivax* mosquito.

11. **For Deeper Thought** A local hospital reports to the county health department that over the past three days it is seeing an increase in admissions of toddlers for dehydration secondary to acute gastroenteritis. As the officer assigned to investigate, what information might you want to obtain from the hospital or cases that will help you identify the cause of the outbreak and institute preventive measures if indicated?

Website Resources

Centers for Disease Control and Prevention: http://www.cdc.gov

Centers for Disease Control and Prevention; FoodNet—Foodborne Disease Active Surveillance Network: http://www.cdc.gov/foodnet

Centers for Disease Control and Prevention: Morbidity and Mortality Weekly Report (MMWR); MMWR: Summary of Notifiable Diseases: http://www.cdc.gov/mmwr

Centers for Disease Control and Prevention, Public Health Image Library (PHIL): http://phil.cdc.gov

Global Health Council: http://www.globalhealth.org

Healthmap: http://www.healthmap.org (gives worldwide map of recent infectious outbreaks)

National Library of Medicine: http://www.nlm.nih.gov

World Health Organization: http://www.who.int/en

References

Carson-DeWitt, R., & Frey, R. (2006). "Typhoid Fever," *Gale Encyclopedia of Medicine* (3rd ed.). 2006. Retrieved from: Encyclopedia.com. http://www.encyclopedia.com/doc/1G2-3451601676.html

Centers for Disease Control and Prevention. (updated February 4, 2011). Estimates of Foodborne Illness in the United States, CDC 2011 Estimates: Findings. Retrieved from http://www.cdc.gov/foodborneburden/2011-foodborne-estimates.html

Centers for Disease Control and Prevention. (April 8, 2011). Measles Imported by Returning U.S. Travelers Aged 6-23 Months, *MMWR* 2001-2011. Retrieved from http://www.cdc.gov/mmwr/preview/mmwrhtml/mm6013a1.htm

Centers for Disease Control and Prevention. (updated December 22, 2010). Norovirus: Technical Fact Sheet. Retrieved from http://www.cdc.gov/ncidod/dvrd/revb/gastro/norovirus-factsheet.htm

Centers for Disease Control and Prevention. (updated December 23, 2010). *Salmonella—Salmonella* Outbreaks. Retrieved from http://www.cdc.gov/salmonella/outbreaks.html

Centers for Disease Control and Prevention. (updated January 12, 2011). CDC Features—Surveillance for Norovirus Outbreaks. Retrieved from http://www.cdc.gov/Features/dsNorovirus

Centers for Disease Control and Prevention. (reviewed November 2, 2010). Parasites—*Giardia*: Epidemiology & Risk Factors. Retrieved from http://www.cdc.gov/parasites/giardia/epi.html

Centers for Disease Control and Prevention. (modified March 5, 2011). *E. coli*: *E. coli* Break Investigations. Retrieved from http://www.cdc.gov/ecoli/outbreaks.html

Centers for Disease Control and Prevention. (reviewed July 1, 2010). Tuberculosis: Basic TB Facts. Retrieved from http://www.cdc.gov/tb/topic/basics/default.htm

Centers for Disease Control and Prevention. (updated November 19, 2010). Tuberculosis (TB): Fact Sheet—Trends in Tuberculosis, 2009. Retrieved from http://www.cdc.gov/tb/publications/factsheets/statistics/TBTrends.htm

Centers for Disease Control and Prevention. (updated February 23, 2010). Meningitis: Meningitis Questions & Answers. Retrieved from http://www.cdc.gov/meningitis/about/faq.html

Centers for Disease Control and Prevention. (reviewed April 28, 2010). Sexually Transmitted Diseases (STDs). Retrieved from http://www.cdc.gov/std

Centers for Disease Control and Prevention. (2009). Health, United States, 2009. Retrieved from http://www.cdc.gov/nchs/data/hus/hus09.pdf#029

Centers for Disease Control and Prevention. (May 13, 2011). Morbidity and Mortality Weekly Report (MMWR): Summary of Notifiable Diseases—United States, 2009. Retrieved from http://www.cdc.gov/mmwr/PDF/wk/mm5853.pdf

Centers for Disease Control and Prevention. (updated December 9, 2010). National Vital Statistics Report (Volume 59, Number 2) Deaths: Preliminary Data for 2008. Retrieved from http://www.cdc.gov/nchs/data/nvsr/nvsr59/nvsr59_02.pdf

Centers for Disease Control and Prevention. (updated February 8, 2010). Malaria: Malaria Facts. Retrieved from http://www.cdc.gov/malaria/about/facts.html

Centers for Disease Control and Prevention. (updated August 11, 2010). Basic Information about HIV and AIDS and Basic Statistics. Retrieved from http://www.cdc.gov/hiv/topics.htm

Heymann, D. L. (ed.). (2008). *Control of Communicable Disease Manual* (19th ed.). Washington, D.C.: American Public Health Association.

National Institute of Allergy and Infectious Diseases. (updated March 11, 2011). HIV/AIDS: Quick Facts. Retrieved from http://www.niaid.nih.gov/topics/HIVAIDS/Understanding/Pages/quickFacts.aspx

World Health Organization. (August 2009). Diarrheal Disease. Retrieved from http://www.who.int/mediacentre/factsheets/fs330/en/index.html

World Health Organization. (April 2005). Media Center: Drug-resistant Salmonella. Retrieved from http://www.who.int/mediacentre/factsheets/fs139/en

World Health Organization. (May 2005). Media Center: Enterohaemorrhagic Escherichia coli (EHEC). Retrieved from http://www.who.int/mediacentre/factsheets/fs125/en

World Health Organization. (May 2005). Media Center: Cholera. Retrieved from http://www.who.int/mediacentre/factsheets/fs107/en/index.html

World Health Organization. (August 2009). Protozoan Parasites (*Cryptosporidium, Giardia, Cyclospora*). Retrieved from http://www.who.int/water_sanitation_health/dwq/en/admicrob5.pdf

World Health Organization. (April 2005). Media Center: Tuberculosis. Retrieved from http://www.who.int/mediacentre/factsheets/fs104/en/index.html

World Health Organization. (n.d.). Health Statistics and Health Information Services: Disease and Injury Regional Estimates for 2004. Retrieved from http://www.who.int/healthinfo/global_burden_disease/estimates_regional/en/index.html

World Health Organization. (April 2010). Media Center: Malaria. Retrieved from http://www.who.int/mediacentre/factsheets/fs094/en/index.html

World Health Organization. (n.d.). Fact File:10 Facts on HIV/AIDS. Retrieved from http://www.who.int/features/factfiles/hiv/en/index.html

World Health Organization. (July 2010). HIV/AIDS Q&A. Retrieved from http://www.who.int/features/qa/71/en/index.html

World Health Organization. (May 2011). Millennium Development Goals: Progress Towards the Health-Related Millennium Development Goals. Retrieved from http://www.who.int/mediacentre/factsheets/fs290/en/index.html

Yorita, C., Krista, L., Holman, R. C., Steiner, C. A, et al. (2009). Infectious disease hospitalizations in the United States. *Clinical Infectious Diseases, 49*(7): 1025–1035. doi:10.1086/605562

Chapter 9

OUTBREAK INVESTIGATIONS

Learning Objectives

Upon completion of this chapter, you should be able to:

1. Define an outbreak of disease and describe how it is the same as or different from an epidemic.
2. Understand the different features of a common source and propagated outbreak.
3. Describe the three main settings in which disease outbreaks occur.
4. Identify the 10 steps of an outbreak investigation and be able to describe some of the features of each step.
5. Describe which of the 10 steps fit into the following categories: Identifying there is a problem, controlling the outbreak/prevention of further cases, measuring the outbreak, and finding the responsible agent.

Key Terms

attack rates

common source
  outbreak

disease outbreak

epidemic curve

food-specific attack rate

propagated outbreak

secondary attack rate

Chapter Outline

INTRODUCTION

Outbreak is a scary word. It implies an "out of control" situation with a "doomsday" expectation. Most people who hear the word only have a negative view of the possible results from an outbreak. Sick people are pictured lined up at hospitals waiting for attention from overwhelmed healthcare workers. Very often, however, outbreaks go unnoticed and do not even make the news. Most are caused by exposure to contaminated food, water, or by direct contact with others who have an infectious disease. Illness in outbreaks can be minor "self-limited" diseases or major deadly diseases. Throughout history, disease outbreaks have had major impacts on large populations, sometimes on a worldwide scale. Although outbreaks are always undesirable, the successful investigation of an outbreak can lead to positive advances in future protection of public health.

No one really knows how many outbreaks occur in the United States each year. There are regulations about reporting outbreaks to health authorities, but many times these outbreaks are not seen in their entirety and never reported. The Centers for Disease Control and Prevention does receive more than 1,000 reported outbreaks per year in the United States. This is usually only the "tip of the iceberg." For example, there are an estimated 75 million food borne illnesses in the United States each year. Many of these illnesses are a part of an outbreak, but it is unclear how many outbreaks these illnesses could represent.

DEFINITION OF AN OUTBREAK OF DISEASE

The World Health Organization defines a **disease outbreak** as the occurrence of cases of disease in excess of what would normally be expected in a defined community, geographical area, or season. An outbreak may occur in a restricted geographical area or may extend over several countries. It may last for a few days, or weeks, or for several years.

The key phrase in this definition is "in excess of what would be normally expected." Without knowing the normally expected (baseline) rate of disease, it is not possible to know whether the disease is in excess of normal. This means that an outbreak is not defined by any specific number of cases of disease. For example, a disease that has been eradicated from human populations has a normal rate of disease that is zero. So for that disease, it would only take a single case of disease to be considered an outbreak. An example would be smallpox. Because smallpox has been eradicated, a single case of smallpox seen in humans would be considered an outbreak. On the other hand, a disease such as hepatitis A may be somewhat common in humans in some populations. In this case, an outbreak of hepatitis A would not be declared unless the number of current cases was higher than normal.

Another definition of an outbreak that has gained popularity is one that is specific to food borne or water borne diseases. This definition establishes that an outbreak occurs whenever more than two cases of a similar illness are seen from the same source. Because the source is usually apparent from the beginning, there often does not need to be a full investigation of this type of outbreak.

How does the definition of an outbreak differ from the definition of an epidemic? In general, an outbreak is the same as an epidemic. The main difference is that an outbreak is an excess of disease that usually occurs in a shorter period of time or in a more localized geographical area. An epidemic may also occur in a shorter period of time, but generally the designation of an epidemic is reserved for a period of months or years and over an entire country or many countries. However, it is not wrong to use the terms "epidemic" and "outbreak" interchangeably. Throughout this chapter, it will be clear that the discussion about an outbreak will be very similar to the discussion of an epidemic in previous chapters.

disease outbreak:
the occurrence of cases of disease in excess of what would normally be expected in a defined community, geographical area, or season

TYPES OF OUTBREAK: COMMON SOURCE AND PROPAGATED

common source outbreak:
occurs when all cases of the infection are acquired from the same source in a limited period of time and in a limited geographical location

Outbreaks are generally classified as one of two types—common source and propagated. In a **common source outbreak**, all cases of the infectious disease are acquired from the same source in a limited period of time and in a limited geographical location. It is also characterized by very minimal (or zero) transmission from person to person. Generally, a common source outbreak has a smaller number of cases than a propagated outbreak and is often caused by contaminated food or water. A typical example of a common source epidemic is a food borne illness caused by exposure to one specific food or restaurant. Common source epidemics are usually characterized by a dramatic single "peak" of cases. Many common source outbreaks go unreported because they are generally small in numbers and often do not come to the attention of public health authorities.

A **propagated outbreak** is characterized by an outbreak that continues over an extended period of time. This outbreak has individuals exposed to the original source, but then it will also have secondary infections in individuals exposed to those initially ill people via person to person spread. The propagated epidemic usually lasts for a longer period of time and has various numbers of "peaks" of cases over time. The initial source often resolves, but the outbreak continues by infected persons infecting other persons. Propagated outbreaks often result in larger numbers of cases than common source outbreaks. Most outbreaks of respiratory diseases, such as influenza, are propagated outbreaks, as well as some food or water borne outbreaks such as those occurring from norovirus infections.

Accurate identification of the type of outbreak is very important in determining the etiologic agent that is causing the outbreak and in developing recommendations for the control of and further prevention of the outbreak. In the discussion of the steps of an outbreak investigation presented later, the methodology for identifying the type of outbreak will be discussed.

Several interesting observations can be made about the list shown in Table 9-1. The major outbreaks are from propagated respiratory outbreaks such as influenza.

propagated outbreak: an outbreak that continues over an extended period of time and includes cases that are transmitted from person to person

Historical Note 9·1

Major Outbreaks

Recorded history has identified a number of major outbreaks from around the world. Table 9-1 lists some of the most historically important outbreaks of disease. These are the events that give the term "outbreak" its deadly reputation. These outbreaks have resulted in hundreds of millions of deaths and considerably more in morbidity and health care costs. Some were only over a period of months and some have lasted for years. The most deadly of the historical outbreaks was the Great Influenza outbreak of 1918–1919. In just six months, this outbreak was estimated to have killed 100 million people worldwide. Although other outbreaks, such as the Black Death, likely killed more people, the Great Influenza outbreak killed all those people in just six months, whereas the Black Death killed people for over 200 years. It is estimated that if an outbreak with the same impact as the Great Influenza outbreak occurred today, it would kill over 350 million people worldwide. That is more people than live in the entire United States!

Check It Out

For an interactive global map showing current epidemics or outbreaks, go to: http://www.healthmap.org/en/

Person to person transmission is usually necessary for an outbreak to include so many people. However, the outbreaks of plague throughout history are noteworthy because plague is very seldom transmitted from person to person. This is the reason that although plague kills large numbers of people, it takes many years. With the exception of the first cholera pandemic in 1817–1823, food and water borne outbreaks are generally absent from this list. Also notice that a "seasonal influenza" outbreak is listed, but this is a recurring outbreak that happens each year. In the United States, the seasonal influenza outbreak kills about 36, 000 people a year, but that has been happening every year for years. In addition, there are ongoing outbreaks such as AIDS and malaria that are noteworthy because they have killed large numbers of people worldwide but are entirely preventable.

These historical outbreaks have been deadly and scary events; however, they are by no means the most frequent types of outbreaks occurring in the past or present around the world. The setting for most outbreaks is a smaller, localized situation that at some point has affected, or will affect, all of us.

TABLE 9-1 Worst Outbreaks in History

- Great Influenza Outbreak of 1918–1919

- The Black Death 1300–1400s (plague)

- HIV/AIDS 1981 to present

- Annual Seasonal Influenza Outbreaks

- The Plague of Justinian 541 AD

- The First Cholera Pandemic 1817–1823

- The Antonine Plague 165–180 AD

- The Asiatic (Russian) Influenza 1889–1890

Based on: Epic Disasters: The World's Worst Disasters; http://www.epicdisasters.com/index.php/site/comments/the_worst_outbreaks_of_disease/

OUTBREAK SETTINGS

Outbreaks of disease occur in many settings. Through the news media, one can regularly read about outbreaks caused by drinking, eating, relaxing, swimming, flying on airplanes, taking cruises, playing on athletic teams, visiting petting zoos, going to school, going to daycare, living in a nursing home, hiking, staying in a hotel, being in a hospital, camping, taking showers, and having sex. Much of our daily lives can be the setting for an outbreak, some for minor illnesses, and others for life-threatening illnesses.

The setting of an outbreak is generally classified into three categories:

1. Food borne outbreaks,

2. Water borne outbreaks, and

3. Community acquired outbreaks.

The most common outbreak is in a food borne setting. A food borne outbreak is generally considered to exist if there are more than two reports of a similar illness from the same food source, frequently in a restaurant or at a community dinner. A food borne outbreak may have a widely varied number of cases and has no seasonal distribution. Although the food borne outbreak is the most common, in only about 50% of the outbreaks is the food culprit identified, so a large number of these outbreaks go unsolved. Although this type of setting is very often a common source outbreak, there is also the possibility of the outbreak being propagated by infected food service workers. So although there may not be direct person to person contact, infected food service workers not using proper food handling techniques can pass their illness on to customers of the facility through food. The most common infectious agents involved in food borne outbreaks are norovirus, *Salmonella*, bacterial toxins from *Staphlyococcus*, *Campylobacter*, *Shigella*, and hepatitis A virus. (See Chapter 8 for further discussion of these agents.)

In disease that occurs from a water borne outbreak, infection occurs by either ingesting water contaminated by pathogens or by swimming in water contaminated by pathogens. Most often these outbreaks are common source types. The numbers of cases in these outbreaks can be variable and often unknown. The most common agents responsible for water borne outbreaks are norovirus, *Shigella, Giardia, Crytosporidiosis*, and *E. coli*.

The most widely varied of the outbreak settings is the community acquired setting. This is because the diseases that occur in this setting include most all types of infectious diseases, such as respiratory diseases and gastrointestinal diseases. The diseases in this setting are transmitted most often by person to person transmission in schools, hospitals, daycare, nursing homes, prisons, and high-density living areas such as military barracks, hotels, and even airplanes. Some common agents that cause the diseases acquired in a community setting include norovirus, varicella, influenza, rhinovirus, parasites, and adenovirus.

By considering these common settings, it is clear that outbreaks can come in all "shapes and sizes" in a wide variety of settings. This variation in the possible diseases acquired and the agents that cause them is the reason that there needs to be a standard method of investigating an outbreak. No assumptions should be made

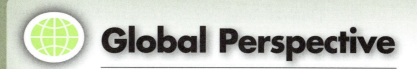

Global Perspective

The CDC

The Centers for Disease Control and Prevention is well known for its role as disease detectives in the United States. CDC also maintains a role in the international outbreak arena, particularly during WASH-related diseases (water, sanitation, and hygiene), providing its expertise in global outbreaks by working with ministries of health, nongovernmental organizations (NGOs), United Nations organizations, and health-related professionals from around the world. The CDC does this by providing assistance with the identification of the cause of an outbreak, identifying possible risk factors, controlling the spread of the outbreak, and assisting with the development of prevention practices. A recent major outbreak that CDC responded to in a major way was the 2010 outbreak of cholera in Haiti following the earlier major earthquake there.

that cannot be confirmed by actual methodology and data. When an outbreak is suspected, the setting in which the outbreak occurs requires recognition to begin to find the cause and to control it.

STEPS IN AN OUTBREAK INVESTIGATION

Wise cooks still refer to a cookbook if they want to ensure perfection. When a possible disease outbreak is occurring, there is no room for error; and although many epidemiologists have had experience with multiple outbreak investigations, the need for an "outbreak cookbook" is critical. The epidemiologist's cookbook for the 10 steps of an outbreak investigation is provided in Table 9-2. If there is a suspected outbreak of a disease in a population, these 10 steps, in this order, will allow investigators to have the best success of determining the cause of the outbreak and preventing future cases of the same disease.

In general, these 10 steps are organized into categories that first identify that a problem exists, then measure it, find the responsible agent, and prevent it from occurring further. Each of these general steps is important to complete fully before moving on to the next step. An outbreak investigation is a process where each step is dependent on the successful completion and information obtained in the previous step(s). For example, it is easy to imagine how problematic it would be through the entire investigation if an accurate diagnosis was not determined and confirmed. Also, it is important to notice that several of the later steps in the investigation involve prevention and control of future disease and preparing a written report of

TABLE 9-2 The Steps of an Outbreak Investigation

1. Confirm the diagnosis.

2. Confirm the existence of an outbreak/epidemic.

3. Define a case and count cases.

4. Orient data in terms of person, place, and time.

5. Determine who is at risk.

6. Develop a hypothesis and test it.

7. Determine control measures.

8. Plan a more systematic study.

9. Execute disease control and prevention measures.

10. Prepare a written report.

© Cengage Learning 2013

the entire process. Although these steps may not seem like part of an "investigation," the ultimate goal of an outbreak investigation is to control existing disease and to prevent future occurrence, as well as to find the cause of the problem.

Step 1: Confirm the Diagnosis

The first step of the outbreak investigation process seems very obvious, but it is very important not to overlook. Table 9-3 includes the considerations that are important to confirming the specific diagnosis of the potential outbreak. When a suspected outbreak is first noticed in a community, the symptoms of the disease need to be reviewed for consistency and accuracy. Ensuring that the disease is properly diagnosed takes knowledge of the suspected medical condition and a "re-look" at the records of the individuals suspected to be early cases of the disease. It is also important to confirm any laboratory results so that any inaccuracies can be ruled out. Also, at this point, if possible, a visit to existing cases to confirm the clinical and laboratory findings, as well as to determine if there is additional information about the illness that patients can provide, may be warranted. Once the potential for diagnosis and laboratory errors has been ruled out, it is important to summarize the clinical findings and laboratory findings. The idea of this summarization is to look at the general symptoms related to the suspect outbreak that are known to that point. This will begin to form the case definition that is to be established in step 3 of the investigation. It is not necessary to have the formal definition at this point. First, it must be decided that there is actually an outbreak to investigate.

TABLE 9-3 Outbreak Investigation
Step 1: Confirm the Diagnosis
• Ensure suspected illness is properly diagnosed.
• Rule out laboratory error.
• Visit/assess patients (cases).
• Summarize clinical findings.

Step 2: Confirm the Existence of an Outbreak/Epidemic

One of the more fundamental errors of an outbreak investigation is the failure to establish that the disease being seen in the community is in fact an outbreak and not just the normal occurrence of the suspected disease. Although it may not seem to be a problem to investigate an occurrence of disease even if it is the normal occurrence of that disease, conducting an outbreak investigation is not without risk for potential backlash from political, medical, and publicity arenas. These investigations can be costly and time-consuming, so the risks and the cost make it necessary to ensure that there is truly an outbreak occurring.

The considerations important to establishing the existence of an outbreak are provided in Table 9-4. The normal rate of the illness/symptoms in a population must be known before it can be determined if there is an excess of disease. For most diseases or conditions, the normal rate of occurrence can be found through a number of the data sources discussed in Chapter 4. It is important to be able to quickly access these data sources such as health department surveillance data, hospital discharge records, vital records, and disease registries. Depending on the disease, one or many of these sources may provide a quick indication of the normal amount of the disease in a community or population. Another option is to use rates of the potential diseases or symptoms in neighboring communities or populations. This may be possible if a similar outbreak investigation has been performed recently in neighboring communities. Notice that the word "quickly/quick" has been used several times in this step. Time is always critical with an outbreak investigation, and often there are only hours or days to find and control the outbreak. If there is time, and no other data are available, an investigator could do a quick survey of the community to establish the normal level of disease in that population.

Establishing the existence of a disease also utilizes the concept of the epidemic threshold discussed in previous chapters. The normal rates of disease over time are used to determine a range of "normal high limits" and "normal low limits," and these establish the ranges of disease over time. The normal high limit of this range is used to determine if there is an excess. If the observed rate of disease is higher than this upper limit of the normal range, then it is considered that the observed rate is in excess of normal. Figure 9-1 is an example of an epidemic threshold established for a fictitious disease.

TABLE 9-4 Outbreak Investigation

Step 2: Establish the Existence of an Outbreak

- What is the expected number of disease?

- Use Health Department surveillance data.

- Use hospital discharge records.

- Use vital records.

- Use registries.

- Use neighboring rates—you may need to.

- Last resort: conduct a survey.

© Cengage Learning 2013

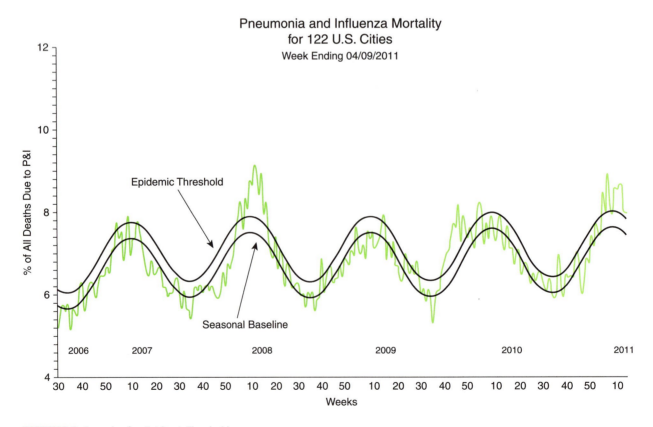

Pneumonia and Influenza Mortality for 122 U.S. Cities
Week Ending 04/09/2011

FIGURE 9-1 Example of an Epidemic Threshold

Courtesy of the Centers for Disease Control and Prevention: http://www.cdc.gov/flu/weekly/pdf/External_F1015.pdf

The actual rate of disease is established from existing records and is represented by the bold green solid line over time. The up and down variation in the line over time establishes the normal range of that disease. The upper and lower limits of the normal range are represented by the upper and lower black parallel lines and are established by statistical methods and generally represent three standard deviations above and below the line. Notice that the black lines of the limits are much smoother than the actual rate of disease, which provides levels that are more standard over time. Any amount of disease that is greater than the upper limit (also known as the "epidemic threshold") is considered to be in excess of normal and, consequently, establishes the existence of an outbreak.

Step 3: Define a Case and Count Cases

Once the outbreak is established, a case definition needs to be formalized, and the number of cases according to the definition needs to be counted. The information necessary to establish a usable and detailed case definition is provided in Table 9-5. Like the other steps of an outbreak investigation, it is important to write down a case definition. The case definition can be simple and short, or it can be complicated and long. This all depends on the disease being investigated. The aspects of the disease that need to be included in a case definition are such things as the clinical symptoms, the laboratory test results necessary, the dates that the

TABLE 9-5 Outbreak Investigation

Step 3: Define and Count Cases

- Case classification (definition) should include:

    a. Clinical symptoms

    b. Laboratory verification

    c. Restrictions of person, place, and time

    d. Confirmed, suspected, possible case criteria

- Count cases

    a. Cast a wide net

    b. Health clinics, hospitals

    c. Advertise

    d. Ask other cases

symptoms appeared, the geographic boundaries of the outbreak, and any specific characteristics of the persons that are important to the definition of a case (such as age or gender). Although on occasion all of this information is not available (such as laboratory results), these aspects of a case's definition should be established and then used to clearly identify who is to be considered a case for the specific outbreak.

One of the most common errors in an outbreak investigation is the failure to utilize a "strict" case definition. As discussed in Chapter 7, the accuracy of any study, including an outbreak investigation, is very dependent on the ability to correctly classify the outcome of a study. If the cases in an outbreak investigation include too many misclassified cases, then the conclusion of the investigation will not be accurate. As an example, very often the disease being investigated in an outbreak is a gastrointestinal disease resulting from food or water contamination. The symptoms of the various possible agents can vary, but many times the inclusion or exclusion of just one symptom can significantly increase the accuracy of the definition. For example, vomiting and diarrhea may seem to coexist in most gastrointestinal diseases, but the reality is that being able to separate cases by those that have only one or both of these symptoms can be a tremendous help in identifying the agent causing the outbreak. So if the case definition does not include vomiting, then it is important to not count anyone with vomiting as a case even if they are sick and the other aspects of the case definition are met.

Another common error in the use of a case definition is ignoring the date of onset of the symptoms. An outbreak is very often a result of specific circumstances that include an "event in time." If someone with the same disease occurring before that time is counted as a case, the ability to make accurate conclusions from the investigation will be harmed.

One other important aspect of a case definition is to decide if the cases need to be classified as "confirmed, suspected, or possible." Once the formal case definition is established, anyone that meets the complete definition is considered a confirmed case. However, often, the ability to assess all aspects of the case definition may be difficult either because of the lack of laboratory support, lack of time, or missing information. So, a formal case definition may also need to include criteria for identifying suspected cases and possible cases. Many times, a *suspected* case is a person who meets the entire case definition with the exception of the laboratory results. This refers to a person with "missing" laboratory information, not laboratory information that contradicts the case definition.

A further deviation from a strict case definition would be the criteria for a *possible* case, which could be a person who is missing additional information such as date of onset or geographic location. A possible case could also be someone who reports the appropriate symptoms but did not seek medical attention so there is no documentation for those symptoms. Clearly, the distinction between a confirmed case, a suspected case, and a possible case can be somewhat variable, but it is necessary to identify these classifications as part of a case definition.

Further, when making these distinctions, it is important for the investigator to decide how these different classifications will be analyzed. The analysis of the outbreak can be performed using only confirmed cases, but it can also be performed using "any" confirmed, suspected, or possible cases. However, the determination of the case group for the analysis must be established prior to beginning the investigation so that the results do not bias the choice of which analysis to perform.

Using the established case definition, it is then important to find and count all cases that exist. In order to find all cases, it may be necessary to look well beyond the suspected source of the event. Although this does not mean violating the geographic limitations of the case definition, it does mean that investigators may need to "cast a wide net" to find as many cases as possible.

For example, a person meeting the case definition may live a long distance from the suspected source of the outbreak but may travel to and from the geographic location identified in the case definition. Investigators may also need to actively search for cases at local hospitals and clinics that might have treated persons with the disease suspected as causing the potential outbreak. Once these potential cases are identified, the investigators may need to contact them to further determine if they meet the case definition. Other methods used to identify additional cases include possible advertisements in local area news media or contacting existing cases and asking about friends or family who may have similar symptoms.

Step 4: Orient Data in Terms of Person, Place, and Time

After identifying and counting all cases, the next step is to "get to know the data." All good data analysis in epidemiology begins by simply organizing and graphically presenting the information. Many investigators would prefer to quickly test for associations between suspected etiologic agents and the disease, but it is unwise to skip this basic step. Table 9-6 provides the basic techniques for orienting the

TABLE 9-6 Outbreak Investigation

Step 4: Orient Data in Person, Place, and Time

- Get to know your data

- Descriptive epidemiology

  - Person: age, race, gender, medical status, exposures

  - Place: map cases (GIS)

  - Map attack rates, not numerators

  - Time: epidemic curve

© Cengage Learning 2013

outbreak data with respect to person, place, and time. These techniques allow the investigator to quickly understand the fundamental information about the outbreak. This fundamental information will likely provide considerable "clues" that will enable the investigator to begin to understand the context and situation of the outbreak.

By definition, at this stage of an outbreak investigation, all of the individuals included are true cases, which mean that they all have the disease under investigation (there is no comparison group yet). There is much that can be learned about those with disease even if only knowing about their cases. For example, are the cases all men or all women or both? What is the age distribution? Is there cultural variation or is the group culturally similar? Is the outbreak among medically impaired people or people in general good health? What activities have the cases been involved with lately that could be related to the disease, such as recent exposures to specific restaurants, food, or water sources? The methodology for assessing this information is to use simple descriptive statistics such as frequencies of these attributes in the cases identified. For example, the investigator should identify the proportion of the cases who are men and the proportion of the cases who are women, and the age distribution of the cases. The investigator should also identify the frequency (proportion) of cases who were exposed to specific restaurants or food during the correct time period. This exposure information about the cases will be very important in determining the next several steps to find the cause of the outbreaks.

The cases should also be organized according to geographic location to determine the potential place of exposure and infection. Developing a graphical map to plot the location is a very simple and extremely valuable step when trying to determine where to focus an investigation in a community setting. Of course, if the outbreak investigation is already focused on a specific location such as a restaurant, the mapping of cases is less useful; but many times the cases are coming from hospitals and clinics, and mapping the cases will help narrow down the places to look for the source of the outbreak. The graphical display of the location of the cases can be a very simple map. Each case can be placed on the map and then any existing clusters of cases can be observed. But the key to a good map is knowing the population "denominators" in the various locations. Knowing the denominators of the locations on a map will allow the investigator to plot attack rates.

An **attack rate** is a special case of an incidence rate where the numerator is the number of new cases in a defined population in a defined period of time and the denominator is the population at risk during the same time period. It is calculated according to the following formula:

$$\text{Attack rate} = \frac{\text{Number of cases in a time period or location}}{\text{Population at risk in the same time period or location}} \times 100$$

attack rates: rates of disease during short periods of time or when the entire population is available to observe

An example of a setting where a calculated attack rate may be helpful would be during an outbreak of diarrheal disease from food served at a specific event. The entire population attending the event can be defined, and all new cases from that defined population would be used to calculate the rate. For example, if 329 guests dined at

Restaurant Getill on the evening of November 7, 2011, and 78 of them became ill with diarrhea within 48 hours, the attack rate would be 78 / 329 or 23.7%.

An example where calculating attack rates for mapping might be helpful would be in investigating an outbreak of hepatitis A in Community Seafud. The numerator could be the number of cases presenting to the small county health clinic over the past month. The denominator could be the populations from various parts of the community. Plotting attack rates on a map can be very helpful to identify the locations where cases were proportionally high. Using the attack rates prevents the misinterpretation of clusters of cases. For example, in a location within a community that has a high population density, it can be expected that more cases would come from that location. So simply seeing a high number of cases in that location could be misleading. Using attack rates allows the investigators to "control" for the size of the population.

Orienting the group of cases by time provides additional information about the outbreak and possible cause. The exercise of graphing the number of cases over a period of time results in the traditional epidemic curve. An **epidemic curve** is the plot of time trends in the number of cases for a defined population and time period. An example of an epidemic curve is provided in Figure 9-2. Notice that along the horizontal x-axis is the time in days and along the vertical y-axis is the number of cases. The shape of the plot of the cases versus time provides several pieces of information to the investigator. First, the earliest set of cases to appear on the graph can be used to identify the likely date of the first exposure in the outbreak. For example, if the outbreak is from cholera, and the typical incubation period for cholera is 1 to 2 days, investigators can back up 1 to 2 days from the earliest cases to identify the approximate date of the first exposure. Further, in the same fashion, investigators can use the highest peak of the graph to identify the most common date of exposure.

The other main piece of information provided by an epidemic curve is the ability to identify the type of outbreak. A single high and short peak in cases represents a common source outbreak. On the other hand, multiple peaks in cases or long plateaus in cases indicate a propagated outbreak. A key measure of a propagated outbreak is a secondary attack rate. A **secondary attack rate** is the rate of disease

epidemic curve: the plot of time trends in the number of cases for a defined population and time period

secondary attack rate: the rate of disease in an outbreak that results from transmission of the disease from person to person

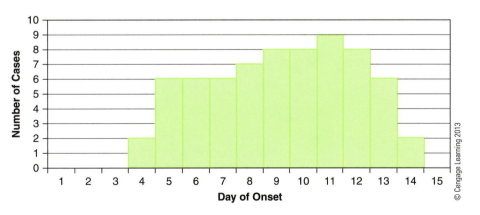

FIGURE 9-2 Example of an Epidemic Curve

in an outbreak that results from transmission of the disease from person to person. It may be used when an outbreak is continuing over a longer period of time and gives an indication of the amount of transmission that is occurring from person to person. The secondary attack rate is calculated using the following formula:

$$\text{Secondary attack rate} = \frac{\text{Number with disease exposed to the primary case(s)}}{\text{Total number exposed to the primary case(s)}} \times 100$$

Step 5: Determine Who Is at Risk

Up to this point in the investigation, the steps have been to identify the outbreak and case definition, then count cases and describe them. But at this point, there is only information about the cases. In order to finally identify the cause of the outbreak, it will be necessary to gather information from subjects who are not cases. The steps to start this comparison between those with the disease (cases) and those without the disease (controls) begin with determining who is at risk for the disease, in other words who does NOT have the disease but is at risk to get the disease. The steps to define and investigate the population at risk are described in Table 9-7.

The population at risk is important for two main reasons. First, this will be the population used as controls to approach subjects for a study to test the hypothesis to find the cause of the outbreak later in the investigation. At this point in the investigation, the cases have been identified, but the comparison group for hypothesis testing will need to come from a population with similar characteristics. Second, the population at risk is important in defining the population for whom prevention and control measures will be targeted.

TABLE 9-7 Outbreak Investigation

Step 5: Define and Investigate the Population at Risk

- Where did the cases come from?

- Using definition of cases, identify population with the same criteria:

  - Geographic location

  - Time period

  - Population characteristic

- Look for any remaining cases in population at risk.

- This population will also be the target of prevention and control measures.

© Cengage Learning 2013

Step 6: Develop a Hypothesis and Test It

Once the population at risk has been identified, it is finally time to develop a formal hypothesis about the suspected cause of the outbreak and to test that hypothesis. Table 9-8 includes the aspects to consider in this step. The hypothesis for the outbreak is a statement that proposes an agent likely to be the cause of the disease. Also included in the hypothesis should be information about the expected mode of transmission of disease, the population affected, and any behaviors or exposures necessary to transmit the disease. The hypothesis should include the information necessary to develop a valid study to confirm or reject the expected source of the outbreak. So, for example, if the disease is a food borne illness, the hypothesis should specify the population who may have eaten the food, the time period during which that food was eaten, the specific food ingredient that is suspected to be contaminated, the food service facility, and if there is person to person transmission.

The hypothesis can now be tested using a valid study design. Most often the initial study designed to test the first hypothesis in an outbreak investigation is a retrospective case control study. The case group has been established and counted; the study will require the enrollment of a group of non-ill controls from the population at risk. The study performed at this stage is usually the routine retrospective study. The cases and controls are often surveyed about their exposures such as foods eaten or water sources. Then the responses in each of the groups are compared. If the hypothesis suggests that a certain food is the culprit, the study is often referred to as an "eaten, not-eaten study" because information about food exposures is the usual comparison.

TABLE 9-8 Outbreak Investigation

Step 6: Develop a Hypothesis and Test It

- Develop a hypothesis to confirm the cause of disease.

  - Include suspected etiologic agent

  - Include mode of transmission

  - Identifies expected exposures

  - Specifies population

- Test the hypothesis using a study design.

  - Retrospective study to compare cases to controls

  - Possible prospective study if exposure is still present

The information from the cases and controls pertaining to the specific exposure, such as food, can be used to calculate specific attack rates, such as a food-specific attack rate. A **food-specific attack rate** is a rate of disease among those who have eaten a specific food item. The food-specific attack rate is unique in that the denominator is only those with the same exposure (food) as the ill people in the numerator, but the denominator includes ill and non-ill eaters of that food. These individual food-specific attack rates for different foods can be compared to indicate which food likely made people sick. The formula for a food-specific attack rate is provided here:

$$\text{Food-specific attack rate} = \frac{\text{Number who ate a specific food and became ill}}{\text{Number who ate the specific food}} \times 100$$

The food-specific attack rate can also be calculated for those who have not eaten the specified food as well (the number who did *not* eat a specific food item and became ill divided by the number who did not eat the specific food × 100). Then the food-specific attack rate for those who did eat the food is compared to the food-specific attack rate for those that did not eat the same food. This is done for all the foods or suspected exposures mentioned in the hypothesis.

Consider the example in Figure 9-3 using a fictitious food and illness in an outbreak investigation. Using the case definition, 46 cases were identified and consented to participate. Then 29 additional subjects who did not have the illness, but were in the population at risk, were approached and consented to participate as controls. Each subject was asked about his or her recent exposure to specific foods. After all subjects were surveyed, a total of 54 subjects ate the specific food, and 21 subjects did not eat the specific food. Using the information in the table, food-specific attack rates can be calculated for those who ate the food and for those who did not eat the food. For those who ate the food, 43 of the 54 subjects were ill for a food-specific attack rate of 79.6%. For those who did not eat the food, 3 of the 21 subjects were ill for a food-specific attack rate of 14.3%.

Clearly, the attack rate is much higher among those who ate the food versus those who did not. At this stage, a measure of association appropriate for this study design would be an odds ratio, which can be calculated from this information to be OR = 23.5. The interpretation of this odds ratio is that those who were ill were 23.5 times more likely to have eaten the food than those who were not ill. This food certainly seems to be associated with the illness.

food-specific attack rate: a rate of disease among those who have eaten a specific food item

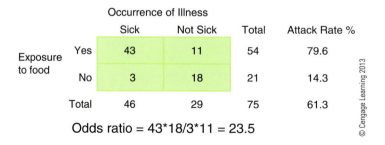

| | | Occurrence of Illness | | | |
		Sick	Not Sick	Total	Attack Rate %
Exposure to food	Yes	43	11	54	79.6
	No	3	18	21	14.3
	Total	46	29	75	61.3

Odds ratio = 43*18/3*11 = 23.5

© Cengage Learning 2013

FIGURE 9-3 Food-Specific 2 × 2 Table for Fictitious Illness and Food

TABLE 9-9 Outbreak Investigation

Step 7: Determine Control Measures

- Destroy implicated food.

- Close water source or beaches.

- Treat carriers.

- Vaccinate susceptible population.

- Develop and implement a comprehensive training program.

Step 7: Determine Control Measures

Many investigators are tempted to consider their job done once the culprit food or exposure has been identified. But remember that the reason an outbreak investigation is performed is not only to identify the cause, but also to control the current outbreak and to prevent future outbreaks. The remaining four steps of the outbreak investigation entail control and prevention, deciding if further study is needed and documenting the findings. The seventh step of an outbreak investigation is to determine appropriate control measures as described in Table 9-9.

In many outbreaks, such as a common source outbreak, the cause may no longer be present and the outbreak is self-controlled. But for an outbreak in which the causative agent is still a risk for causing more cases of disease, it is important to consider and then institute control measures to stop the current outbreak. Many times, the control measures can be as simple as destroying the implicated food or shutting down an identified contaminated water source. In a propagated epidemic with person to person transmission, control measures may include treating the carriers and vaccinating the population at risk. For those outbreaks caused by behaviors in the food service process, there may need to be a comprehensive training program to ensure that good food service processes are maintained or established when needed. Control measures are completely dependent on the identified source of the outbreak.

Step 8: Plan a More Systematic Study

Once identified control measures have been implemented to limit the spread of the current outbreak, it may be necessary to continue to study the outbreak with a more comprehensive design as described in Table 9-10. The goal of the initial hypothesis and study in step 6 was to quickly find the source of the outbreak in order to be

TABLE 9-10 Outbreak Investigation

Step 8: Perform a More Systematic Study

- Initial study may be inconclusive.

- Reconsider hypothesis.

- Revisit patients.

- Expand exposures.

- Utilize additional lab specimens.

- Identify an additional or more refined control group.

- Use a more comprehensive design.

- Perform research to expand knowledge.

© Cengage Learning 2013

able to control it. But often the initial information enabling control of the outbreak is not enough to enable complete prevention of future outbreaks. For example, the initial study may identify a specific restaurant as the source of the outbreak, but the specific food was not identified. Further, it may be only a single supplier of the food versus other suppliers. It may also be a specific ingredient used in multiple foods that may still need to be identified. Or if the outbreak was a community-based outbreak, it still may be necessary to look for the specific exposure or additional exposures. There may be the opportunity to use more comprehensive laboratory techniques. Another reason to do a more systematic study would be to watch for future disease in a prospective study.

The study designs used for outbreak investigations are the same designs used in the observational studies discussed in Chapter 5. Although the outbreak scenario makes the study implementation more imminent, the design should be developed with equal planning and care as a research study. In an outbreak, a retrospective design is the quickest study to complete because the investigator usually has access to a group of cases from the outbreak itself. So to do the initial test of the hypothesis in step 6, most investigators choose a retrospective (case control) design. However, if a more systematic study is determined to be necessary, it makes more sense for the investigators to perform a prospective study beginning with healthy individuals with their exposures initially identified. The prospective study also allows investigators to see if control and prevention measures are working. Further, using a prospective study design allows investigators to make additional prevention interventions and to evaluate the success of those interventions.

Steps 9 & 10: Execute Disease Control and Prevention Methods and Prepare a Written Report

The last two steps of an outbreak investigation are listed in Table 9-11. Throughout the investigation, the goal has been to find the problem and fix it. Now, as the investigation is wrapping up, it is important to use all the information available to prevent the spread or resurgence of the outbreak. This includes many of the same activities as in step 7, but these activities should be ongoing and constant. Added activities for the longer term could include surveillance for the future occurrence of the disease and regular communication with the affected population about the control of the outbreak. Another important method would include communication with health care workers and facilities to be on the lookout for further symptoms of the disease.

There should be a written report of the outbreak investigation. The report should include information about the setting, the methods used, the results of any data

TABLE 9-11 Outbreak Investigation

Step 9: Execute Prevention Measures

- Treat carriers.

- Vaccinate susceptible population.

- Conduct training programs.

- Keep surveillance for future disease.

- Communicate with the population and health officials.

Step 10: Prepare a Written Report

- Describe setting.

- Document methods.

- Present results.

- Document the specific causative agent and source.

- List recommendations for control and prevention.

© Cengage Learning 2013

collection and analysis, the identified causative agent, and recommendations for control and prevention. The report should be written so that members of the affected community can understand the issues, especially the recommendations for control and prevention. Any report provided to the community should be written with the coordination of the appropriate health authorities who will be responsible for following up with the ongoing public health activities. Finally, the investigators may want to consider whether to develop the report for a scientific report in a medical journal or epidemiologic bulletin.

Summary

Disease outbreaks occur commonly in human populations. These outbreaks can be large or small, with minor disease or deadly disease, and can be seen in a variety of settings. In order to determine the source of the outbreak, there are a number of standard steps that should be undertaken to identify the definition of disease, the etiologic cause of the disease, the location of the source, and prevention measures for the disease.

A Closer Look

A Systems Approach for a Food Borne Outbreak Investigation

Food borne illnesses, many of which are preventable, represent an important disease burden in the United States. CDC collects data on food borne disease outbreaks submitted from all states and territories through the Foodborne Disease Outbreak Surveillance System. Since 1992, CDC has defined a food borne disease outbreak as the occurrence of two or more similar illnesses resulting from ingestion of a common food. State, local, and territorial health department officials use a standard, Internet-based form to voluntarily submit reports of food borne outbreaks to CDC. An online toolkit of clinical and laboratory information is available to support investigation and reporting of outbreaks.

During 2008, the most recent year for which data are finalized, 1,034 food borne disease outbreaks were reported, which resulted in 23,152 cases of illness, 1,276 hospitalizations, and 22 deaths (http://www.cdc.gov/mmwr/pdf/wk/mm6035.pdf). The public health system and its various public health agencies play a major role in investigating and coordinating activities related to outbreaks of food borne illnesses. The ultimate goal is to facilitate the transfer of information to identify the cause of the outbreak and its subsequent control. This is essential so that more people do not get sick in the outbreak and similar outbreaks are prevented from happening in the future.

The established procedures described in this chapter are usually conducted by an outbreak investigation team. Depending on the location and size of an outbreak, this team can consist of a few or many individuals. In this section, the process of investigating a food borne illness is described from a systems level. Similar processes are used for other types of outbreaks such as water borne and infectious disease outbreaks.

Role of Local, State, and Federal Agencies

Public health agencies that identify and investigate food borne illnesses operate on several levels. Which agency or agencies participate in an investigation depends on the size and scope of the outbreak. Sometimes one agency starts an investigation and then calls on other agencies as more illnesses are reported across county or state lines.

- *Local agencies:* Most food borne outbreaks are local events. Public health officials in just one city or county health department investigate these outbreaks.

Continues

- *State agencies:* Typically the state health department investigates outbreaks that spread across several cities or counties. This health department often works in collaboration with the state department of agriculture and with federal food safety agencies.

- *Federal agencies:* For outbreaks that involve large numbers of people or severe or unusual illness, a state may ask for help from the Centers for Disease Control and Prevention (CDC). CDC usually leads investigations of widespread outbreaks—those that affect many states at once. States communicate regularly with one another and with CDC about outbreaks and ongoing investigations through established surveillance systems. For food borne outbreaks, CDC routinely collaborates with federal food safety agencies, such as the Food and Drug Administration (FDA) or Food Safety and Inspection Service (FSIS), part of the U.S. Department of Agriculture, throughout all phases of an outbreak investigation. FDA and FSIS, by law, oversee U.S. food safety and regulate the food industry with inspection and enforcement. In the case of an outbreak of food borne illness, they work to find out why it occurred, take steps to control it, and look for ways to prevent future outbreaks. They may trace foods to their origins, test foods, assess food safety measures in restaurants and food processing facilities, lead farm investigations, and announce food recalls.

Outbreak Investigation Teams

When a suspected outbreak comes to the attention of an agency, a special team of experts is identified to conduct an investigation. Outbreak investigative teams are usually made up of a variety of professionals, including:

- Epidemiologists are the disease detectives who initially investigate the outbreak, decide what additional information is needed, and which specialists to involve.

- Microbiologists are laboratory scientists who study germs. Their job is to identify pathogens.

- Environmental health specialists, sometimes called "sanitarians," study conditions in the field that may lead to disease.

- Regulatory compliance officers and inspectors are the officials who make sure food safety laws are followed.

A team may add other professionals as the investigation proceeds. For small outbreaks in a locally defined area, the team may include fewer people but would use the services of other specialists or laboratories, as needed.

Food Industry's Role

The food industry itself plays an important role in preventing and responding to outbreaks of food borne illness. Larger companies that produce, process, and package foods often have food safety managers on staff to identify and prevent problems. Some companies require their suppliers to meet specific food safety standards. They may also inspect their suppliers or hire outside auditors to inspect them. Based on findings of an outbreak investigation, the food company involved often takes steps to help stop the outbreak and avoid a similar one in the future. Such measures include stopping processing, cleaning and disinfecting facilities and equipment, training or retraining employees, recalling food, and changing industry-wide practices.

Summary

A large number of people become ill from food borne illnesses every year, many of which are preventable. The ability of the public health system to quickly identify and respond to these outbreaks can prevent others from becoming ill. Outbreaks are handled initially by the local health agency. If outbreaks cross county or state boundaries, other agencies become involved. Widespread food borne outbreaks are reported to the Foodborne Disease Outbreak Surveillance System. A variety of scientists participate in the investigative team to look for causes of the outbreak, which leads, with help from the food industry, to control of the current outbreak and methods to prevent future outbreaks.

Review Questions

1. Which term best describes an outbreak that spreads from person to person?

    a. Epidemic
    b. Common source outbreak
    c. Person to person attack rate
    d. Propagated outbreak

2. Outbreaks can be caused by:

    a. Contaminated food
    b. Contaminated water
    c. Exposure to ill people
    d. All of the above

3. The first study design used in an outbreak investigation is usually a:

    a. Prospective study
    b. Observational study
    c. Case control study
    d. Prevalence study

4. **True or False** The ultimate goal of an outbreak investigation is to control the spread of the disease.

5. **True or False** The first step in an outbreak investigation is to develop a hypothesis.

6. Which of the following terms is NOT part of a case definition?

    a. Possible case
    b. Confirmed case
    c. Likely case
    d. Suspected case

7. Outbreaks are usually classified into which of these categories:

    a. Food borne
    b. Water borne
    c. Community acquired
    d. All of the above

8. **True or False** An outbreak is not defined by a specific number of cases of disease.

9. An example where only one case of a particular disease would be considered an outbreak would be:

    a. Influenza
    b. Smallpox
    c. Norovirus
    d. Hepatitis A

10. Name the three common categories of outbreak settings.

    1. _____
    2. _____
    3. _____

11. **For Deeper Thought** The county health department has received a number of reports from hospitals regarding young children reporting vomiting and diarrhea. How would you go about investigating this problem?

Website Resources

Centers for Disease Control and Prevention: http://www.cdc.gov

Global Health Map: http://www.healthmap.org

Chapter 10

VACCINE PREVENTABLE DISEASES

Learning Objectives

Upon completion of this chapter, you should be able to:

1. List four situations in which immunization is indicated.
2. Describe the difference between active and passive immunity and give an example of each.
3. List one advantage and one disadvantage of herd immunity.
4. List three major reasons people refuse vaccines.
5. Be able to describe the concept of the antigenic shift and antigenic drift of the influenza virus and the impact on the vaccine.

Key Terms

active immunity

adverse event

adverse reaction

antibodies

antigen

antigenic drift

antigenic shift

bacille Calmette-Guérin (BCG)

cell-mediated immunity

efficacy

herd immunity

immunity

immunization

immunoglobulins

inactivated vaccines

inoculation

live, attenuated vaccine

passive immunity

recombinant

rubeola

vaccination

vaccine-associated paralytic polio (VAPP)

wild virus

Chapter Outline

INTRODUCTION

Along with sanitation improvements and the discovery of antibiotics, vaccines had the largest impact on infectious diseases in the twentieth century (see Table 10-1). Although eradication of disease is the ultimate goal of immunizations programs, the immediate goal is the prevention of disease in the community. Once leading causes of morbidity and mortality, diseases such as polio, measles, diphtheria, and smallpox have now either completely disappeared or almost disappeared (see the historical timeline in Table 10-2). The World Health Organization recognized the success of immunization programs and selected three diseases—smallpox, polio, and measles—as targets for eradication. Success was achieved with the eradication of smallpox worldwide declared in 1980. Improved, safer vaccines and vaccines against new infections are a focus of intense research. This chapter focuses on the principles of immunization, factors that impact the use and success of vaccine programs and, therefore, impact the epidemiology of the diseases they are meant to prevent. This chapter will also present a selection of current vaccine preventable diseases.

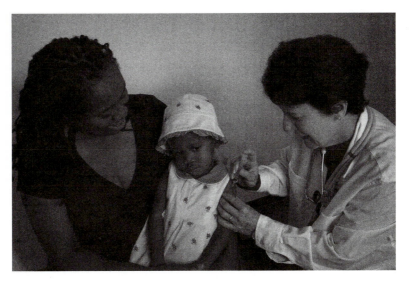

Immunizations, Especially in Young Children, Minimize the Spread and/or Contraction of Some Infectious Diseases
Courtesy of Centers for Disease Control and Prevention Public Health Image Library (PHIL): http://phil.cdc.gov/Phil/details.asp

TABLE 10-1 Current Vaccine Preventable Diseases

Anthrax

Cervical cancer

Diphtheria

Haemophilus influenza type b (Hib)

Hepatitis A

Hepatitis B

Herpes zoster (Shingles)

Human papillomavirus (HPV)

H1N1 flu (Swine flu)

Influenza (Seasonal flu)

Japanese encephalitis (JE)

Lyme disease

Measles

Continues

TABLE 10-1 Current Vaccine Preventable Diseases (Continued)

Meningococcal
Monkeypox
Mumps
Pertussis (Whooping cough)
Pneumococcal
Poliomyelitis (Polio)
Rabies
Rotavirus
Rubella (German measles)
Smallpox
Tetanus (Lockjaw)
Tuberculosis
Typhoid fever
Varicella (Chickenpox)
Yellow fever

© Cengage Learning 2013

TABLE 10-2 Historical Timeline of Important Events in the History of Vaccines

First Generation of Vaccines (pre-1950s):

1798	Smallpox vaccine
1885	Rabies vaccine
1897	Plague vaccine
1917	Cholera vaccine
	Typhoid vaccine
1918-19	Spanish flu epidemic

1923	Diphtheria vaccine
1926	Pertussis vaccine
1927	Tetanus vaccine
	Tuberculosis vaccine
1935	Yellow fever vaccine
1940s	DTP vaccine
1945	Influenza vaccine

1950s- 1960s:

1952	Peak of polio infections in the United States
1955	Inactivated Salk polio vaccine (IPV) licensed
1959	Call for global smallpox eradication
1963	Oral Sabin polio vaccine (OPV) licensed
1963	Measles vaccine licensed
1964	Advisory Committee on Immunization Practices holds its first U.S. meeting
1964-65	Largest rubella epidemic in the United States
1966	U.S. measles eradication goal announced
1967	Mumps vaccine licensed
1969	Rubella vaccine licensed

1970s-1990s:

1971	Routine smallpox immunization ceases in United States Measles/mumps/rubella vaccine licensed
1975	Largest public vaccination program in United States against Swine flu
1977	Last indigenous case of smallpox in the world (Somalia)
1979	Last case of (wild virus) polio in the United States
1980	Smallpox declared eradicated from the world
1988	Worldwide Polio Eradication Initiative launched
1989-1991	Major resurgence of measles in United States
1990	Vaccine Adverse Event Reporting System (VAERS) instituted
1994	Polio elimination certified in the Americas

Continues

TABLE 10-2 Historical Timeline of Important Events in the History of Vaccines (Continued)	
1996	Change to use of IPV in the United States because of vaccine associated paralytic polio
1999	FDA recommends removing mercury from all vaccines
2000s:	
2000	Worldwide measles initiative launched
2001	September 11th results in increased concern of bioterrorism
2003	Measles declared no longer endemic in the Americas
2005	Rubella no longer endemic in the United States
2008	Measles outbreaks across the United States as vaccination rates drop

© Cengage Learning 2013

THE SCOPE OF THE PROBLEM

Infectious diseases are targeted for prevention or eradication based on their impact on the population. High case-fatality rates (e.g., AIDS), high economic costs (e.g., chickenpox), or significant potential complications (e.g., measles) may all be reasons to consider the benefits of a vaccination program to minimize the effects of a particular infectious disease. The incidence of an infection may be used to determine whether the immunization should be administered routinely or only to high-risk persons or in high-risk situations.

Why Immunize?

The economic, public health, and personal advantages of having safe, effective immunization practices are clear when evaluating the diseases that are currently vaccine preventable. In the early 1940s, there was an average of 175,000 cases of pertussis per year, resulting in the deaths of 8,000 children annually. In 1976, the nadir of this disease occurred with only 1,010 cases reported. Since that time, the number of cases has been increasing and in 2004, there were 25,827 cases reported; but this is still far fewer than in the pre-vaccine era. A recent change in vaccine recommendations that now includes routine administration of the vaccine to adolescents may show further decreases when that data becomes available because adolescents and adults have accounted for at least half of this increase.

In the 1920s, there were 100,000-200,000 cases of diphtheria, a respiratory infection, each year with 13,000 deaths. With the current immunization practice in the United States, there is an average of only one case per year. In regions of the world such as Russia, where immunizations are not routine, there are still tens of thousands of cases per year.

A major rubella (German measles) outbreak occurred in 1963-1964 prior to the availability of the vaccine. Twelve million persons became infected with the disease. Many were pregnant women, and as a result, 11,000 fetuses died and 20,000 babies were born with congenital rubella syndrome that causes severe lifelong complications. Now there are fewer than 1,000 cases of rubella each year with fewer than 10 cases of the congenital syndrome.

Before the polio vaccine, 13,000-20,000 persons were paralyzed each year from the polio virus infection, and about 1,000 deaths occurred. The last case of **wild virus** disease in the United States occurred in 1979.

These are examples of the impact these diseases had on the public health of our nation prior to widespread immunization practices.

> **wild virus:** the virus as it occurs in its natural form and causes the disease

When to Immunize?

Besides the routine use of vaccines to prevent certain diseases in children and adults (see Figures 10-1, 10-2, and 10-3), there are several other circumstances that warrant the use of specific vaccines. Travel to areas where a disease is endemic constitutes an indication for vaccine use. For example, typhoid fever caused by *Salmonella typhi* remains a public health issue in Southeast Asia, Africa, and South America; and vaccine use prior to travel to these areas is common. Exposure of susceptible hosts to certain diseases warrants post-exposure immunization to prevent or minimize the effects of the disease. The rabies vaccine is the one most associated with this situation, yet measles and varicella vaccines are useful in these cases as well. Certain vaccines are used only for people considered at a particularly high risk of a disease. A classic example of this is when the anthrax vaccine is given to veterinarians and military personnel at risk of biological warfare attacks.

Recommended Immunization Schedule for Persons Aged 0 Through 6 Years—United States * 2011
For those who fall behind or start late, see the catch-up schedule

Vaccine ▼ Age ▶	Birth	1 month	2 months	4 months	6 months	12 months	15 months	18 months	19–23 months	2–3 years	4–6 years
Hepatitis B	HepB	HepB				HepB					
Rotavirus			RV	RV	RV						
Diphtheria, Tetanus, Pertussis			DTaP	DTaP	DTaP	see footnote	DTaP				DTaP
Haemophilus influenzae type b			Hib	Hib	Hib	Hib					
Pneumococcal			PCV	PCV	PCV	PCV					PPSV
Inactivated Poliovirus			IPV	IPV	IPV						IPV
Influenza					Influenza (Yearly)						
Measles, Mumps, Rubella						MMR		see footnote			MMR
Varicella						Varicella		see footnote			Varicella
Hepatitis A						HepA (2 doses)				HepA Series	
Menungococcal										MCV4	

Range of recommended ages for all childern

Range of recommended ages for certain high-risk groups

FIGURE 10-1 Recommended Immunization Schedule for Persons Aged 0 through 6 Years
Courtesy of Centers for Disease Control and Prevention: 2011 Child & Adolescent Immunization Schedules: http://www.cdc.gov/vaccines/recs/images/0-6yrs_chart_only.jpg

Recommended Immunization Schedule for Persons Aged 7 Through 18 Years—United States * 2011

For those who fall behind or start late, see the schedule below and the catch-up schedule

Vaccine ▼ Age ▶	7–10 years	11–12 years	13–18 years
Tetanus, Diphtheria, Pertussis		Tdap	Tdap
Human Papillomavirus	*see footnote*	HPV (3 doses)(females)	HPV series
Meningococcal	MCV4	MCV4	MCV4
Influenza	Influenza (Yearly)		
Pneumococcal	Pneumococcal		
Hepatitis A	HepA Series		
Hepatitis B	HepB Series		
Inactivated Poliovirus	IPV Series		
Measles, Mumps, Rubella	MMR Series		
Varicella	Varicella Series		

Range of recommended ages for all children

Range of recommended ages for catch-up immunization

Range of recommended ages for certain high-risk groups

FIGURE 10-2 Recommended Immunization Schedule for Persons Aged 7 through 18 Years
Courtesy of Centers for Disease Control and Prevention: 2011 Child & Adolescent Immunization Schedules: http://www.cdc.gov/vaccines/recs/images/7-18yrs_chart_only.jpg

Recommended Immunization Schedule for Adults, Aged 19 Years and Up—United States * 2011

For those who fall behind or start late, see the schedule below and the catch-up schedule

VACCINE ▼ AGE GROUP ▶	19–26 years	27–49 years	50–59 years	60–64 years	≥65 years
Influenza*	1 dose annually				
Tetanus, diphtheria, pertussis (Td/Tdap)*	Substitute 1-time dose of Tdap for Td booster; then boost with Td every 10 years				Td booster every 10 years
Varicella*	2 doses				
Human Papillomavirus (HPV)*	3 doses (females)				
Zoster				1 dose	
Measles, Mumps, Rubella (MMR)*	1 or 2 doses		1 dose		
Pneumococcal (polysaccharide)	1 or 2 doses				1 dose
Meningococcal*	1 or more doses				
Hepatitis A*	2 doses				
Hepatitis B*	3 doses				

*Covered by the Vaccine Injury Compensation Program

For all persons in this category who meet the age requirements and who lack evidence of immunity (e.g., lack documentation of vaccination or have no evidence of previous infection)

Recommended if some other risk factor is present (e.g., based on medical, occupational, lifestyle, or other indications)

No recommendation

FIGURE 10-3 Recommended Immunization Schedule for Adults, Aged 19 Years and Up (2011)
Courtesy of Centers for Disease Control and Prevention: Morbidity and Mortality Weekly Report (MMWR)—Recommended Adult Immunization Schedule—United States, 2011: http://www.cdc.gov/mmwr/preview/mmwrhtml/mm6004a10.htm?s_cid=mm6004a10_e

There are currently two vaccines in use that not only prevent the infection against which they are targeted, but also have a role in cancer prevention. Hepatitis B vaccine has been shown to prevent the long-term complication of liver cancer, and human papillomavirus vaccine has been shown to minimize the risk of cervical cancer in women. These are further discussed in Chapter 12, Cancer.

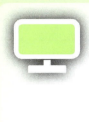

Check It Out

To find required/recommended immunizations for global travel, go to: http://cdc.gov. Click on "T" across the top of the Home Page, and then select "Travelers' Required Immunizations."

PRINCIPLES OF VACCINATION

This section explains the basics of how vaccines work, including a discussion of some immunology concepts related to vaccines, types of immunity, classifications of vaccines, and risks of both immunizing and not immunizing.

Basic Immunology

immunity: the ability of the human body to accept the presence of substances that are part of the body ("self") and attempt to eliminate substances that are foreign to the body ("nonself")

antigen: substance that is capable of producing an immune response; may be live or inactivated

antibodies: protein molecules produced by B lymphocytes in response to an antigen

immunoglobulins: protein molecules produced by B lymphocytes in response to an antigen

cell-mediated immunity: the system that eliminates antigens with specific cells, but not antibodies

Immunity is the ability of the human body to accept the presence of substances that are part of the body ("self") and to attempt to eliminate substances that are foreign to the body ("nonself"). This is the "self versus nonself" concept of immunity. This process allows for protection from infectious diseases because the body is able to recognize invading infectious agents as foreign and proceed to eliminate the organism. Immunity is specific to the currently invading organism or to a group of organisms that are closely related to that invading agent and is usually indicated by the presence of a specific antibody to that agent.

A substance capable of producing an immune response may be live or inactivated and is referred to as an **antigen**. Examples of live antigens include viruses and bacteria. On occasion, only a small portion of the infectious agent is the attracting antigen, and this would be considered an inactivated antigen. Examples of inactivated antigens include the surface protein on a hepatitis B virus or the polysaccharide cell coat on certain bacterium. Some inactivated antigens produce strong immune responses, whereas others produce weak responses. Once the immune system recognizes a foreign antigen, it surmounts a response that is purposed to eliminate the invader. This usually involves the production of **antibodies** or **immunoglobulins**, which are protein molecules produced by B lymphocytes. In some cases, there are specific cells, like T-helper cells, that facilitate the elimination of the antigen, and this is referred to as **cell-mediated immunity**.

Types of Immunity

Immunity is acquired by two different mechanisms—active and passive. A third method of protection is herd immunity.

Active immunity is achieved when a person's own immune system responds to a foreign substance. An antigen-specific antibody is produced during the initial invasion, and if the infection is survived, this response can be elicited on future invasions with the same or similar organisms. Immunity against that organism usually lasts for many years or sometimes even a lifetime and is considered permanent immunity. There are two basic mechanisms to obtain active immunity—when a person becomes infected with the organism and when a person is immunized. Vaccines stimulate the immune system similar to the natural disease but without the illness or complications. Many vaccines will also produce the immunologic memory that the natural disease does as well.

Passive immunity is achieved when immune response products—antibodies—produced by an animal or person, are transferred to another human. This mechanism provides short-term protection against an invading organism, but the protection wanes over time as the antibodies naturally degrade. There is no ongoing production of the antibodies by the body; therefore, this protection is temporary. There are several mechanisms for obtaining passive immunity, the most common being an infant's immune protection provided by maternal antibodies that cross the placenta or when a mother breastfeeds. These antibodies may be present and protective for up to the first 12 months of the infant's life. Another mechanism of passive immunity is the transfusion of large amounts of pooled antibodies (immune globulin).

With **herd immunity**, the host does *not* have the immunity against a specific disease but depends on the immunity of those around him in the community for protection. If enough people are vaccinated against a specific infection, then the disease tends not to spread in that community. This type of protection can be helpful for persons who, for health reasons, cannot be vaccinated. This type of immunity will *not* protect hosts if they are exposed to the disease. Those persons who refuse immunizations for any reason depend on herd immunity for their own protection.

active immunity: when the host's immune system responds to an invading organism or antigen and produces its own immune response

passive immunity: when immune response products like antibodies, produced by another animal or person, are transferred to another human to provide immune protection

herd immunity: when hosts depend on the immunity of those around them in the community for their protection

Classification of Vaccines

inoculation or **vaccination:** the procedure of administering the substance that will stimulate the immune response; used interchangeably with the term "immunization"

immunization: the stimulation of the immune system; used interchangeably with the terms "inoculation" and "vaccination"

live, attenuated vaccine: a vaccine made with the wild type organism—or an organism that occurs in nature and causes disease—and modified such that it is no longer capable of producing significant disease in the host

There are two basic types of vaccines—those that contain live organisms and those that contain inactivated portions of an organism. The terms **inoculation** and **vaccination** generally refer to the procedure of administering the substance that will stimulate the immune response, whereas **immunization** technically refers to stimulation of the immune system. In practicality and for the purposes of this discussion, all three terms are used interchangeably.

With **live, attenuated vaccines**, the wild type organism—or an organism that occurs in nature and causes disease—is modified such that it is still a live organism but is no longer capable of producing significant disease in the host, although a milder case of the original wild type infection may still occur. This weakened organism is still able to replicate and must replicate to provoke an immune response. The immune response that occurs is similar to what would occur with the natural organism infecting a host; and thus most live vaccines only require one dose to stimulate a response. A small number of persons may not respond to the first dose, and for this reason, a second dose of a live virus vaccine is often recommended to produce a higher level of immunity in the community. Examples of live virus vaccines include the mumps-measles-rubella (MMR), chickenpox (varicella), nasal influenza, and **bacille Calmette-Guérin (BCG)** (for tuberculosis).

Inactivated vaccines are made by inactivating the organism with heat or chemicals. The active ingredient used in the vaccine is what is known to elicit the desired immune response and may consist of the whole cell of the organism, a piece of the organism, the bacterial toxin rendered harmless, or genetically engineered antigens. These vaccines are generally not as effective as live vaccines, and multiple doses are required. Antibodies against the specific antigen wane over time, and therefore, booster doses may be required at periodic intervals.

bacille Calmette-Guérin vaccine (BCG): a live, attenuated vaccine using *Mycobacterium bovis*, or a cow tuberculin bacterium, as the antigen; used globally to prevent TB meningitis and disseminated TB in infants worldwide in high-risk areas

inactivated vaccines: vaccines made from inactivating the organism with heat or chemicals

Risks

With regards to vaccines, there are risks to immunizing persons and risks for not immunizing them. This section will briefly address these issues and discuss the reasons some people refuse recommended vaccines.

Risks for Immunizing

As with any medication, vaccines have risks for causing negative effects. These are classified into two different types. An **adverse event** includes *any* event that occurs following an immunization. This includes true adverse reactions, plus reactions that are only coincidental to the vaccine. An **adverse reaction** is an event that is actually *caused by* the vaccine and may also be referred to as a "side effect" of the vaccine.

Examples of adverse reactions would be nonspecific systemic reactions such as fever or headache, allergic reactions to a component in the vaccine, or the rashes that can be seen with the live measles or chickenpox vaccines after an appropriate incubation period. There may also be more severe reactions. Localized adverse reactions such as pain or swelling at the site of the injection are also possible. Adverse reactions and events are reported by patients or their physicians through the Vaccine Adverse Event Reporting System (VAERS) cosponsored by the Centers for Disease Control and Prevention and the Food and Drug Association. This is a national vaccine safety surveillance program that collects information on vaccines licensed for use in the United States because "rare reactions, delayed reactions, or reactions within subpopulations" may not be identified prior to licensure.

The National Vaccine Injury Compensation Program (VICP) was created in 1986 to protect the vaccine makers from legal actions and thus to ensure continued vaccine supplies and stable costs while maintaining a process to compensate those who had been injured by vaccines. The U.S. Department of Health and Human Services, the U. S. Department of Justice, and the U.S. Court of Federal Claims all maintain roles in managing the VICP. In February 2011, the U.S. Supreme Court upheld the role of these regulatory agencies in protecting the vaccine makers from direct lawsuits. See Table 10-3 for a summary of claims filed against various vaccines

adverse event: includes *any* event that occurs following an immunization

adverse reaction: an event that occurs following immunization and that is actually *caused by* the vaccine; also known as a "side effect"

TABLE 10-3 Claims Filed against Various Vaccines

Claims Filed and Compensated or Dismissed by Vaccine[1] January 3, 2012 Vaccines Listed in Claims as Reported by Petitioners

Vaccine(s)	Filed			Compensated	Dismissed
	Injury	Death	Total		
DT (diphtheria-tetanus)	64	9	73	22	50
DTP (diphtheria-tetanus-whole cell pertussis)	3,282	696	3,978	1,266	2,696
DTP-HIB	16	8	24	3	19
DTaP (diphtheria-tetanus-acellular pertussis)	321	75	396	141	166
DTaP-Hep B-IPV	49	22	71	20	19
DTaP-HIB	6	1	7	4	2
DTaP-IPV-HIB	5	4	9	0	3
Td (tetanus-diphtheria)	163	3	166	84	62
Tdap	72	0	72	23	4
Tetanus	79	2	81	30	34
Hepatitis A (Hep A)	43	2	45	12	13
Hepatitis B (Hep B)	569	49	618	207	339
Hep A- Hep B	9	0	9	6	1
Hep B-HIB	8	0	8	3	2
HIB (*Haemophilus influenzae* type b)	22	3	25	9	9

HPV (human papillomarvirus)	160	9	169	23	32
Influenza (Trivalent)	719	42	761	334	84
IPV (Inactivated Polio)	262	14	276	7	266
OPV (Oral Polio)	280	28	308	158	149
Measles	143	19	162	55	107
Meningococcal	23	1	24	6	2
MMR (measles-mumps-rubella)	837	56	893	322	424
MMR-Varicella	21	1	22	7	3
MR	15	0	15	6	9
Mumps	10	0	10	1	9
Pertussis	5	3	8	2	6
Pneumococcal Conjugate	28	4	32	7	19
Rotavirus	50	1	51	25	15
Rubella	189	4	193	70	123
Varicella	66	5	71	36	18
Nonqualified[2]	71	9	80	0	79
Unspecified[3]	5,405	7	5,412	3	3,721
TOTAL	**12,992**	**1,077**	**14,069**	**2,892**	**8,035**

[1] The number of claims filed by vaccine as reported by petitioners in claims since the VICP began on October 1, 1988, which have been compensated or dismissed by the U.S. Court of Federal Claims (Court). Claims can be compensated by a settlement between parties or a decision by the Court.

[2] Claims filed for vaccines which are not covered under the VICP.

[3] Insufficient information submitted to make a determination. The majority of these claims are part of the Omnibus Autism Proceedings.

Source: U.S. Department of Health and Human Services; National Vaccine Injury Compensation Program: http://www.hrsa.gov/vaccinecompensation/statisticsreports.html#Claims

over the past 30 years. In 2008, the Health Resources and Services Administration section of the Department of Health and Human Services contracted with the Institute of Medicine to review biological, epidemiologic, and clinical evidence of adverse events associated with certain vaccines covered by the VCIP.

Risks for Not Immunizing

The public health impact of vaccines on the diseases they prevent was discussed in the previous section "Why Immunize?" Those are the risks for not immunizing. This section looks to further assess the risk of not immunizing. The risk of a couple of infections will be compared with the risk of the vaccines that prevent them.

The DTP vaccine protects against diphtheria, tetanus, and pertussis. Prior to the use of this vaccine, diphtheria caused death in 1 in 20 cases of the disease, and tetanus caused death in 2 in 10 cases. Pertussis caused death in 1 in 1,150 infections, but caused pneumonia in 1 in 8 cases and encephalitis in 1 in 20 cases. The vaccine has had no reports of deaths caused by its use. Acute encephalopathy has occurred in 0-10.5 in 1,000,000 doses (far less than the disease), convulsions or shock with full recovery in 1 in 14,000, and continuous crying with full recovery in 1 in 1,000.

Rubella vaccine is given in combination with the vaccines for mumps and measles. The rubella epidemic in 1964-1965 caused 12 million cases of the German measles and, subsequently, 20,000 cases of congenital rubella syndrome. Congenital rubella syndrome causes deafness, blindness, heart disease, and severe mental retardation and will occur in 1 in 4 women who become infected early in their pregnancy. Natural infection with the measles vaccine caused death in 2 of 1,000 infections, encephalitis 1 in 1,000 cases, and pneumonia in 6 of 100 cases. The vaccine has been associated with encephalitis or severe allergic reactions in 1 in 1,000,000 (still less than the natural measles virus).

Reasons for Refusal

Current immunization practices have had a demonstrable impact on the diseases they have been developed against. Despite that, each year outbreaks of various vaccine preventable diseases occur. Worldwide, often this occurs because of a lack of vaccines, the inability of developing countries to financially afford vaccines, or the lack of vaccine programs in developing countries. In the United States, the reason for outbreaks of preventable diseases is often related to voluntary refusal to be immunized. Objections to vaccinations that are widely accepted as reasonable or allowable include immunosuppression, allergy to a component of the vaccine, and religious objections. Other reasons for refusal that are not considered acceptable include:

- *There is a sense there is no longer a threat from that disease.* When there is no vaccine for a disease and the number of persons getting the disease is high, people are worried about the disease and its effects. When a vaccine becomes available, the number of persons vaccinated increases and adverse reactions become more apparent at the same time that the disease cases are decreasing. Now people

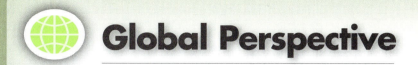

Global Perspective

Worldwide Immunization Programs

Over the past decade, the World Health Organization and UNICEF (previously the United Nations International Children's Emergency Fund, but now known simply as the United Nations Children's Fund) have focused on worldwide immunization programs in order to decrease the overall childhood mortality in children under 5 years of age. The WHO reports that immunizations would be expected to avert 2.5 million deaths in children per year, according to the Third Edition of the *State of the World's Vaccines and Immunization, Executive Summary* (2009). It is still reported that about 20% of the children, most from developing countries, fail to get the recommended immunizations against six major childhood diseases—diphtheria, tetanus, pertussis, measles, polio, and tuberculosis. Pneumonia and diarrheal disease account for a majority of deaths in young children worldwide, and with the development of newer vaccines such as those against rotavirus, pneumococcal disease, and others, WHO and the United Nations are pushing to expand the immunization practices particularly in those countries that have the higher mortality rates for children.

Children are not the only focus for worldwide vaccine programs however. A major effort is being made to ensure that all mothers and neonates are immunized against tetanus. Vaccines for use in adults are increasingly being instituted worldwide. Also, in regards to the efforts to eradicate polio, for the first time, India has gone a whole year without a case of wild type polio (World Health Organization, http://www.searo.who.int/, dated 23 January 2012). This is a major accomplishment.

The major barriers found in instituting immunization practices worldwide are three-fold—(1) deficiencies in health care delivery, (2) weaknesses in the health care infrastructure and logistics, and (3) a lack of education regarding the importance and benefits of vaccines. In addition, as in the United States, more recently there have been more and more objections to immunization programs based on fears of perceived adverse effects.

begin to worry more about the adverse effects of the vaccine than the disease it protects against. If enough people refuse immunization, outbreaks occur and they are reminded of the consequences of the disease. Vaccinations rates then start to increase again. Ultimately, the goal is that enough people are immunized so that the disease disappears completely.

- *There is concern over possible side effects of the vaccine.* In 1998, Dr. Andrew Wakefield, a British physician, published what he reported as his data showing an association of the mumps-measles-rubella (MMR) vaccine with the increasing rates of autism. These data have since been identified as fraudulent but not without causing a major scare that caused MMR vaccination rates to plummet and outbreaks of the disease to soar. Other concerns over a possible link between the preservative, thimerosal (mercury), and autism were raised in several studies that subsequently led to the removal of this agent from vaccines. Since that time, the incidence of autism has not changed, and further reviews have shown no causal association.

- *There is apprehension that the increasing number of recommended vaccines will overload the immune system.* In actuality, although there are more diseases that are now vaccine preventable, the total number of antigens that are presented in these vaccines is less than previously. Vaccine components have become more pure.

- *There are political objections.* This concern primarily manifests as the question of whether the government has the right to dictate the mandatory use of immunizations for school entry or for other circumstances.

EXAMPLES OF VACCINE PREVENTABLE DISEASES

This section contains a brief description of several representative diseases that are preventable with the use of vaccines. Each listing discusses the infectious agent, worldwide and U.S. statistics, mode of transmission, clinical disease with complications, vaccine type, vaccine efficacy and vaccine recommendations, and high-risk groups, if any. Excellent resources for further information about these and other infectious diseases and their vaccines include the Centers for Disease Control and Prevention publication, *The Pink Book—Epidemiology and Prevention of Vaccine Preventable Diseases,* and *Control of Communicable Diseases Manual* (19th ed.) published by the American Public Health Association.

Anthrax

Anthrax is caused by *Bacillus anthracis*, a Gram-positive, spore-producing bacillus. The spores, rather than the bacteria, are the infectious agents. This infection causes disease in animals, with humans being incidental hosts. It occurs most frequently as an occupational hazard—in persons exposed to infected animals, such as veterinarians, or in persons exposed to contaminated animal products, such as tannery workers. In 2001, anthrax spores were sent through the postal system as a bioterrorism agent and caused 22 cases of anthrax in humans with a 50% case fatality rate.

There are three forms of the clinical disease, according to the type of exposure and transmission. (Figure 10-4A shows skin exposure to anthrax, and Figure 10-4B is a chest X-ray of a person exposed to the agent.) The incubation period is 7 days for all forms, but it may be up to 42 days for the inhalation form. Greater than 95% of natural infections that occur worldwide are of the *cutaneous form* that is spread when the organism comes into direct contact with a cut or break in the skin during the handling of contaminated animal products. The case fatality rate is 5-20% if untreated, but death is rare if the disease is treated. The *inhalation form*, spread when spores are inhaled into the respiratory system, starts with mild respiratory symptoms but rapidly progresses to severe disease within 3-4 days, leading to shock and death. Case fatality rates are extremely high at 85% in this form, but that rate may be reduced with aggressive antibiotic and supportive medical therapy. This is the form that has raised international concerns about its use as a biological terrorism agent. The third form of anthrax, the *gastrointestinal form*, is transmitted by eating infected meats in endemic areas. This form causes severe gastrointestinal disease and death in 25-50% of cases.

efficacy: the measure of how well a vaccine performs by calculating the reduction of disease of vaccinated persons over unvaccinated persons as a percentage of those at risk (unvaccinated)

The vaccine in use is an inactivated subunit vaccine that is administered with five doses. **Efficacy** (the measure of how well a vaccine performs) after the full course is reported to be at 95%. Current recommendations for this vaccine are to immunize only those at highest risk for exposure to the anthrax disease or spores. This includes veterinarians at risk, workers exposed to infected hides, persons who

A
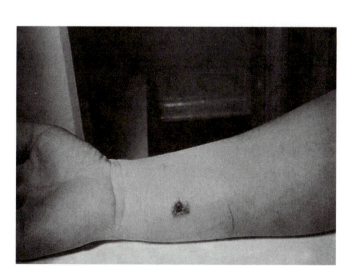
B
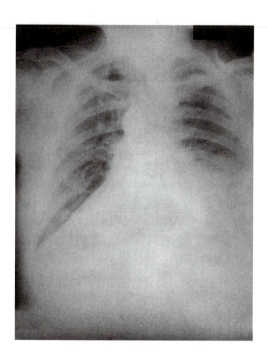

FIGURE 10-4 Anthrax. (A) Cutaneous Anthrax, 7th Day (B) Chest X-ray of Inhalation Anthrax, 4th day
Courtesy of Centers for Disease Control and Prevention Public Health Image Library (PHIL): http://phil.cdc.gov/Phil/details.asp

work directly with the organism, and military members deployed to high-risk areas. There was much controversy when the universal anthrax vaccination program was initiated in the U.S. Armed Forces in 1998. The Department of Defense has continued its anthrax program and has set up a website specific to the program (www. anthrax.osd.mil). The FDA has verified the vaccine's effectiveness against inhalation anthrax.

Hepatitis B (HBV)

HBV is a DNA virus that causes acute and chronic hepatitis, cirrhosis of the liver, and is responsible for up to 80% of the cases of liver cancer. Approximately 2 billion persons worldwide are infected with hepatitis B, and about one-third of these will go on to have chronic disease. Hepatitis B causes about 600,000 deaths worldwide each year. In the United States, up to 1.4 million people have chronic hepatitis. According to data from the CDC (2008), the incidence rate of hepatitis in the United States was down to 1.3 per 100,000 persons overall (1.7 cases per 100,000 men and 1.0 cases per 100,000 women), the lowest ever. Rates varied by ethnicity with blacks having the highest rate at 2.2 cases per 100,000; whites, 0.9 cases per 100,000; Hispanics, 0.8 cases per 100,000; and Asian/Pacific Islanders, the lowest rates at 0.7 cases per 100,000. Rates also varied across the country with the highest rates found in West Virginia (4.6 per 100,000) and the lowest found in Montana (0.2 per 100,000).

The HBV virus is transmitted through contact with infected blood or body fluids. Activities that promote transmission include sexual contact, IV drug use, infants born to infected mothers, needle sticks in health care environments, contact with blood or open sores of an infected person, or sharing personal items such as razors or toothbrushes. It is infectious on fomites for more than 7 days at room temperature. The incubation period is about 90 days with a range of 60–150 days. Only about one-half of those persons infected will show any symptoms with acute disease—nausea, vomiting, abdominal pain, and dark urine. Later an infected person may develop jaundice causing a generalized yellow color to their skin and eyes.

The case fatality rate of the acute infection is 1%. The risk for chronic infection with this virus is highest in the youngest population—90% in infants, 25-50% in children 1–5 years old, and only about 5% in adults. Of those who develop chronic hepatitis, 15–25% will die prematurely from liver cancer or cirrhosis. This rate is also related to age with the youngest children at highest risk. Approximately 3,000–4,000 persons in the United States die each year from cirrhosis, and 1,000–1,500 persons die with liver cancer.

The vaccine manufactured against hepatitis B is a **recombinant** vaccine of hepatitis B surface antigen (HBsAg) produced in yeast cells. After receiving the recommended three doses of vaccine, more than 95% of infants and more than 90% of teens and adults will have adequate circulating antibodies; but this response diminishes with older patients, thus making the vaccine effectiveness 80-100%. Recommendations are for universal immunization of all newborns/infants, adolescents who have not previously been immunized, and adults at high risk for infection. Adults considered at high risk for HBV infection include those persons with multiple sex partners, household contacts and sexual partners of HBsAg-positive persons, persons with other sexually transmitted infections, and men having sex with men (MSM). Other high-risk adults include IV drug users, health care workers, persons with severe kidney disease, and international travelers to areas with high endemic rates of HBV infection. In China and other parts of Asia, 8-10% of the population has chronic infections starting in childhood. Other areas of endemic disease include the Amazon and Eastern and Central Europe. Less than 1% of the population in North America and Western Europe is chronically infected.

recombinant: genetically engineered vaccine that combines DNA sequences from multiple sources

Human Papillomavirus (HPV)

Human papillomavirus (HPV) is a DNA virus that infects the skin or mucosal epithelium. There are over 100 different types, most of which cause the common skin warts; but HPV is also responsible for the most common sexually transmitted infection worldwide. About 40 types affect mucosal surfaces and are associated with varying risks for future anogenital (anus or genital area) cancers in both males and females. Worldwide, there are about 529,000 new cases of cervical cancer each year, resulting in 274,000 deaths. More than 85% of these deaths are in developing countries. (See discussion of cervical cancer in Chapter 12, Cancer.) HPV has also been associated with other cancers such as anal, penile, vulvar, and vaginal; but these occur much less frequently than cervical cancers. In the United States, about 20 million men and women are infected with HPV for a prevalence rate of about 6.7% overall, although about 50% of sexually active persons will become infected at some time in their life. Each year about 6 million new infections (2,000 cases per 100,000 persons) occur, and 12,000 women develop cervical cancer.

HPV is transmitted via genital, oral, or anal sexual contact, and most people who are infected are not aware they have the infection. Most of the time (> 90%), the immune system will fight off the infection and no change in the cells occurs. Other times genital warts similar to skin warts will occur. These warts may disappear on their own within 1-2 years, or sooner with treatment, but do not turn into cancer. In a third scenario, the HPV infection causes anogenital cancer, most commonly cervical. HPV type 16 causes about 50% of cervical cancers, and types 16 and 18 together account for about 70%. Infection with one type of HPV does not prevent infection with another type. Other anogenital cancers associated with infections by HPV include cancer of the vulva, vagina, penis, and anus.

There are two licensed vaccines currently on the market to protect against HPV. Both are inactivated recombinant vaccines, and both are effective against the common types 16 and 18 that cause cervical cancer. One is also effective against the more common types that cause genital warts. Efficacy is between 95–99% against cervical cancers after a three-dose regimen to women who have not yet become sexually active. There is less benefit to sexually active women who have already been infected with one or more of the HPV virus types contained in the current vaccines. Therefore, current recommendations are aimed at immunizing persons prior to sexual activity, and the vaccine is routinely given to adolescent girls at 11–12 years of age, although it can be given to women aged 9–26 years. In October 2009, the vaccine against HPV types that cause both cancer and genital warts was approved for use in males age 9–26, and it is now being given also to this target group.

Measles

Measles, also known as **rubeola** or the "10-day measles," is an extremely contagious respiratory disease that is caused by a RNA paramyxovirus. (See the historical timeline in Table 10-2 for important events related to measles.) Approximately 10 million cases occur worldwide each year. Measles remains a leading cause of death among children worldwide, particularly in developing countries. The Measles Initiative of 2001, led by the WHO, CDC, the UN, and other international organizations, established a goal to reduce global measles mortality by 90% by 2010. It costs less than $1 to vaccinate a child against measles; but in countries with poor nutrition and limited access to health care, the mortality rates for measles are as high as 10–30%. By 2008, 83% of the world's children had received at least one dose of measles vaccine, and mortality had decreased by 78%; but there were still 164,000 deaths, the majority of them in Africa and Asia.

As of November 2002, measles was no longer endemic in the Americas; however, in 2008, more cases of measles were reported in the United States than in any year since 1997. The CDC reported that more than 90% were acquired abroad or linked to imported cases, and more than 90% of cases were in persons who were not vaccinated. An example was a 7-year-old unimmunized boy and his family who traveled to Switzerland where he was exposed to the measles virus. On return to his home in San Diego, he exposed 839 people to the disease (48 were infants too young to be immunized and required quarantine). Eleven unvaccinated children, three of them young infants, developed the disease. The subsequent cost of this outbreak in direct medical cost, as well as the cost of the health personnel involved in controlling the outbreak, was $177,000. At the time of this writing, there are two possible measles outbreaks being investigated—one in Boston where three cases have been reported over the month related to a worker at the French consulate and a second alert of an infected person traveling on an airplane from Baltimore to San Diego, causing an investigation there.

rubeola: the common measles; also known as the "10-day measles"

Transmission of the measles virus is by respiratory droplets from breathing, coughing, or sneezing. It is *very* easily spread. The incubation period is usually about 10 days from exposure to fever and 14 days from exposure to rash. Symptoms include cough, runny nose, conjunctivitis, lesions in the oral mucosa, and fever, followed by the rash (shown in Figure 10-5) that begins on the face, spreads to the entire body, and lasts about one week. A person is contagious from 3–5 days before the rash appears to about 4 days after the rash appears. Complications occur in about 30% of cases and include ear infections, pneumonia, diarrhea, encephalitis, and death. Those at highest risk include those with poor nutrition and Vitamin A deficiency. Measles during pregnancy can cause miscarriages, stillbirths, or babies born with low birth weights.

The first vaccine licensed in the United States was in 1963. Persons born before 1957 are considered universally immune because prior to the widespread use of the vaccine, more than 90% of children were exposed and immune by 15 years of age. The current vaccine used (MMR) is a live, attenuated vaccine that is combined with antigens for mumps and rubella (note that rubella is also known as "German measles" or the "3-day measles" and is distinct from the measles discussed in this section). Vaccine efficacy is 99% after the two-dose series is completed. MMR is considered a routine vaccination with the first dose given at, but not before, the first birthday. Persistent circulating maternal antibodies that may be present could interfere with the immune response to the vaccine if it is given before the first birthday. Adults without prior immunization should be considered candidates for vaccine if they attend college, are international travelers, or work in medical facilities.

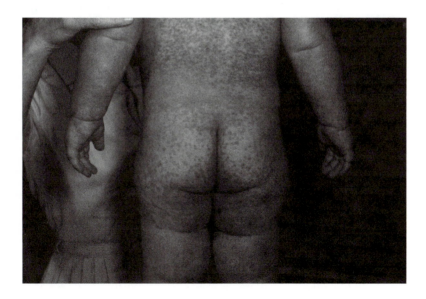

FIGURE 10-5 Young Child with a Measles Rash
Courtesy of Centers for Disease Control and Prevention Public Health Image Library (PHIL): http://phil.cdc.gov/Phil/details.asp

Meningococcal Disease

Neisseria meningitidis, a Gram-negative diplococcus (two cocci that pair together), is the major cause of bacterial meningitis in infants and adolescents and is also the organism with the most potential to cause meningitis epidemics. Different serotypes predominate in different geographical locations and among different age groups. Meningococcal meningitis occurs sporadically throughout the world, but the highest burden occurs in sub-Saharan Africa in an area referred to as the "African meningitis belt," which stretches from Senegal to Ethiopia. During the 2009 epidemic season, 88,199 cases were reported with 5,352 deaths (case fatality rate of 6.1%). In the United States, there are 1,000–3,000 cases of meningococcal disease each year (0.4–1.3 cases per 100,000 persons), but they tend to be sporadic rather than epidemic as occurs in Africa.

Meningococcal disease is transmitted by respiratory droplets or direct mucosal contact with the organism. Of the U.S. population, 5 to 10% are asymptomatic carriers who may harbor the organism in their nose or throat and transmit the disease unknowingly to others. Infections peak in the late winter to early spring. The incubation period is 3–4 days, and an infected person is contagious until 24 hours after appropriate antibiotics have been started. The organism gets into the bloodstream and then spreads to the meninges, the membranes that cover the brain and spinal cord. As with all types of meningitis, the clinical symptoms include sudden onset of fever, headache, stiff neck, and photophobia (sensitivity to light). Vomiting and a specific rash may also occur. Complications occur in about 20% of survivors and include permanent hearing loss, neurologic deficiency, or loss of a limb. The case fatality rate of meningococcemia (*Neisseria meningococcus* in the blood) is as high as 17%, even with appropriate antibiotic therapy. A study in 2001 found that college freshmen living in dormitories were at a moderately increased risk for developing meningococcal disease, and this study prompted the requirement for vaccination in this population prior to starting college.

The meningococcal vaccine currently in use is a polysaccharide conjugate vaccine, a type of inactivated vaccine, that contains antigens against four of the five most common serogroups. Efficacy after the single recommended dose is greater than 98%. This vaccine is routinely recommended for adolescents at 11–12 years old, for college students not previously immunized, and for adults at higher risk of disease. Those considered at higher risk include microbiologists who work with the infecting agent, travelers to endemic areas such as sub-Saharan Africa, military recruits, and persons with certain immunodeficiencies. In 2008, there were 33 reports of Guillain-Barré syndrome, a neurologic condition that causes muscle weakness and paralysis, that occurred following vaccination with the conjugate meningococcal vaccine. The occurrence was rare, and it is still not known if it was a true adverse reaction rather than an adverse event.

Pertussis

Bordetella pertussis, a Gram-negative bacillus that causes pertussis, is also known as "whooping cough." A highly contagious respiratory disease, pertussis was a major cause of childhood mortality in the United States prior to the availability of the

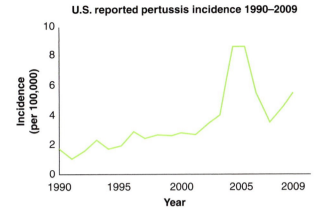

U.S. reported pertussis incidence 1990–2009

FIGURE 10-6 Pertussis Incidence, United States, 1990-2009
This graph shows incidence per 100,000 persons of reported pertussis in the United States from 1990-2009. Although the incidence of reported pertussis is substantially lower than the peak in 2004, incidence has been increasing since 2007 and continues to remain higher than in the 1990s.

Courtesy of Centers for Disease Control and Prevention; Pertussis (Whooping Cough)—Surveillance and Reporting: http://www.cdc.gov/pertussis/surv-reporting.html

vaccine in the 1940s. In 2008, there were 16,000,000 cases of pertussis worldwide, most in developing countries, with 195,000 resultant deaths. It is estimated that 82% of the world's population has been covered with the three recommended doses of the vaccine. In 2009, there were 17,000 cases of pertussis reported in the United States (see Figure 10-6).

Transmission of pertussis is via respiratory droplets, and the incubation period is 7–10 days before onset of symptoms. The disease is characterized by an initial mild acute respiratory illness (catarrhal stage), followed by paroxysms of cough that terminate with the characteristic "whoop" noise heard when gasping for air after a coughing fit (paroxysmal stage). The cough frequently lasts weeks to months (convalescent stage). The disease is particularly severe in young infants who frequently also have episodes of apnea (no breathing) and who, because of the coughing and vomiting, have difficulty maintaining their nutritional state. Over half of infected infants require hospitalization. Adolescents and adults typically have much milder courses that are not unlike the common cold and may not be recognized as pertussis. Because neither infection nor immunization provides lifelong protection, immunity wanes and adolescents and adults became the frequent source of infections to infants. An infected person is contagious for the first 2–3 weeks or until 5 days after appropriate antibiotic treatment. Complications include pneumonia (22%), apnea in infants (almost 50% of hospitalized infants), encephalopathy (<0.5%), seizures (2%) and death (0.5–1%).

As this text was being written, an epidemic had been occurring in California since the beginning of 2010. There have been 8,383 confirmed or suspected cases of pertussis (incidence rate of 21.4 cases per 100,000 residents of California), the highest year of reported cases since 1947 when 9,394 cases were reported. The rates are highest among infants under 6 months of age (417.8 cases per 100,000) and therefore without the benefit of protection of the initial three doses of vaccine. Of those requiring hospitalization, 70% of those have been less than 6 months old. There have been 10 infant deaths, all under 2 months of age, and 9 of the 10 had not yet received their first dose of vaccine. By race/ethnicity, the rates are highest in the Hispanic population (22.5 cases per 100,000), followed by the whites (18.0 cases per 100,000). The epidemic is not over, but the number of new cases reported each week is slowing.

The previous vaccine used in the United States contained the whole *Bordetella* cell, and although efficacious, there were more side effects associated with it. The current U.S. licensed vaccine is an acellular subunit vaccine that contains inactivated components of the *Bordetella* bacterium. It is always combined with antigens against tetanus and diphtheria (DTaP = Diphtheria, Tetanus toxoid, acellular pertussis). Efficacy rates for the vaccine used in the United States are from 80-85%. The current recommendations are for the vaccine to be given in 3 doses to infants 2–6 months old with boosters at 15 months and before entering kindergarten. Because adolescents were frequently a source of infection for young infants, a booster dose with a reduced dose of diphtheria (Tdap = Tetanus, diphtheria, acellular pertussis) is now recommended at 11–12 years of age. With the epidemic currently occurring in California, a single dose of the same vaccine used in adolescents is being recommended for adults.

Polio

Poliomyelitis is an infectious disease caused by a RNA virus of the enterovirus group that attacks the nervous system. In 1988, the World Health Organization spearheaded the Global Polio Eradication Initiative. (See the historical timeline in Table 10-2 for important events related to polio.) Since that time, cases of polio worldwide have dropped 99% from 350,000 cases to 1,604 cases in 2009. By 2010, there were only four countries left in the world still endemic with the disease—Afghanistan, Pakistan, India, and Nigeria. The peak of this disease in the United States occurred in 1952 with over 21,000 paralytic cases, but the incidence declined rapidly after the introduction of the vaccines. The last wild case of disease in the United States occurred in 1979 in the Amish population of the Midwest. It had been imported from the Netherlands.

Transmission of the virus occurs through the fecal-oral route. The virus multiplies in the intestines and can later attack the nerve tissues of the spinal cord, leading to paralysis. It is excreted in the stools of infected persons and can be transmitted to other susceptible hosts who have contact with those feces. The incubation period is 6–20 days. Up to 95% of those infected will have no symptoms, and another 4–8% will have minor flu-like symptoms. Less than 1% will develop paralysis, usually of the legs; and of those who do develop paralysis, 5–10% die from the resultant paralysis of the respiratory muscles (see Figure 10-7).

The live oral vaccine, previously in use in the United States, simulated the wild virus in that it replicated in the gastrointestinal system and was excreted in the stools of the immunized host. It had the subsequent advantage of then stimulating

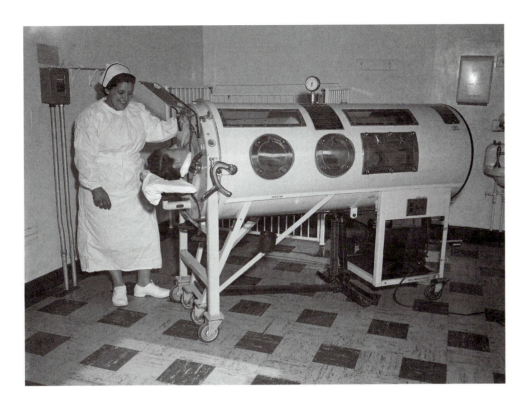

FIGURE 10-7 "Iron Lung" for Respiratory Paralysis of Polio
Courtesy of Centers for Disease Control and Prevention Public Health Image Library (PHIL): http://phil.cdc.gov/Phil/details.asp

an immune response in anyone who came into contact with those feces. Since the immunized were usually young infants and children, anyone who changed their diapers had a secondary exposure to the vaccine virus. During the predominant use of the live oral vaccine, there were about 8 cases per year of **vaccine-associated paralytic polio (VAPP)**; so in 1996, the United States changed over to exclusive use of the inactivated polio vaccine (IPV). Worldwide, however, the oral vaccine is still used for the advantages mentioned previously. Efficacy of OPV after three doses is 95%; of IPV after three doses is 99%. Recommendations currently in the United States are for three doses from 2–6 months old with a booster given before entrance to kindergarten.

> **vaccine-associated paralytic polio (VAPP):** polio disease caused by the live, attenuated virus, rather than the wild virus, contained in the oral polio vaccine

Smallpox

Smallpox is a serious, contagious, and potentially fatal skin infection caused by the variola virus, a DNA virus belonging to the Orthopoxvirus family. The variola virus is stable in the environment, can be aerosolized, and would be infective for several hours. It is for this reason that smallpox is considered a potential bioterrorism agent. Smallpox is transmitted by respiratory droplet, direct contact with the blister fluid, and contact with contaminated objects such as bedding. The incubation period of smallpox is usually 12–14 days and is followed by a flu-like illness with fever that

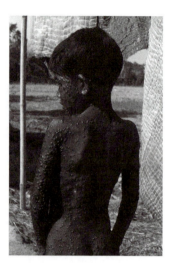

FIGURE 10-8 Smallpox
Courtesy of Centers for Disease Control and Prevention Public Health Image Library (PHIL): http://phil.cdc.gov/Phil/details.asp

lasts only 2–3 days. As those symptoms subside, the classic rash (see Figure 10-8) of blisters appears, starting on the extremities and then spreading to the trunk. The contagious period is between when the fever starts and the rash has been present for about a week. As with chickenpox, an infected host is no longer infectious after all the lesions have crusted. There were two main forms of the disease—the milder course of variola minor (case fatality rate of less than 1%) and the more severe form of variola major (case fatality rate of 30%). Most survivors were left with deep scars on their bodies. No effective treatment has been developed.

The smallpox vaccine, no longer in widespread use, contains live vaccinia virus, an Orthopoxvirus similar to variola. The two viruses are so similar that immunity to vaccinia protects against smallpox. The vaccine has been found to be protective for at least 10 years.

Because of its potential use in bioterrorism, the World Health Organization has directed that no facilities, other than their collaborating centers in Russia and the United States, be allowed to store the smallpox virus. The vaccine seed virus is kept in the Netherlands with a stockpile of the vaccine to be used in case of an outbreak.

Historical Note 10·1

Smallpox

Smallpox is thought to have originated about 3,000 years ago in Egypt or India and was introduced into Europe between the fifth and seventh centuries. Spanish and Portuguese explorers introduced the disease to the New World . Epidemics occurred across continents and depleted populations. It killed such rulers as Queen Mary II of England, King Louis XV of France, and Tsar Peter II of Russia. The word "variola" came from the Latin word for "stained" or "mark on the skin" in 570 AD. The term "small pockes" was first used in England in the fifteenth century.

It was known that survivors of the disease became immune to later disease. Inoculating the skin of a susceptible host with fluid from the pustule of someone with smallpox was practiced long before the eighteenth century in Africa, China, and India. In 1670, it became a practice in the Turkish Ottoman Empire, and later reports of variolation (inoculation with the smallpox fluid) were sent to England. Lady Mary Montague, the wife of a British ambassador to Turkey, had suffered from an infection and had lost her brother to the disease. She saw the variolations being done there and had her 5-year-old son inoculated. She was instrumental in bringing the practice to England and later to all of Europe where it gained widespread acceptance. Variolation was brought to the New World in 1721. Reverend Cotton Mather was one of the first to conduct an epidemiological study to compare the death rates among those who were variolated (2%) as compared to those who were not (14%) during a smallpox epidemic in Boston in 1721.

In 1757, an 8-year-old boy, Edward Jenner, was variolated. He later became a physician in England and was interested in the fact that the dairymaids who became infected with cowpox never developed smallpox during the epidemics. In 1796, he removed fluid from a cowpox pustule from a dairymaid, Sarah Nelms, and inoculated it onto an 8-year-old boy, James Phipps. James developed a minor illness from which he recovered quickly. Two months later, Dr. Jenner inoculated James with material from a smallpox pustule, and no disease developed. After repeating this procedure a few more times, Jenner published his findings in 1798. The Latin for cow is "vacca" and for cowpox was "vaccinia," so Jenner called his procedure "vaccination."

The last wild type case in the United States occurred in 1949, and the last worldwide case occurred in Somalia in 1977. Smallpox is the first vaccine preventable disease to be eradicated globally.

Tuberculosis

The disease caused by *Mycobacterium tuberculosis* was discussed in Chapter 8, Infectious Diseases. The bacille Calmette-Guérin vaccine (BCG) is a live, attenuated vaccine using *Mycobacterium bovis*, or a cow tuberculin bacterium, as the antigen, and it has been around for more than 80 years. This vaccine is generally *not* considered effective against the primary pulmonary infection, nor does it prevent latent TB disease from being activated in the host. Therefore, it is not considered useful in breaking the transmission of pulmonary spread. However, the vaccine *has* been found to be effective in preventing TB meningitis and disseminated disease in newborns and infants. Because of this, the WHO recommends routine immunization of all infants born in high endemic areas as soon as possible after birth with a single dose of BCG. The rationale is that there is risk for early exposure to the organism, and the incubation period for development of TB meningitis and miliary (disseminated) TB is brief after exposure. More than 100,000,000 infants per year are immunized with BCG worldwide, which accounts for about 80% of infants born in high-risk countries. This immunization dose causes ulceration at the site of the injection and ultimately forms a scar, which is used as a marker for prior immunization.

In a meta-analysis study, the vaccine has been found to be about 86% effective against developing these two forms of TB and 65% effective in reducing subsequent deaths from TB disease. Immunity wanes over time and is nonsignificant after 10–20 years. The WHO recommends considering using this vaccine in high-risk infants and children who are skin-test negative and who are born or living in low-risk countries. Because of low endemic levels and lack of consistent protective levels against pulmonary infections, the United States does not routinely use BCG, but rather screens high-risk persons and treats them when infection is found.

The BCG vaccine has also been found to be effective in preventing infection by the organism that causes leprosy and in treating bladder cancer.

Varicella

Varicella, more commonly known as "chickenpox," is caused by the herpes zoster virus, a DNA virus and member of the herpes virus family. This same virus causes herpes zoster infections, or "shingles," in adults. Chickenpox continues to occur worldwide with a slightly higher incidence in the tropics, particularly in adults. Prior to the routine use of a vaccine against varicella in the United States, universal infection occurred in children, and there were about 4 million cases per year. It was a major cause of indirect economic costs from loss of school/work days by children and their parents. Hospitalization rates in the pre- vaccine era were higher for adults with the disease (8 per 1,000 cases) than in children (2–3 per 1,000 cases). Deaths before the institution of vaccine use in 1995 occurred in 1 of 60,000 cases, or about 103 per year. This has decreased by 90% since the vaccine has been widely used. It is estimated that 500,000–1,000,000 cases of herpes zoster occur each year primarily in older persons and persons with immunosuppression. The lifetime risk of developing shingles is 32%.

Most transmission of the organism is through spread in respiratory droplets, but the risk also occurs with direct contact with fluid from the typical vesicles (blisters) of the disease (see Figure 10-9A) or with inhalation of the vesicular fluid. The incubation period is about 14–16 days and is followed by 1–2 days of fever before the onset of the rash, which typically consists of crops of blisters that occur starting on the head and spreading to the trunk and then to the extremities. An infected person will normally have 200–500 lesions during the course of the infection. A person with the disease is contagious from 2–3 days before the rash appears until all blisters have broken and crusted, usually 5–7 days. This accounts for prolonged loss of work/school days. The most common complication and reason for most hospitalizations related to chickenpox is secondary bacterial infection. Other complications of the primary disease include pneumonia and secondary central nervous system infections. Reye's syndrome, a severe condition that affects the liver and other organ systems, has been seen in patients with varicella who also use aspirin or aspirin products. The incidence of Reye's syndrome has decreased markedly since this association was recognized and the use of aspirin during infection was discouraged.

Complete recovery from chickenpox usually provides lifelong immunity, but in some, the virus will remain latent in the nerve roots. This virus can then become reactivated later in life causing recurrent disease that presents as herpes zoster or shingles (see Figure 10-9B). Shingles is preceded by several days of pain along the pattern of a sensory nerve, usually involving one side of the face or trunk. Shingles is frequently complicated by severe persistent pain in the region of the lesions even after all the lesions have resolved, a condition called "postherpetic neuralgia."

The varicella vaccine is a live, attenuated vaccine. Vaccine efficacy after one dose is 70–90% against all disease and 90–100% against moderate to severe disease. A second dose is now recommended to boost immunity and reduce breakthrough chickenpox. The zoster vaccine contains the same live, attenuated virus as the varicella vaccine but in higher concentrations. Efficacy of the zoster vaccine after the single recommended dose is only 64% in persons aged 60–69 and 51% overall, but disease when it occurs, is much milder. The vaccine also has been associated with a 66% decrease in the development of postherpetic neuralgia among those who do develop the disease.

A 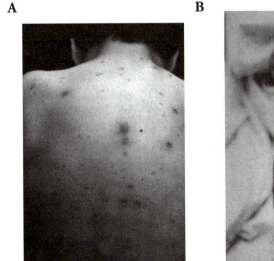   **B**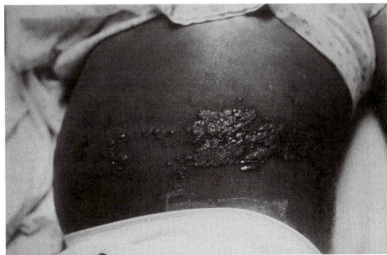

FIGURE 10-9 Varicella. (A) Classical Lesions of Chickenpox (B) Classical Herpes Zoster (Shingles)
Courtesy of Centers for Disease Control and Prevention Public Health Image Library (PHIL): http://phil.cdc.gov/Phil/details.asp

THE FUTURE

The World Health Organization is continuing the push with its initiatives to eradicate polio and measles worldwide. In addition, there is a major focus on developing effective vaccines against two other of the world's major pandemics—HIV/AIDS and malaria. More than 60 million persons have been infected with HIV since its start, and more than 20 million of them have died. The lack of knowledge as to what markers will be associated with immune protection, the marked genetic variability of the virus and the lack of animal models all complicate the search for a safe and effective vaccine. Multiple trials with various products have been unsuccessful until recently. Researchers from the U.S. Military HIV Research Program (MHRP) announced in October 2009 that their vaccine reduced the risk of HIV infection by about 31% in a trial conducted in Thailand. This is the first vaccine that has shown any promise, and further work is ongoing to improve and learn from these data.

Malaria is a life-threatening disease that is endemic in many parts of the world. It is caused by a protozoan, *Plasmodium*, which is transmitted to humans via the bite of a mosquito. According to the World Health Organization, in 2008, there were 247 million cases of malaria and one million deaths, mostly in Africa. Malaria accounts for 20% of deaths in children in Africa. A large-scale clinical trial in infants and toddlers is currently underway in seven sub-Saharan countries using the most advanced malaria vaccine currently available. Initial results are expected in late 2011 with follow-up results expected in 2013. This is the first vaccine to show promise with substantial, but not complete, protection in children.

Summary

For more than 300 years, people have researched ways to combat the major infections of the time, such as smallpox, measles, and polio. Along with improved sanitation practices, vaccines have had the largest impact on improved public health in the United States and worldwide. Targeted vaccine use in various specific situations, as well as the routine use of vaccines in children, adolescents, and adults, has reduced the morbidity and mortality of vaccine preventable diseases. This chapter discussed the basics of the immune system, active and passive immunity, and the advantages and limitations of herd immunity. The distinguishing features between the live, attenuated vaccines and various types of inactivated vaccines were delineated. The risks of immunizing (adverse events and reactions) and the risks of not immunizing (versus the risks of the natural disease), as well as several reasons people currently refuse vaccines that are known to prevent disease, were covered. These issues impact the use and success of vaccine programs and, therefore, impact the epidemiology of the diseases they are meant to prevent. The last half of the chapter discussed some examples of the infections that are currently vaccine preventable—their occurrence in the United States and worldwide, the clinical picture, and the vaccines used for protection. Vaccines have had a major impact in preventing infections that caused severe diseases in the past and will continue to have this impact in the future as new vaccines are developed. However, almost half of the deaths worldwide are still caused by infectious diseases. Having a basic understanding of the principles of vaccines is important to be able to understand how they work in the public health setting. And to know a little about the disease is important to know how to interrupt its transmission or to prevent it.

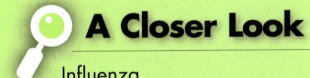

A Closer Look

Influenza

Hippocrates described an influenza-like illness more than 2,400 years ago. Since that time, there have been many descriptions of flu-like epidemics, but the first widely accepted influenza epidemic occurred in 1580 and spread from its origin in Asia to Europe and Africa. More than 8,000 deaths occurred in Rome alone. Since that time, influenza has been well known to cause seasonal disease, as well as to cause epidemics and pandemics.

The Organism and Its Clinical Picture

The "flu," as it is commonly known, is a respiratory illness caused by one of several types of influenza virus. This virus is an RNA virus that occurs as three different primary types—A, B, and C. Type A influenza virus is further classified into subtypes based on two surface protein antigens—hemagglutinin (HA or H) and neuraminidase (NA or N). There are 16 known hemagglutinin and 9 known neuraminidase proteins. An example of this is the recent H1N1 influenza outbreak in 2010. Influenza A causes sporadic cases of disease, seasonal epidemics, and pandemics. Humans are the usual reservoir for human influenza A virus; wild birds are

Continues

the natural hosts for avian influenza, but the virus can also be found in animals such as pigs, horses, and others. On occasion, an animal influenza A virus will infect a human and mutate enough so that it is able to cause human to human infection. The swine influenza virus is an example. Influenza B is found only in humans and is frequently a cause of seasonal flu. It can cause epidemics but has not been the source of any pandemics. Type C causes sporadic milder infections and is not associated with epidemics or pandemics.

Transmission of the virus is by respiratory droplet directly or on fomites. The incubation period is only 2 days and symptoms begin suddenly with fever, chills, headache, body aches, and cough. This is followed by nasal congestion, sore throat, and worsening cough accompanied by vomiting and possibly diarrhea. An infected adult is contagious for 3–5 days, whereas an infected child can be contagious for 7–10 days. Rapid tests are available that have a sensitivity of less than70% but specificity of 95%. Those who test positive can be isolated from those at risk and thus help prevent spread. Those at highest risk for severe disease include the young (less than 2 years old) and the older (more than 64 years old), those with poor nutrition, and those with certain underlying medical conditions (heart disease, asthma or other respiratory disease, pregnancy, and diabetes). Possible complications of influenza infections include pneumonia, ear infections, and encephalopathy. As with chickenpox, if aspirin or aspirin products are used during influenza disease, there is a small but real risk of Reye's syndrome.

Epidemiology

When seasonal epidemics occur in the United States, attack rates range from 5–20% in the general population, but can be as high as 50% in closed populations such as nursing homes. Influenza accounts for more than 200,000 hospitalizations and 36,000 deaths each year, mostly in those persons over 65 years old. Annual epidemics usually last 8–10 weeks and begin as early as October and last as late as May, but usually peak in January-February. The severity of seasonal flu is dependent on several factors: natural or vaccine-induced levels of immunity, age and health of the population, strain virulence, and extent of antigenic variation of new viruses. One or more strains or subtypes of influenza A may circulate in one season. Infection induces immunity to the infecting virus and antigenically similar influenza viruses.

In the hemagglutinin or neuraminidase protein antigens of influenza A, minor mutations occur continuously and result in new strains of the virus. This is called **antigenic drift**, and it is for this reason the seasonal influenza disease can vary each year. This is why people can have more than one influenza infection and why global surveillance is critical to monitor virus strains for production of the annual vaccine. New strains are named based on type, geographic location, laboratory number, year of isolation, and subtype—e.g., A/Brisbane/10/2007(H3N2). **Antigenic shift** is an abrupt, major change that produces a novel influenza A virus subtype in humans that was not currently in circulation. This major mutation can occur directly from animal to human transmission or through genetic reassortment of animal and human viral genes that produces a new human subtype. Antigenic drifts happen all the time; shifts happen occasionally.

For global influenza pandemics to occur, three conditions must be met. A new subtype of influenza A virus (antigenic shift) must be introduced into the human population. No immunity exists for this new virus, and therefore, all are susceptible. Secondly, this new virus must cause severe disease in humans. If only mild disease occurs, or if infected persons remain asymptomatic, there are no major consequences. Lastly, the virus must be able to spread easily from person to person in a sustained manner. Without easy spread,

antigenic drift: minor mutations in the hemagglutinin or neuraminidase protein antigens of influenza A virus that occur continuously; results in new strains of the virus

antigenic shift: an abrupt, major change in the protein antigens that produces a novel influenza A virus subtype in humans that was not currently in circulation

there is no risk of worldwide spread. These conditions were met, and this is what occurred with the 1918 influenza outbreak that is discussed later.

Vaccine

There are two types of influenza vaccine—the inactivated injectable form and the live, attenuated nasal spray form. Each vaccine form contains the antigenic components of three virus strains—two influenza A and one influenza B. The hemagglutinin antigens of influenza A are more protective, and the neuraminidase antigens lessen severity of disease. The different strains contained in each flu vaccine are reviewed each year based on surveillance and scientist's recommendations. Most years one or two of the three virus strains in the influenza vaccine are updated to keep up with the changes in the circulating influenza viruses. Protective antibodies are present two weeks after the single recommended dose. The efficacy of the vaccine is 70–90%.

Influenza Outbreaks

- *Influenza (Spanish flu) outbreak of 1918:* The animal origin of the H1N1 pandemic of 1918 is not known, but it was clearly a novel virus with no circulating immunity. This pandemic was the most serious and deadly known in modern times. It was called the "Spanish flu" because of its high incidence in Spain, not because it started there. This pandemic began in the spring of 1918 and then resurfaced with more severe disease in the fall of that year. A third wave occurred in the winter months of 1919. Overall, one-third to one-half of the world's population became infected and 20–50 million people died. It was complicated by the massive troop movements that help spread the infection across the Atlantic as World War I was coming to an end.

- *Avian influenza:* Avian influenza (H5N1) is a zoonotic infection that is endemic in Asia, Africa, the Near East, and parts of Europe. There are only a few types that have crossed over to infect humans. One of these types, the highly pathogenic avian influenza (HPAI), has caused the largest number of severe disease and deaths since 1997. Although it is difficult for a human to become infected with this avian virus, and human to human spread is even less likely, the mortality rate associated with this flu is greater than 60%. There is no cross protection from exposure to other influenza A viruses. When the initial human cases began to be noted, it was thought that this virus would be the cause of the next pandemic, but this did not occur. Sporadic cases do still occur and are monitored by WHO and CDC.

- *Swine flu outbreak of 2009–2010:* In March 2009, the first cases of a new, more severe influenza began to appear in Mexico. By April, the first cases were reported in the United States; and by June, after there had been more than 1 million Americans infected, the World Health Organization proclaimed it a pandemic. By August, more than 170 countries had reported swine flu cases. By the time President Obama declared a national emergency in October, there had been over 1,000 deaths in the United States with 10% occurring in children. This new influenza A virus strain (H1N1) contained genes from swine (pig) influenza viruses, bird virus genes, and human influenza genes. About one-third of the adults over 60 years old had circulating antibodies to this H1N1 outbreak, suggesting an earlier exposure in their lives. Clinically, the disease was similar to the normal seasonal flu, except that symptoms were more severe and infected hosts were more likely to have vomiting and diarrhea. A vaccine separate from the routine annual flu vaccine was rapidly developed and deployed to combat the epidemic. The U.S. Public Health Emergency ended in June 2010, and the WHO declared an end of the pandemic in August 2010. CDC reported that from April 2009 to April 2010, there were 43–89 million U.S. cases of influenza with 195,000–403,000 related hospitalizations and 8,870–18,300 deaths.

Review Questions

1. All of the following are reasons to immunize EXCEPT:
    a. Routine childhood immunizations
    b. Cancer prevention
    c. Moving to Botswana, Africa
    d. At-risk circumstances such as veterinarians or animal workers or for military personnel at risk for bioterrorism
    e. All of the above are reasons to immunize.

2. List three reasons people/parents refuse immunizations.

    _____

    _____

    _____

3. Match the following terms in Column A with their corresponding terms in Column B. (Each answer must be used at least once.)

Column A	**Column B**
_____ Oral polio virus vaccine (OPV)	a. Active immunity
_____ Breast feeding	
_____ Flu shots	b. Herd immunity
_____ Measles	
_____ Rabies	c. Passive immunity

4. For which of the following diseases did Dr. Jenner develop the first "vaccine"?
    a. Measles
    b. Smallpox
    c. Polio
    d. Hepatitis

5. **True or False** Smallpox was a good candidate for eradication because infection and communicability were obvious as they occurred with the presence of obvious skin lesions.

6. An example of a live, attenuated vaccine is _____, and an example of an inactivated (killed) vaccine is _____.

7. The first disease eradicated worldwide by the use of vaccine was:

    a. Polio
    b. Smallpox
    c. Measles
    d. Whooping cough (pertussis)

8. Vaccines being used in cancer prevention include:

    a. Human papilloma virus vaccine
    b. Measles vaccine
    c. Hepatitis B vaccine
    d. A and C

9. All the following diseases are no longer endemic in the United States because of our immunization program EXCEPT:

    a. Pertussis
    b. Measles
    c. Smallpox
    d. Polio

10. Of the following diseases, which two vaccine preventable diseases may be used as bioterrorism agents? (Circle two answers.)

    a. Polio
    b. Smallpox
    c. Anthrax
    d. Meningococcus

11. **For Deeper Thought** Infection with virus X causes severe diarrheal disease, particularly in infants and children, and is spread via the fecal-oral route, via respiratory droplets, and possibly via fomites. Globally, it is responsible for about 524,000 deaths in children less than 5 years old each year; in the United States, almost all children have had the disease by the time they reach 5 years old. In the United States, virus X causes 400,000 visits to doctors' offices, 200,000 visits to the Emergency Room, and 55,000–70,000 hospitalizations for dehydration each year. The estimated annual direct costs of medical care are approximately $210 million annually. Briefly list pros and cons of developing a vaccine program against viral X disease and make your final hypothesis on whether it is desirable as a vaccine preventable disease and how you might test your hypothesis.

Website Resources

Centers for Disease Control and Prevention: http://www.cdc.gov

Centers for Disease Control and Prevention; search "Seasonal Influenza" to locate information about Flu Activity & Surveillance: http://www.cdc.gov

Centers for Disease Control and Prevention, Public Health Image Library (PHIL): http://phil.cdc.gov/phil

Centers for Disease Control and Prevention, *The Pink Book—Epidemiology and Prevention of Vaccine Preventable Diseases* (11th ed.) (May 2009): http://www.cdc.gov; locate the Vaccines homepage and click on "Publications."

Centers for Disease Control and Prevention, Vaccines: http://www.cdc.gov/vaccines

National Library of Medicine: www.nlm.nih.gov

National Network for Immunization Information: http://www.immunizationinfo.org

World Health Organization: www.who.int

References

Bloomberg Businessweek. (March 22, 2010). Measles outbreak triggered by unvaccinated child. Retrieved from http://www.businessweek.com/lifestyle/content/healthday/637218.html

Boston Herald—News and Opinions. (February 26, 2011). Third suspected case of measles surfaces. Retrieved from http://news.bostonherald.com/news/regional/view/2011_0226third_suspected_case_of_measles_surfaces

California Department of Public Health. (2011, January 7). Pertussis Report. Retrieved from http://www.cdph.ca.gov/programs/immunize/Documents/PertussisReport2011-01-07.pdf

Centers for Disease Control and Prevention. (May 2009). The Pink Book: Chapters; Epidemiology and Prevention of Vaccine Preventable Diseases. Retrieved from http://www.cdc.gov/vaccines/pubs/pinkbook/pink-chapters.htm

Centers for Disease Control and Prevention. (2009). H1N1 Flu: 2009 H1N1 Flu: Situation Update: Retrieved from http://www.cdc.gov/h1n1flu/update.htm

Centers for Disease Control and Prevention. (updated June 25, 2010). Viral Hepatitis Statistics and Surveillance. Retrieved from http://www.cdc.gov/hepatitis/Statistics/2008Surveillance/Table1b.htm

Centers for Disease Control and Prevention. (updated November 24, 2009). Sexually Transmitted Diseases. Retrieved from http://www.cdc.gov/std/HPV/STDFact-HPV.htm

Centers for Disease Control and Prevention. (reviewed January 4, 2010). Vaccines and Immunizations. Retrieved from http://www.cdc.gov/vaccines/default.htm

Centers for Disease Control and Prevention. (updated August 31, 2009). Measles (Rubeola)—Measles Outbreaks. Retrieved from http://www.cdc.gov/measles/outbreaks.html

Centers for Disease Control and Prevention. (updated August 27, 2010). Pertussis (Whooping Cough)—Fast Facts. Retrieved from http://www.cdc.gov/pertussis/fast-facts.html

Centers for Disease Control and Prevention. (updated January 11, 2011). Pertussis (Whooping Cough)—Outbreaks. Retrieved from http://www.cdc.gov/pertussis/outbreaks.html

Centers for Disease Control and Prevention. (n.d.). Emergency Preparedness and Response—Anthrax. Retrieved from http://emergency.cdc.gov/agent/anthrax

Chen, R. T., Rastogi, S. C., Mullen, J. R., Hayes, S., Cochi, S. L., Donlon, J. A., & Wassilak, S. G. (1994). The Vaccine Adverse Event Reporting System (VAERS). *Vaccine, 12*, 542–550.

Malaria Vaccine Initiative. (January 31, 2011). Full enrollment achieved in large-scale Phase 3 malaria vaccine candidate trial. Retrieved from http://www.malariavaccine.org/RTSSenrollment.php

National Center for Biotechnology Information. (January 2005). National Library of Medicine, National Institute of Health; Baylor University Medical Center Proceedings, *Edward Jenner and the history of smallpox and vaccination*. Retrieved from http://www.ncbi.nlm.nih.gov/pmc/articles/PMC1200696

National Network for Immunization Information. (n.d.). Vaccine Information. Retrieved from http://www.immunizationinfo.org/vaccines

U.S. Department of Health and Human Services. (n.d.). Health Resources and Services Administration. National Vaccine Injury Compensation Program (VICP). Retrieved from http://www.hrsa.gov/vaccinecompensation/default.htm

Vaccine Adverse Event Reporting System. (February 25, 2011). VAERS-Vaccine Adverse Event Reporting System. Retrieved from http://vaers.hhs.gov/index 2/25/11

World Health Organization. (revised August 2008). Media Center: Factsheets: Hepatitis B. Retrieved from http://www.who.int/mediacentre/factsheets/fs204/en/index.html

World Health Organization. (updated July 2010). Programmes and Projects—New and Under-utilized Vaccines Implementation (NUVI)—Human Papillomavirus (HPV). Retrieved from http://www.who.int/nuvi/hpv/en

World Health Organization. (November 26, 2009). Global Eradication of Measles—Report by the Secretariat. Retrieved from http://apps.who.int/gb/ebwha/pdf_files/EB126/B126_17-en.pdf

World Health Organization. (January 23, 2004). Weekly Epidemiologic Record—Position Paper on BCG. Retrieved from http://www.who.int/immunization/wer7904BCG_Jan04_position_paper.pdf

World Health Organization. (n.d.). Media Center: Factsheets: Meningococcal Meningitis. Retrieved from http://www.who.int/mediacentre/factsheets/fs141/en

World Health Organization. (October 11, 2010). Immunization, Vaccines and Biologicals—Pertussis. Retrieved from http://www.who.int/immunization/topics/pertussis/en/index.html

World Health Organization. (November 2010). Media Center: Factsheets: Poliomyelitis. Retrieved from http://www.who.int/mediacentre/factsheets/fs114/en/index.html

World Health Organization. (n.d.). Media Center: Factsheets: Smallpox—Historical Significance. Retrieved from http://www.who.int/mediacentre/factsheets/smallpox/en

Chapter 11

CARDIOVASCULAR DISEASE

Learning Objectives

Upon completion of this chapter, you should be able to:

1. Describe the Framingham Heart Study—its purpose, cohorts, and major findings.
2. Describe the process of atherosclerosis and how it causes cardiovascular disease.
3. Be able to identify the impact of gender and race/ethnicity on the prevalence and mortality of cardiovascular disease.
4. Describe the measurement of blood pressure, its normal values, high values, and the impact of gender, age, and race on its prevalence and mortality.
5. Name six major risk factors (two non-modifiable and four modifiable) for cardiovascular disease and give an example of the impact of each on this disease.

Key Terms

aerobic exercise
angina
arrhythmia
atherosclerosis
blood pressure
cardiac arrest

cardiopulmonary
  resuscitation (CPR)
cardiovascular disease
  (CVD)
cerebrovascular
  accident (CVA)

cerebrovascular
  disease
cholesterol
congenital heart
  defects
coronary arteries

coronary artery disease (CAD)

coronary heart disease (CHD)

diastolic blood pressure

exercise

Framingham Heart Study

heart attack

heart failure

hemorrhagic stroke

high blood pressure (HBP)

high-density lipoproteins (HDL)

hypertension

intima

ischemic stroke

low-density lipoproteins (LDL)

metabolic equivalent (MET)

moderate intensity

myocardial infarction (MI)

peripheral artery disease (PAD)

physical activity

physical fitness

plaque

sedentary

stroke

systolic pressure

transient ischemic attack (TIA)

valvular disease

vigorous intensity

Chapter Outline

INTRODUCTION

Cardiovascular disease (CVD), a generic term that includes several different conditions that affect the heart (*cardio-*) and blood vessels (*-vascular*), is the leading cause of death for both men and women in the United States across all races and ethnicity except Asian Americans. Stoke is the fourth most common cause of death in the United States. The current goal of the American Heart Association is "to improve the cardiovascular health of all Americans by 20%, while reducing deaths from cardiovascular disease and stroke by 20%" by 2020.

Although technically not a cardiovascular disease but a **cerebrovascular disease** (*cerebro-* = brain), stroke is often considered at the same time as cardiovascular disease because both conditions share the same risk factors and underlying processes. In fact, the WHO considers strokes in the broad group of cardiovascular diseases because it is "a disease of the blood vessels that supply the brain." Many will use the category of "cardiovascular" disease to discuss all diseases with a similar underlying etiology. The Centers for Disease Control and Prevention reports heart disease and stroke statistics separately. They are therefore discussed as separate entities in this chapter. It is important, however, when reviewing literature or statistics related to cardiovascular diseases that you know if stroke is included or if it is separate.

cardiovascular disease (CVD): a generic term that includes several different conditions that affect the heart and blood vessels

cerebrovascular disease: disease that involves the blood vessels of the brain; stroke

Framingham Heart Study: a study designed by Boston University and the National Heart Institute in 1948 to study cardiovascular disease and its risk factors; has involved multiple generational cohorts

Historical Note 11·1

The Framingham Heart Study

As the incidence and mortality of infectious diseases began their decline from the early 1900s, the incidence of cardiovascular disease began its rapid incline. Because the focus in the United States had been on the control of infectious disease through improved sanitation, vaccine development, and the production of antibiotics, little was known about the causes and control of this new epidemic of diseases affecting the heart. In 1948, the National Heart Institute (now the National Heart, Lung, and Blood Institute or NHLBI) and Boston University began an ambitious project to follow over time a large number of persons who had not yet developed cardiovascular disease to study the characteristics of the disease and to determine the risk factors. This project is commonly known today as the **Framingham Heart Study**, named for the city in Massachusetts that was the home of the study participants. The original cohort involved 5,209 enrollees, with the age and sex distribution as shown in Table 11-1, who underwent complete physical examinations, extensive medical and lifestyle histories, and laboratory testing

TABLE 11-1 Original Cohort of the Framingham Heart Study (1948)

Age and Sex at Entry to Study

Age	29-39	40-49	50-62	Totals
Men	835	779	722	**2,336**
Women	1,042	962	869	**2,873**
Totals	**1,877**	**1,741**	**1,591**	**5,209**

Based on: The Framingham Heart Study; Original cohort: http://www.framinghamheartstudy.org/participants/original.html

every two years. In 1971, the study enrolled its second cohort—5,124 offspring of the original cohort and their spouses with ages ranging from less than 10 years old to 70 years old. In 2002, the third generation of study participants was enrolled. This cohort consists of the grandchildren of the original cohort and involves 4,095 persons from ages 19-79. All three cohorts have similar numbers of men and women.

Over the years since the study began, the diversity of the town of Framingham has changed. In 1994, the Framingham study enrolled 506 men and women from diverse ethnic backgrounds into the Omni cohort study. The second generation of this group was enrolled in 2002. The proportion of men and women and their age ranges approximated the original Framingham cohorts. Out of these original studies, the stored blood samples are now being used to study genetics and other diseases.

The results of this study have changed the way medicine is practiced. Whereas when the study started in 1948, very little was known about the causes, risk factors, or processes involved in the development of cardiovascular disease, now because of the study, much is known. In addition to identifying the events leading to disease, interventions have also been studied. See Table 11-2 for some of the major milestones of the study. Most of these will be discussed later in this chapter, when discussing either the diseases or the risk factors. The proposed objectives of the Framingham Heart Study in the mid-1900s was an enormous undertaking, not only for that time, but for

Continues

the present as well. To follow such a large cohort over a long period of time is difficult; to follow multiple generations, like this study does, is phenomenal.

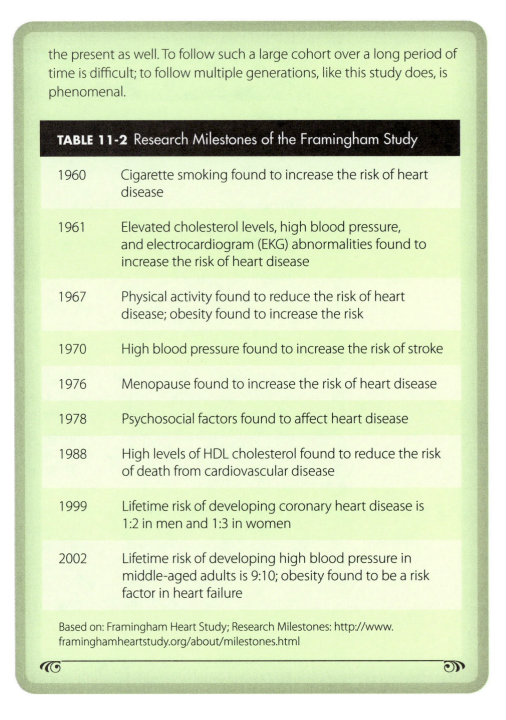

TABLE 11-2	Research Milestones of the Framingham Study
1960	Cigarette smoking found to increase the risk of heart disease
1961	Elevated cholesterol levels, high blood pressure, and electrocardiogram (EKG) abnormalities found to increase the risk of heart disease
1967	Physical activity found to reduce the risk of heart disease; obesity found to increase the risk
1970	High blood pressure found to increase the risk of stroke
1976	Menopause found to increase the risk of heart disease
1978	Psychosocial factors found to affect heart disease
1988	High levels of HDL cholesterol found to reduce the risk of death from cardiovascular disease
1999	Lifetime risk of developing coronary heart disease is 1:2 in men and 1:3 in women
2002	Lifetime risk of developing high blood pressure in middle-aged adults is 9:10; obesity found to be a risk factor in heart failure

Based on: Framingham Heart Study; Research Milestones: http://www.framinghamheartstudy.org/about/milestones.html

atherosclerosis: fat, other cells, and debris deposits under the lining of the arteries, causing narrowing of the vessels; also known as "hardening of the arteries"

The Framingham Heart Study resulted in the understanding of the characteristics and risk factors associated with cardiovascular disease. More recent studies are now focusing on the benefits of choosing healthy lifestyles such as low-fat diets, increased physical activity, and smoking cessation. It is now well documented that **atherosclerosis**, or "hardening of the arteries," has its beginning in childhood; and therefore the public health emphasis on prevention and public policies need to focus on earlier intensive interventions.

THE SCOPE OF THE PROBLEM

Annually, the American Heart Association (AHA), along with the Centers for Disease Control and Prevention, the National Institutes of Health, and others, gather the most recent data available on the wide array of cardiovascular diseases, as well as the associated risk factors, and publish this information in a report entitled *Heart Disease and Stroke Statistics*. The most recent update available at the time of this writing is the 2011 update published online on December 15, 2010. The statistics in the current report are primarily from 2005-2008, which reflect the multitude of information that must be collected, compiled, and analyzed prior to its publication. All of the information used in this section of the chapter comes from this report unless otherwise specified. Statistics given in this section are for cardiovascular diseases as a group. Statistics for individual diseases will be presented in the section on the selected diseases later in the chapter.

Prevalence

In 2008, there were approximately 82,600,000 adults in the United States with cardiovascular disease (including people with high blood pressure). This means slightly more than 1 in 3 Americans has some form of CVD. The actual number of cardiovascular diseases is higher because a person may have more than one disease—e.g., someone may have both high blood pressure and heart failure. Also in 2008, 7 million Americans over the age of 20 years, or about 2.5% of the U.S. population, had a stroke.

1. *Age:* Excluding congenital heart defects, the prevalence of CVD in the United States increases with a person's age. For persons between the ages of 40–59 years old (the "baby boomers"), 39.6% of men and 39.6% of women have CVD. For persons between the ages of 60–79 years old, the rate has almost doubled to 73.6% of men and 73.1% of women with CVD. Over 40 million American adults with CVD are over the age of 60 years. The prevalence of stroke also increases with age, ranging from around 2% among persons 40–59 to 7.5% among persons 60–79 and over 14% among persons 80 years of age or older.

2. *Gender:* Once thought of as a disease primarily of men, the rates of CVD are about equal among men and women. In 2004, the American Heart Association created the *Go Red for Women* campaign to raise the awareness of women's risk of CVD. Women had not been aware that CVD could present differently in women than in men and that it had become the number one killer of American women as it was in men. Overall, the prevalence of stroke is 2.7% and similar among men and women over 18 years of age.

3. *Race/Ethnicity:* The prevalence of CVD varies among the different races and ethnicities. Focusing on heart disease only, whites (11.9%) and blacks (11.2%) have the highest prevalence, whereas Asian Americans (6.3%) have the lowest. Hispanics (8.5%) and American Indians/Alaskan Natives (8.0%) fall

in between. There is variation even among the various Asian ethnicities with Asian Indians (9%) over twice that of Asian Koreans (4%). Ethnic differences also exist among those persons who have had strokes. In order of decreasing prevalence, American Indian/Alaskan Natives have a prevalence of 6.0%, blacks (4.0%), Hispanics (2.6%), whites (2.3%), and Asian/Pacific Islanders (1.6%).

Incidence

As published in the *Heart Disease and Stroke Statistics: Update 2011*, men aged 35–44 years have an average annual rate for a first major CVD event of 3 per 1,000 men. This rate increases to 74 per 1,000 as men age to 85–94 years of life. Women have these same rates, but they occur about 10 years later than in men. Before the age of 75, men have more CVD events related to coronary heart disease than women, but women have more events related to stroke than men. After age 75, these differences narrow. The lifetime risk of CVD at age 40, if currently disease-free, is 2 in 3 for men and 1 in 2 for women. If still disease-free at age 50, the lifetime risk for men is 51.7%; for women, 39.2%.

There are about 795,000 stroke episodes per year with 610,000 of them being first-time strokes, and the rest are recurrent strokes. The incidence of stroke has been decreasing for whites but not for blacks since the 1990s. Black men have an age-adjusted incidence rate at age 45–84 of 6.6 per 1,000. For white men this age range, the rate is almost half that at 3.6 per 1,000. The same is true for black women (4.9 per 1,000) and white women (2.3 per 1,000). It is supposed that this racial difference results from socioeconomic status differences. Hispanics also have a higher rate of strokes than whites, but not as high as blacks.

Death Rates

As mentioned previously, CVD is the leading cause of death in the United States for all but Asian Americans for whom cancer is the leading cause of death. In 2007, the latest year from which statistics are available and presented in the *Heart Disease and Stroke Statistics 2011 Update*, there were 813,804 U.S. deaths (34% of all U.S. deaths) from cardiovascular disease as the primary cause of death. However, there were 1,342,314 deaths (55% of all deaths) with cardiovascular disease mentioned as a primary or underlying cause on the death certificate. This shows that 1 of every 2–3 deaths are related to CVD. This is an average of more than 2,200 American deaths per day or one death every 39 seconds! The overall death rate as a result of CVD was 251.2 per 100,000 Americans in 2007.

For a breakdown of the death rates among gender and race/ethnicity see Table 11-3. This table shows that the death rate in men is almost 50% higher than the death rate in women. In regards to race/ethnicity, blacks have the highest rates, followed by whites. Far lower rates are associated with Hispanics and American Indian/Alaska Natives, with the former having a slightly higher rate than the latter. Asians/Pacific

TABLE 11-3 Age-Adjusted Cardiovascular Disease Death Rates, 2007, United States (per 100,000 Americans)		
	Men	**Women**
Total	300.3	211.6
White	294.0	205.7
Black	405.9	286.1
Hispanics	165.0	111.8
American Indians/Alaska Natives	159.8	99.8
Asians/Pacific Islanders	126.0	82.0

Based on: American Heart Association; Heart Disease and Stroke Statistics—2011 Update: A Report from the American Heart Association published in *Circulation* 2011; 123; e18-e209 online (December 15, 2010): http://circ.ahajournals.org/cgi/reprint/CIR.0b013e3182009701

Islanders have the lowest rates and are the only ethnicity where CVD is not the leading cause of death. As one might expect, the risk of CVD mortality increases with increasing age, but over 150,000 deaths (18.4% of all CVD deaths) occurred in persons less than 65 years old, and almost one-third of the CVD-related deaths occurred before the age of 75 years. The average life expectancy in the U.S. is 77.9 years.

Deaths as a result of CVD showed an increase from 1900 to its peak in 1968. Since 1968, CVD-related deaths have continued to decline across all ethnicities and both genders. Lifestyle/environmental changes that impacted the major risk factors and increased use of evidence-based medical practices were about equally responsible for the decline in the death rates.

Strokes account for 1:18 deaths in the United States, making it the fourth leading cause of death. (It was previously the third leading cause of death, but chronic lower respiratory diseases now outrank stroke because of a reclassification of lung diseases.) Regardless of whether strokes rank third or fourth as a leading cause of death, someone dies of stroke about every 4 minutes on average. Deaths resulting from stroke in 2007 totaled 135,952 for an overall death rate of 42.2 per 100,000. See Table 11-4 for a breakdown of rates among both genders and across the races/ethnicities. As can be seen in the table, death rates resulting from stroke were highest in blacks by far, followed by whites, then Asians/Pacific Islanders, and then Hispanics. American Indians/Alaska Natives had the lowest rates. Men had a slightly higher death rate across all ethnicities except whites, for whom rates were similar for both genders.

TABLE 11-4 Age-Adjusted Death Rates for Stroke, United States, 2007 (per 100,000)

	Men	Women
Whites	40.2	39.9
Blacks	67.1	55.0
Hispanics	34.4	30.8
Asians/Pacific Islanders	35.5	33.2
American Indians/Alaska Natives	31.1	28.4

Based on: American Heart Association; Heart Disease and Stroke Statistics—2011 Update: A Report from the American Heart Association published in *Circulation* 2011; 123; e18-e209 online (December 15, 2010): http://circ.ahajournals.org/cgi/reprint/CIR.0b013e3182009701

The mean age of death from stroke overall was 79.6 years in 2007, but men had a younger mean age than females. More women die of stroke each year than men because there are more elderly women than men. Women accounted for 60.6% of deaths as a result of stroke in the United States in 2007. A general decline in annual stroke death rates has occurred since 1997. Although much of this decline is thought to be because of improved detection and treatment of high blood pressure, some decrease may be the result of improved care immediately after strokes occur.

Financial Costs

In 2007, there were almost 7 million procedures or operations performed because of CVD in the United States. The estimated total costs of CVD for the same year were $286.6 billion for both direct medical costs and the associated indirect costs from loss of productivity, and so forth. According to the 2009 Factbook from the National Heart Lung and Blood Institute, the estimated direct health care costs for the year 2010 were expected to be $324 billion; the indirect costs of loss of productivity were expected to be $42 billion; and the indirect costs of early death were expected to be $137 billion. The total economic cost related to cardiovascular disease in the year 2010 would be $503 billion! In 2009, the direct and indirect costs related to stroke were an estimated $80 billion! An effective education program to promote healthy lifestyle choices and public policies to support these choices would be expected to have a major impact on these diseases and save billions in health care costs.

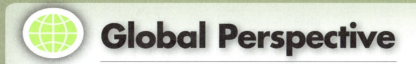

Global Perspective

CVD—Leading Cause of Deaths Worldwide

Not only are cardiovascular diseases the number one killer of Americans, but they are also the leading cause of deaths worldwide according to the World Health Organization. They report that 30% of deaths in 2008, or 17.3 million deaths worldwide, were the result of cardiovascular disease (64%) and stroke (36%). Again, like in the United States, coronary heart disease is the most common CVD and caused 42% of the deaths in this group of diseases. Globally, CVD affects women as equally as men. Persons in low- and middle-income countries are at highest risk for death, with over 80% of worldwide deaths from CVD occurring in this group. The reasons given for this disparity include: higher exposure to risk factors (behavioral) and less exposure to prevention and less access to appropriate health care. Premature death of this high-risk group contributes to poverty levels and reductions in productivity of 1-5% in these countries. WHO is focusing preventive strategies in combating tobacco use, physical inactivity, and unhealthy diets similar to the focus in America. World Heart Day is celebrated annually on September 29 and World Stroke Day on October 29.

BASIC PHYSIOLOGY AND PATHOPHYSIOLOGY

A brief description of the normal anatomy and physiology of the cardiovascular and cerebrovascular systems follows in this section. This will assist in understanding the diseases as they are discussed later in the chapter.

Normal Anatomy and Physiology

The cardiovascular system is made up of the heart and blood vessels (veins, arteries, and capillaries). Veins carry blood *to* the heart, and arteries carry blood *from* the heart. See Figure 11-1 for a diagram of the anatomy of the heart. Blood returns to the heart from the upper body via the superior vena cava and from the lower body through the inferior vena cava, both of which are large veins. These major veins collect blood from the smaller veins throughout the body. Blood then passes into the right atrium of the heart, through the tricuspid valve into

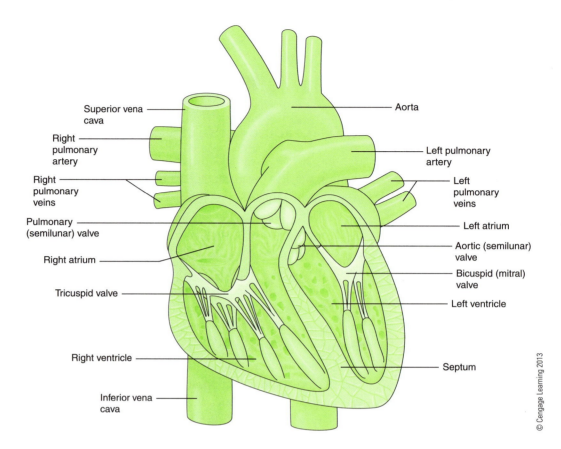

FIGURE 11-1 Anatomy of the Heart

© Cengage Learning 2013

the right ventricle, and then through the pulmonary valve into the pulmonary artery to the lungs. As blood passes through the lungs, it picks up the oxygen required by the cells of the body and releases carbon dioxide into the airways to be released from the body. Blood then returns to the heart via the pulmonary veins, which empty into the left atrium. From there, blood passes through the mitral valve into the left ventricle and then through the bicuspid valve into the aorta to be transported to the rest of the body. Small arteries branch off the aorta as soon as it leaves the heart to turn back to supply the heart muscle itself. These vessels are called the **coronary arteries**. See Figure 11-2 to view the coronary arteries.

The brain is divided into the cerebrum, the largest part of the brain, the cerebellum, which is located below the cerebrum, and the brainstem that connects the cerebellum and cerebrum to the spinal cord. Figure 11-3 shows the anatomy of the brain. The cerebellum controls muscle movements, sensation, emotions, and intellectual processes. It consists of two major hemispheres, the right and the left, that are joined by tissue called the corpus callosum. The right hemisphere controls movements of the left side of the body, and the left hemisphere controls movements of the right side of the body. That is why a stroke that occurs on the right side of the cerebrum causes paralysis on the left side of the body. The cerebrum is

coronary arteries: the arteries that supply the heart muscle

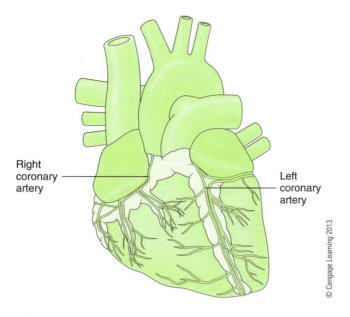

Right coronary artery

Left coronary artery

© Cengage Learning 2013

FIGURE 11-2 Coronary Arteries

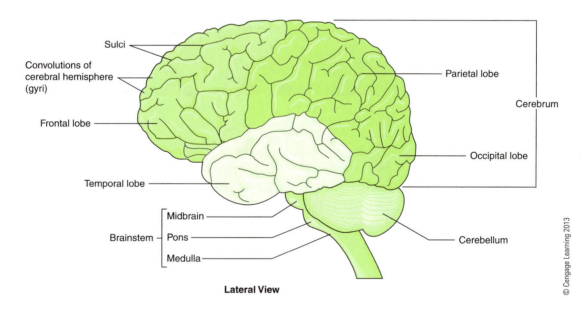

Sulci

Convolutions of cerebral hemisphere (gyri)

Frontal lobe

Temporal lobe

Brainstem — Midbrain
Pons
Medulla

Parietal lobe

Cerebrum

Occipital lobe

Cerebellum

Lateral View

© Cengage Learning 2013

FIGURE 11-3 Anatomy of the Brain

also made up of four different lobes on each hemisphere. The frontal lobes control personality and emotions; the temporal lobes are associated with speech and hearing; the parietal lobes control motor and sensory functions; and vision is controlled in the occipital lobes. The manifestations of a stroke or other brain trauma are dependent, therefore, not only on the hemisphere involved, but also on the lobe involved. The cerebellum is the control center for balance and coordination. The brainstem controls the functions such as the heart rate, breathing, body temperature, and other functions.

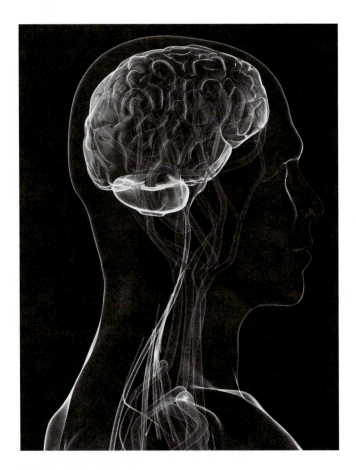

FIGURE 11-4 Arteries of the Brain
© Sebastian Kaulitzki/www.Shutterstock.com

The arterial supply of the brain comes from the carotid arteries anteriorly and the vertebral arteries posteriorly. These major vessels divide multiple times to supply blood to the entire brain. These blood vessels (shown in Figure 11-4) are involved in strokes.

Basic Pathophysiology of Atherosclerosis

intima: inner layer of the wall of an artery made up of the endothelium

plaque: formed by cholesterol, fatty acids, immune cells, and debris that collect under the intima of an arterial wall

The normal walls of an artery are made up of three layers. The outer layer is mainly a fibrous layer. The middle later is made up of smooth muscle, and the inner layer is endothelium, known as **intima**, or a thin layer of cells. When a person has excess cholesterol, high blood pressure, or smokes, the endothelium can be damaged. This allows excess cholesterol to accumulate under the inner layer. This in turn elicits a response from the immune system to clear out the invasion of this bad cholesterol. The combination of the cholesterol, fatty acids, immune cells, and debris form a **plaque**. Plaques can increase in size over time and grow into the lumen of the artery, causing blockage of the artery. Plaques can also rupture into the lumen, and in response, a clot forms that may obstruct further blood flow. See Figure 11-5 for

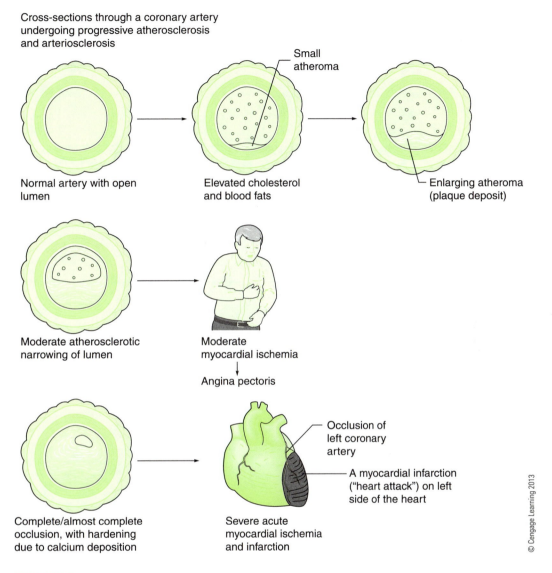

Cross-sections through a coronary artery undergoing progressive atherosclerosis and arteriosclerosis

Normal artery with open lumen

Small atheroma

Elevated cholesterol and blood fats

Enlarging atheroma (plaque deposit)

Moderate atherosclerotic narrowing of lumen

Moderate myocardial ischemia

Angina pectoris

Complete/almost complete occlusion, with hardening due to calcium deposition

Occlusion of left coronary artery

A myocardial infarction ("heart attack") on left side of the heart

Severe acute myocardial ischemia and infarction

© Cengage Learning 2013

FIGURE 11-5 Process of Atherosclerosis

an illustration of the process of plaque formation and atherosclerosis. If this occurs in an artery of the brain, a stroke occurs. If it occurs in one of the coronary arteries, a heart attack occurs, demonstrated in Figure 11-6. Atherosclerotic plaque is the underlying cause of the three main types of cardiovascular disease—coronary artery disease, stroke, and peripheral vascular disease.

TYPES OF CARDIOVASCULAR DISEASES

There are several different types of heart disease. Coronary artery disease and heart failure are the most common and are the types generally referred to when one hears about "preventable" heart diseases. Although prevention is not possible in all cases, it has been well documented that a healthier lifestyle will positively impact the risk

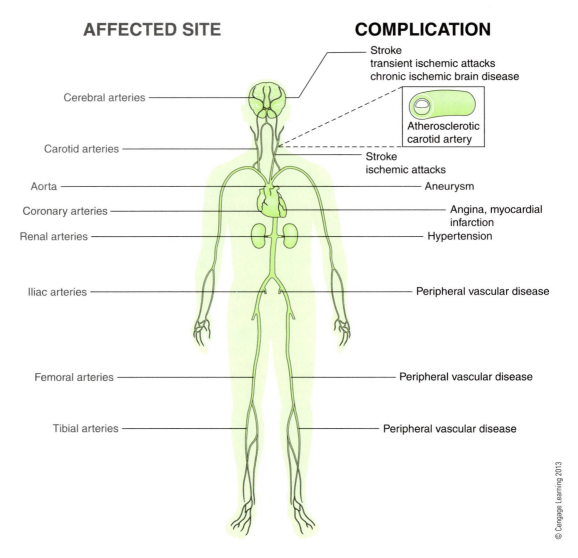

AFFECTED SITE

COMPLICATION

- Cerebral arteries — Stroke / transient ischemic attacks / chronic ischemic brain disease
- Atherosclerotic carotid artery
- Carotid arteries — Stroke / ischemic attacks
- Aorta — Aneurysm
- Coronary arteries — Angina, myocardial infarction
- Renal arteries — Hypertension
- Iliac arteries — Peripheral vascular disease
- Femoral arteries — Peripheral vascular disease
- Tibial arteries — Peripheral vascular disease

© Cengage Learning 2013

FIGURE 11-6 Areas Affected by Atherosclerosis

for these diseases. Other conditions, such as rheumatic heart disease, secondary to the well-known "strep throat," have no lifestyle changes that impact their progression. There are many other cardiovascular diseases that are not discussed in this section, but the purpose was to discuss those with the largest potential for prevention or those with special considerations.

Cardiac Diseases

This section will discuss cardiovascular diseases that primarily affect the heart and its blood vessels. There are multiple cardiac diseases, but only a few are discussed based on the frequency of occurrence and potential for prevention.

Coronary Artery Disease (CAD)

Coronary artery disease (CAD) or **coronary heart disease (CHD)** is the *most common type of heart disease* and causes about two-thirds of all deaths resulting from cardiovascular disease. It occurs when the coronary arteries that supply the heart muscle become stiffened and narrowed by atherosclerotic plaque. Blood flow and oxygen supply to the heart muscle are reduced or blocked with growing plaque. This causes **angina**, the most common symptom of coronary artery disease, which manifests as chest pain. There is a continuum of CHD such that the atherosclerosis in the coronary arteries can lead to heart attacks, heart failure, abnormal heart rhythms, and death.

Myocardial Infarction (MI)/ Cardiac Arrest

Over time chronic atherosclerosis can lead to a **heart attack**, also known as a **myocardial infarction (MI)**. This is caused when blood supply to the heart is severely reduced or completely blocked either by a chronically enlarging plaque or a plaque that ruptures and causes a blood clot that obstructs the artery. When heart cells do not receive enough oxygen, a section of the heart muscle becomes damaged or may die as shown in Figure 11-5. Less frequently, a heart attack can be caused by a spasm of a coronary artery, which also impedes blood supply to the heart muscle. Without treatment to restore flow, the heart muscle continues to die, causing irregular heart rhythms (arrhythmias) or sudden cardiac arrest and possible death. The ultimate degree of damage is determined by the area supplied by the particular artery that is blocked and how long before treatment is started. Sudden **cardiac arrest** is different from a heart attack in that it is total stoppage of all heart function and will result in death within 4-6 minutes if not treated. One-half of all deaths resulting from myocardial infarction occur within the first hour.

According to the *Heart Disease and Stroke Statistics 2011 Update*, there are an estimated 16,300,000 Americans over 20 years old with coronary heart disease. Total prevalence is 7.0% among all adults over 20 years old; 8.3% in men and 6.1% in women. By ethnicity, black men (7.9%) have the highest prevalence, followed by black women (7.6%), white men (7.0%), Mexican American men (6.3%), white women (6.1%), Mexican American women (5.6%), American Indians/Alaska Natives (4.1%), and Asian Americans (3.9%). In 2010, it was estimated that 785,000 Americans would have a new coronary attack of which about 470,000 would be a recurrent attack. An additional 195,000 will have a silent MI, or heart attack that is not recognized at the time it is occurring but evidence of a past attack shows up at a later examination. Women have similar incidence rates as men but about 10 years later. The age-adjusted coronary heart disease incidence rates (per 1,000 person-years) in persons 45–64 years old are highest in white men (12.5), followed by black men (10.6), black women (5.1), and white women (4.0). Age-adjusted incidence rates (per 1,000 population) of first MI were highest in black men, followed by white men (3.9), black women (2.8), and then white women (1.7).

As previously noted, cardiovascular disease is the number one killer of American adults, and coronary heart disease is the most common cardiovascular disease. An American will experience a coronary event approximately every 25 seconds, and

coronary artery disease (CAD)/coronary heart disease (CHD): the most common type of cardiovascular disease; occurs when the coronary arteries that supply the heart muscle become stiffened and narrowed by atherosclerotic plaque

angina: the most common symptom of coronary artery disease; caused by reduced blood supply to the heart muscle and manifested as chest pain

heart attack: also known as a "myocardial infarction (MI)"; caused when blood supply to the heart is severely reduced or completely blocked; the muscle cells do not receive enough oxygen and begin to die

myocardial infarction (MI): caused when blood supply to the heart is severely reduced or completely blocked; the muscle cells do not receive enough oxygen and begin to die; also known as a "heart attack"

cardiac arrest: total stoppage of all heart function

TABLE 11-5 Age-Adjusted Death Rates as a Result of CHD, United States, 2007

	Men	Women
Whites	165.6	94.2
Blacks	191.6	121.5
Hispanics	122.3	77.8
American Indians/ Alaska Natives	112.2	65.6
Asians/Pacific Islanders	91.7	55.0

Based on: American Heart Association; Heart Disease and Stroke Statistics—2011 Update: A Report from the American Heart Association published in *Circulation* 2011; 123; e18–e209 online (December 15, 2010): http://circ.ahajournals.org/cgi/reprint/CIR.0b013e3182009701

about every minute someone will die from one. One of every 6 deaths in the United States is caused by coronary heart disease. About 15% of those who have a MI will die from it. Annual death rates from CHD have been declining steadily since the mid-twentieth century, with almost half of that decline found to be secondary to improved medical management and another 44% was found to be attributable to changes in risk factors. The death rate as a result of CHD overall in 2007 was 126.0 per 100,000. To understand the differences of gender and ethnicity, see Table 11-5. Across all ethnicities, males had rates 57–75% higher than their female counterparts. In the past, women's lower death rates were thought to be a protective mechanism of estrogen, but studies using estrogen in men showed no difference in their mortality rates. Now research is looking to see if male hormones on their own increase the risk. Death rates by ethnicity were highest in blacks, followed by whites,

Check It Out

To assess your own risk for having a heart attack in the next 10 years, go to: http://www.heart.org

From the home page, click on "Conditions" and then "Heart Attack." The link for the risk assessment can be found there.

Hispanics, American Indians/Alaska Natives, and then Asians/Pacific Islanders for both men and women. It is not clear why prevalence rates and mortality rates are higher in black men and incidence rates are higher in white men.

Heart Failure

Heart failure is not complete failure of the heart but is said to occur when the heart muscle becomes ineffective at pumping enough blood and oxygen to meet the needs of the lungs and other body parts. It is most often because of damage to the left ventricle but may also occur as right-sided failure when there is lung disease or pulmonary artery disease. Failure may be acute such as happens when a portion of the muscle dies during a myocardial infarction, but it is more commonly a chronic disorder. Other medical conditions strongly associated with heart failure include coronary artery disease, hypertension, and diabetes, as well as others.

The incidence of heart failure is about 10 in 1,000 population after the age of 65 years old. This markedly increases with increased age. The rates in white women are about one-half of those in white men, but the rates in black women are only slightly less than those in black men. Over all, blacks had the highest risk of developing heart failure (4.6 per 1,000 person-years), followed by Hispanics (3.5 per 1,000 person-years), whites (2.4 per 1,000 person-years), and Asian Americans (1.0 per 1,000 person-years). The higher rates among certain ethnicities are reflective of differences in the prevalence of hypertension and diabetes, as well as socioeconomic status. The overall mortality rate is 85.4 per 100,000 population, or 1 in 9 deaths are related to heart failure. The gender and ethnicity differences for mortality are the same as those reported in relation to incidence.

Other Cardiac Diseases

Arrhythmias occur whenever there is a change in the normal electrical impulses of the heart that cause a change in the heartbeat and, therefore, a change in the heart's ability to pump blood effectively. Arrhythmias result when the normal pacemaker of the heart changes its rate, when the normal electrical conduction pathway is interrupted, or if another part of the heart takes over as pacemaker. Prior heart disease, certain medications, certain cardiac infections, and congenital heart defects may all be associated with a higher risk of developing an abnormal heart rate or rhythm.

Valvular disease is disease that affects any of the four major valves of the heart. It may be from stenosis or narrowing of the opening either naturally or from calcific narrowing or from loose valves that permit regurgitation of the blood instead of the normal forward propulsion. An example of valvular disease is rheumatic heart disease, a complication of "strep throat." Seen frequently in the United States and worldwide prior to the discovery of penicillin in the mid-1900s, rheumatic heart disease now occurs rarely in the United States but is still reported as a major problem in other parts of the world and considered a cardiovascular disease by WHO.

Congenital heart defects are malformations of the heart or large blood vessels that are present at birth. They are the most common type of major birth defects and are present in about 9 per 1,000 live births, resulting in about 36,000 cases each year. These vary from minor holes between two chambers that may close

heart failure: occurs when the heart muscle becomes ineffective at pumping enough blood and oxygen to meet the needs of the body

arrhythmia: a change in the normal electrical impulses of the heart that cause a change in rate or rhythm of the heart beat

valvular disease: disease that affects any of the four major valves of the heart

congenital heart defects: malformations of the heart or major blood vessels that are present at birth

spontaneously to severe heart defects that may require multiple major surgeries or be ultimately fatal. Because some heart defects are minor and not detected until later in life, calculating true prevalence and incidence data is difficult. Congenital heart defects are the most common cause of neonatal mortality as a result of birth defects. The majority of defects have no identifiable cause. The few causes that have been identified or are known to be associated with a higher risk of heart defects in the newborn include certain drugs (alcohol), certain maternal diseases (diabetes) or infections (rubella), and genetic syndromes (Down syndrome).

Vascular Diseases

hypertension: high blood pressure

blood pressure: a measurement of the force the circulating blood exerts on the arterial walls

systolic pressure: the pressure circulating blood exerts on the arterial walls when the heart is contracting

diastolic blood pressure: the pressure circulating blood exerts on the arterial walls when the heart is at rest

This section will discuss the two main vascular diseases that occur: hypertension and peripheral artery disease. Again, there are others, but these are the more common and most preventable. These diseases primarily affect the blood vessels but also have effects on the heart.

High Blood Pressure (HBP) or Hypertension

High blood pressure is also known as **hypertension**. **Blood pressure** is a measurement of the force the circulating blood exerts on the arterial walls. It is recorded as one number over another number, for example, 120/70. The number on the top is called the **systolic pressure**, or the pressure on the arterial walls when the heart is contracting. Ideally, systolic pressure is expected to be less than 120 mmHg. The number on the bottom is the **diastolic blood pressure**, or the pressure on the arterial walls after the contraction when the heart is at rest. Normal diastolic pressure is less than 80mmHg. A single blood pressure measurement is not as indicative as are serial readings at different times of day. See Table 11-6 for an interpretation of various blood pressure values.

TABLE 11-6 Interpretation of Blood Pressure Readings (in mmHg)

	Systolic	Diastolic
Normal Blood Pressure	< 120	< 80
Low Blood Pressure	< 90	< 60
Prehypertension	120-139	80-89
Mild High Blood Pressure	140-159	90-99
Moderate to Severe High Blood Pressure	≥ 160	≥ 100

Based on: Medline Plus—Blood Pressure: http://www.nlm.nih.gov/medlineplus/highbloodpressure.html

There are generally no physical symptoms from mild high blood pressure. Complications of untreated, long-standing disease or severe disease include coronary artery disease, heart failure, stroke, kidney failure, vision loss, erectile dysfunction, and others.

For the purpose of the following statistics, **high blood pressure (HBP)** is defined as systolic pressure above 140 and/or diastolic pressure above 90. About 1 in 3 persons, or 29% of American adults, have high blood pressure, but an additional 8% of adults have undiagnosed hypertension. About 77% of persons with their first stroke have high blood pressure, as well as 69% with their first heart attack, and 74% with their first episode of heart failure. Up to 45 years of age, more men have HBP than women. From 45–64 years old, men and women have similar rates, but after 65 years old, a higher percentage of women have HBP. Black Americans have the highest prevalence rates in the world for HBP, and it is still increasing. Blacks develop HBP earlier in life and have higher blood pressures than their white counterparts and, therefore, have a 1–4 times greater rate of the various complications of HBP. The death rate for HBP in 2007 was 17.8 per 100,000 population. The financial costs associated with HBP for 2007 were $43.5 billion.

Peripheral Artery Disease (PAD)

Peripheral artery disease (PAD) is caused by atherosclerotic plaque that occurs in the peripheral arteries, primarily those of the legs and or pelvis. See Figure 11-6. It can also involve arteries to the arms, kidneys, stomach, and male genitalia. It is similar to coronary artery disease that occurs in the heart and cerebrovascular disease of the brain.

Symptoms of PAD are vague and include cramping, pain, or leg fatigue that resolve with rest and can be easily misdiagnosed. Smoking is a primary risk factor for PAD with others being high blood pressure, diabetes, and high cholesterol. These are all also the major risk factors for atherosclerosis. Lack of treatment may lead to gangrene of a limb. It is not surprising that persons with PAD have a higher risk of having coronary heart disease, myocardial infarctions, and stroke—other diseases associated with atherosclerosis.

Peripheral artery disease affects about 8 million persons in the United States, and its prevalence increases with age. In persons over 65 years of age, approximately

high blood pressure (HBP): defined as systolic pressure above 140 and diastolic pressure above 90

peripheral artery disease (PAD): caused by atherosclerotic plaque that occurs in the peripheral arteries (arteries distal to the main arteries such as the aorta), primarily those of the legs and or pelvis

Check It Out

To assess your own risk for high blood pressure, go to: http://www.heart.org

From the home page, click on "Conditions" and then "High Blood Pressure." The link for the risk assessment can be found there under "Related Tools"—"HBP Risk Calculator."

12–20% are affected. Because the symptoms are so vague, about 20–30% of persons with PAD are not on appropriate medical treatment despite its significant risk of other cardiovascular diseases and increased risk of mortality. Men and women have similar prevalence rates. Blacks are much more likely to have PAD than whites or Hispanics, with the prevalence in Hispanics similar to or slightly higher than in whites.

Cerebrovascular Accident (CVA) or Stroke

Cerebrovascular *disease* is the underlying atherosclerosis that affects the vessels that supply the brain. **Cerebrovascular accident (CVA)** or **stroke** is caused by a sudden impairment of cerebral (brain) circulation. This may be the result of local bleeding into brain tissue from a weakened blood vessel, known as a **hemorrhagic stroke**, or the result of a blood clot that causes obstruction to cerebral blood flow, known as an **ischemic stroke**. Ischemic stroke is the most common type and accounts for about 85% of all strokes. Stroke is to cerebrovascular disease as a myocardial infarction is to cardiovascular disease—a potentially catastrophic event as the result of atherosclerosis. Hemorrhagic stroke is commonly a result of hypertension in local aneurysms or vessel malformations. A blood vessel ruptures and blood accumulates and compresses the surrounding brain tissue. See Figure 11-7 for examples of each type of stroke.

cerebrovascular accident (CVA): caused by a sudden impairment of cerebral circulation; also called a "stroke"

stroke: caused by a sudden impairment of cerebral circulation; also known as a "cerebrovascular accident"

hemorrhagic stroke: a stroke caused by local bleeding into brain tissue from a weakened blood vessel

ischemic stroke: a stroke resulting from a blood clot that causes obstruction to cerebral blood flow

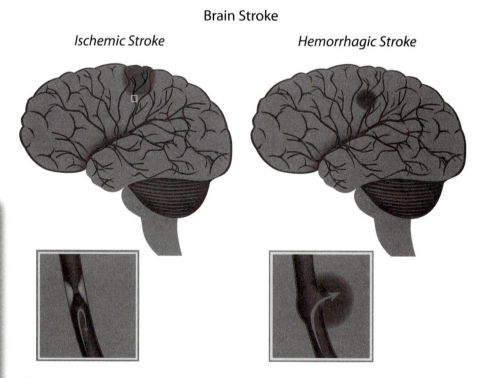

Brain Stroke

Ischemic Stroke   *Hemorrhagic Stroke*

Blockage of blood vessels; lack of blood flow to affected area   Rupture of blood vessels; leakage of blood

FIGURE 11-7 Types of Stroke
© Alila Sao Mai/www.Shutterstock.com

On occasion there is a clot that causes temporary obstruction lasting only minutes to a few hours. This is called a **transient ischemic attack (TIA)** or mini-stroke.

Although the symptoms may be only temporary, the warning signs must be taken seriously. Whatever the cause of the stroke, the interruption of blood flow and oxygen supply to the brain causes serious damage and death of brain cells. Stroke is the fourth leading cause of death in the United States and the most common cause of neurologic disabilities. Specific epidemiologic statistics were discussed in the Scope of the Problem section.

> **transient ischemic attack (TIA):** a clot that causes temporary obstruction in the brain causing symptoms that last only minutes to a few hours; also called a "mini-stroke"

RISK FACTORS AND PREVENTION

When looking at the implementation of prevention strategies, one must consider whether the risk factor has the potential for intervention. As mentioned in Chapter 1, modifiable risk factors are those that can be changed or eradicated with lifestyle changes; therefore, there is potential for decreasing the amount of disease attributable to that risk factor. For example, if all smokers were to stop smoking, about 80% of lung cancer deaths in women and 90% of these deaths in men could be prevented. Other examples of modifiable risk factors include diet, alcohol use, obesity, and physical activity. Nonmodifiable risk factors are those that cannot be changed or eradicated to impact the likelihood of later disease. The most common nonmodifiable risk factors include gender, age, genetics, or family history. There are additional risk factors that may be partially modifiable and may improve with lifestyle changes but cannot be completely eradicated. Examples of partially modifiable risk factors include high blood pressure that can be lowered with lifestyle changes or medications, diabetes mellitus that can be controlled with medications and diet, and high cholesterol that can be moderated with diet and medications.

Risk Factors for Cardiovascular Diseases

The specific risk factors listed for the most common cardiovascular diseases—coronary artery disease, heart failure, hypertension, peripheral artery disease, and stroke—are similar and interrelated. Some are also important risk factors for other diseases. For this reason, three of the major modifiable risk factors (physical inactivity, obesity, and tobacco use) are discussed in more detail in "A Closer Look" at the end of this chapter and in Chapters 12 and 13.

Physical Inactivity

Physical inactivity is not only important on its own as a risk factor, but it also has an impact on other risk factors such as obesity, hypertension, high triglycerides, and diabetes. The recommendation for children 6–17 years of age is for 60 minutes of moderate to vigorous physical activity per day. For adults 18 and up, the recommendation is for 2 hours and 30 minutes of moderate-intensity activity per week and muscle strengthening at least 2 days a week. The relative risk of coronary artery disease associated with physical inactivity is 1.5–2.4. Physical inactivity is the risk factor discussed in "A Closer Look" at the end of this chapter. Please refer to this section for more details.

Obesity

Obesity is not based on weight alone, but on a body mass index (BMI) that is also dependent on height. A BMI greater than 30 is considered obese. Obesity puts an extra strain on the heart to pump the blood and increases blood pressure. And although it is a risk factor on its own, obesity is also linked to higher cholesterol and triglyceride levels, as well as to diabetes, hypertension, and coronary artery disease. Please refer to "A Closer Look" at the end of Chapter 13, Diabetes Mellitus, for details.

Diet

Diets high in saturated fats and cholesterol promote atherosclerosis and obesity. Diets high in salt (sodium) raise blood pressure. Unrefined whole grain foods and oily fish that contain omega-3 fatty acids have been shown to lower cholesterol. Fruits and vegetables with fewer calories help maintain a healthy weight to prevent obesity and control blood pressure.

High Blood Pressure

Hypertension was discussed as a cardiovascular disease, but it is also considered an independent risk factor for cardiovascular disease and stroke. High blood pressure is defined as systolic pressure above 140 and/or diastolic pressure above 90. It is considered a partially modifiable risk factor in that it may be partly the result of genetics and partly the result of lifestyle choices. The interrelationship with obesity and physical inactivity has already been discussed. When blood pressure is lowered with the use of medications and/or lifestyle changes, the risk of developing heart disease is lowered.

Cigarette Smoking

Tobacco use, including exposure to secondhand smoke, promotes atherosclerosis, increases levels of blood clotting factors, raises blood pressure, raises carbon monoxide, and reduces the amount of oxygen that the blood can carry. It is discussed in some detail in "A Closer Look" at the end of Chapter 12, Cancer. One year after someone quits smoking, the risk of artery disease is half the risk of an active smoker. After 5 years, the risk of stroke is markedly decreased; and after 15 years, the risk of coronary artery disease is the same as a nonsmoker.

High Cholesterol

cholesterol: a waxy, fat-like substance needed by the body in certain quantities

low-density lipoproteins (LDL): make up the majority of the cholesterol circulating in the body; also known as the "bad cholesterol" because high levels are responsible for atherosclerosis

Cholesterol is a waxy, fat-like substance that is needed by the body in certain quantities for the production of cell membranes, hormones, vitamin D, and bile acids. It is produced by the body in the liver (1,000 mg/day) and consumed in the diet (200-500 mg/day). Excess cholesterol is deposited in arteries as plaque leading to atherosclerosis and narrowing of the arterial lumen. Cholesterol is carried in the blood by lipoproteins. **Low-density lipoproteins (LDL)**, the majority of cholesterol, are known as the "bad cholesterol" because when levels are high, these are the cholesterol particles that deposit under the arterial endothelium to produce plaque.

High-density lipoproteins (HDL) carry cholesterol back to the liver to be removed from the body, and high levels are protective from cardiovascular disease and stroke. An easy way to remember which is which is: "H"DL is "H"appy cholesterol because it does a good job and "L"DL is "L"ousy cholesterol because it is bad for the body. Triglycerides are another form of fat made in the body and often found elevated when cholesterol levels are high.

Current recommendations are for all adults over 20 years old and children at risk because of personal medical history or with a significant family history to have a fasting lipid panel every 5 years. This panel checks for several lipids—total cholesterol, HDL, LDL, and triglycerides. Desired levels are shown in Table 11-7. HDL levels can be lowered (not a good thing!) by smoking, obesity, physical inactivity, high triglycerides, progesterone, testosterone, and anabolic steroids. Estrogen actually raises HDL levels. LDL levels are increased by diet and in people who are obese. Triglyceride levels are increased in obesity, excess alcohol consumption, diets high in carbohydrates, physical inactivity, and obesity. They can also be elevated as part of a genetic condition.

Approximately 16% of all American adults have high total cholesterol levels (defined as > 240mg/dL), or almost 1 in 6 adults. More women (16.9%) than men (15.6%) have high levels. The percentage of men with high cholesterol peaks in the 45–54-year-olds (20.8%) before beginning a decline and in the 55–64-year-olds for women (30.5%). In men, Mexican American men (17.7%) have the highest levels, followed by white men (16.0%) and then black men (11.2%). For women, white women (17.9%) have the highest levels, followed by Mexican American women (13.8%) who have levels only slightly higher than black women (13%).

> **high-density lipoproteins (HDL):** carry cholesterol back to the liver to be removed from the body; high levels are protective from cardiovascular disease and stroke

Diabetes Mellitus

Diabetes mellitus is discussed in detail in Chapter 13, Diabetes Mellitus. Like hypertension, diabetes is considered a partially modifiable risk factor in that it is partly the result of genetics and partly the result of lifestyle choices. There is also an interrelationship between diabetes and high blood pressure and high cholesterol. Seventy-five percent of those with diabetes will die from heart disease.

Table 11-8 shows the prevalence of these major risk factors for cardiovascular diseases and the relative risk each factor is associated with among adults in the United States.

TABLE 11-7 Optimal Levels of Various Lipids

Lipid	Desired Levels (mg/dL)
Total Cholesterol	< 200
Low-Density Lipoprotein (LDL)	< 100
High-Density Lipoprotein (HDL)	≥ 40 (men) ≥ 50 (women)
Triglycerides	< 150

© Cengage Learning 2013

TABLE 11-8 Risk Factors in American Adults, 2006

Risk Factor	% American Adults with This Risk Factor	Increased Relative Risk for CHD
Physical Inactivity	39.5%	1.5-2.4
Obesity	33.9%	na
High Blood Pressure	30.5%	1.7-2.1
Cigarette Smoking	20.8%	2-3
High Cholesterol	15.6%	1.3-2.6
Diabetes	10.1%	2-4

na = not available

Based on: Centers for Disease Control and Prevention; Stroke Facts: http://www.cdc.gov/stroke/facts.htm; and American Heart Disease—*Circulation,*1998; 97:1837-1847: http://circ.ahajournals.org/cgi/content/full/97/18/1837#T3

Other Risk Factors

Other risk factors that increase the risk for developing cardiovascular disease or stroke include increasing age, male gender, black race, and a family history of high lipids, cardiovascular disease, and/or stroke. These are nonmodifiable but make screening for these diseases at medical evaluations extremely important. Even though disease in the persons with these risk factors may not be preventable, early recognition leads to decreased morbidity (occurrence and complications of the disease) and possibly mortality (death from the disease).

Strategies for Preventing Cardiovascular Diseases

Of importance to remember is that although most of the cardiovascular diseases and stroke discussed occur in adults, the process of atherosclerosis begins in childhood. With the recent trend of increasing obesity in children and adolescents, preventive strategies must be directed at the younger U.S. population, as well as at the older. Given the modifiable risk factors, one can deduce the aims for preventive measures:

1. *Prevent and control high blood cholesterol.* Although genetics can be the cause of high cholesterol, this strategy will help even those persons minimize their risks. A diet low in saturated fat and cholesterol and high in fiber is helpful, as is maintaining a healthy weight and participating in regular moderate to vigorous physical activity. Screening when indicated is helpful to identify those persons in whom intervention with medications and diet is likely to help.

2. *Prevent and control high blood pressure.* Lifestyle changes such as a healthy diet, regular physical activity, and maintenance of a healthy weight are the mainstay of prevention. Not smoking is a major preventive measure, and current smokers can even decrease their risk by quitting. When indicated, the use of medications may be used to lower blood pressure that is still elevated after the above measures have been instituted.

3. *Prevent and control diabetes, when present.* Lifestyle changes with weight loss and increased physical activity may help control diabetes, and in prediabetes, these changes may also delay or prevent onset of the disease. Medications are usually indicated for control as well.

4. *No tobacco use.* Not only does this impact blood pressure, but smoking itself increases the risk for heart disease and stroke.

5. *Moderate alcohol use.* Excessive use of alcoholic beverages increases the risk of high blood pressure, heart attack, and stroke.

6. *Maintain a healthy weight.* Maintaining a body mass index (BMI) in the normal range (18-25) can decrease the risk of cardiovascular disease and stroke, as well as impact the risk factors of diabetes and high blood pressure. This should begin in childhood for its best results.

7. *Regular physical activity.* A moderate level of physical activity for at least 30 minutes for most days of the week will decrease the risk of cardiovascular disease and stroke, as well as improve other risk factors such as obesity, diabetes, and hypertension. This should begin in childhood.

8. *Diet and nutrition.* This is a major intervention that should begin in childhood with increasing fruits and vegetables to the diet, as well as avoiding added salt to foods, and minimizing intake of saturated fats and cholesterol.

Increase Survival Rates with Cardiopulmonary Resuscitation

cardiopulmonary resuscitation (CPR): the method of doing chest compressions and rescue breathing to resuscitate a person who has had a heart attack

Although not a technique that *prevents* cardiovascular disease, bystander **cardiopulmonary resuscitation (CPR)**, the intervention of rescue breathing and chest compressions, has been shown to increase survival from heart attacks. Communities that routinely promote the training of its members in CPR have found improved survival rates.

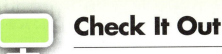

Check It Out

For a personalized nutritional plan, go to: http://www. choosemyplate.gov/ This plan has been promoted by First Lady Michelle Obama and replaces the previous nutritional "pyramid."

Check It Out

To assess your long-term heart health and receive a plan to maintain heart health, go to: http://mylifecheck. heart.org/

Changes recommended by the American Heart Association in 2010 have changed the order of performing CPR steps from the traditional order of "A, B, C" or "Airway, Breathing, Chest Compressions" to "C, A, B" or "Chest Compressions, Airway, Breathing" based on newer studies. It is also hoped that this change will encourage more bystanders to intervene knowing that even chest compressions alone are better than no intervention at all. The median survival rate of out-of-hospital heart attacks is 7.9%, and about 70% of all cardiac deaths occur out of hospital. It is not surprising that bystander CPR can have an impact on mortality from heart disease. See the "Website Resources" section at the end of this chapter to find out how to obtain training in CPR.

THE FUTURE

The Framingham Heart Study has been instrumental in identifying the major risk factors of cardiovascular disease, but lifestyle changes have been slow to follow. A major focus of ongoing efforts in the prevention of cardiovascular disease and stroke is on public education. American people are now being educated on the nutritional contents of foods bought in the grocery store, as well as those in fast-food facilities and restaurants. Awareness of the fat, salt, and caloric intakes of foods has been shown to be effective in changing behavior. The *Go Red for Women* program of the American Heart Association is focusing on public recognition of the different symptoms experienced by women with cardiovascular disease to effect stabilization of the rates of disease in women. The Framingham Heart Study is ongoing and now looking more at the genetic component of heart disease and stroke.

Research being conducted by the National Institute of Neurological Disorders and Stroke (NINDS) at the National Institute of Health is focusing on the genetics of stroke and stroke risk factors. In addition, as the process of brain damage resulting from stroke is better understood, new and better ways to help the brain repair itself to restore important functions are being addressed. Advances in imaging and rehabilitation have shown the brain can compensate for some of these lost functions.

Summary

Cardiovascular diseases are the leading cause of death in the United States, and coronary heart disease is the most common cardiovascular disease. Stroke is the fourth leading cause of death of Americans. Combined, they also account for a significant amount of morbidity and cost this country billions of health care dollars each year. In this chapter, the prevalence, incidence, and mortality differences based on gender, ethnicity, and age were discussed. Atherosclerotic plaque is the common underlying cause among several of the cardiovascular diseases. Several representative heart and vascular conditions, as well as stroke, were discussed for a basic understanding of the disease. The risk factors for CVD were discussed with emphasis on the modifiable risk factors that are the focus of preventive strategies and public health policy.

A Closer Look

Risk Factors—Physical Activity

physical activity: refers to any bodily movement produced by the contraction of skeletal muscle that increases energy expenditure

exercise: a subcategory of physical activity that is planned, structured, and repetitive

physical fitness: includes health-related aspects such as cardiorespiratory fitness, muscular strength and endurance, body composition, flexibility, and balance

aerobic exercise: includes activities that improve cardiorespiratory capacity and endurance

moderate intensity: includes activities that cause some increase in breathing or heart rate such as walking

vigorous intensity: includes activities that cause large increases in breathing or heart rate such as running

metabolic equivalent (MET): refers to a way to classify physical activities by their intensity of energy expenditure, with sitting at rest equal to 1 MET

sedentary: refers to individuals who do not obtain enough physical activity to achieve health benefits

The field of physical activity epidemiology is emerging because of the profound effects this behavior has on health and longevity. There are a few definitions that are important to understand when delving into this field.

First of all, **physical activity** refers to any bodily movement produced by muscle contraction that increases energy expenditure. Often it is used synonymously with the term **exercise**, which is a planned, structured, and repetitive activity designed to improve some aspect of **physical fitness**, which includes health-related aspects such as cardiorespiratory fitness, muscular strength and endurance, body composition, flexibility, and balance. The term **aerobic exercise** is often used to mean the target of the activity is to improve the cardiorespiratory system.

The energy expenditure of an activity is usually converted to an intensity level by type of activity or by self-reported effort. **Moderate intensity** activities include those that cause some increase in breathing or heart rate such as walking, whereas **vigorous intensity** activities include those that cause large increases in breathing or heart rate such as running. To obtain more detail, specific activities can be converted into **metabolic equivalents (METs)** where sitting at rest is equal to 1 MET. It is common to convert types of physical activities to METs using a standard compendium (Ainsworth et al., 2011).

And, finally, the term for people who are not physically active enough to obtain health benefits is **sedentary**. For surveillance issues and for providing recommendations to the general public, it is often easier to use self-report effort measures, combined with examples of the activities that generate the appropriate level, than to specify MET levels.

Continues

Background

Although it is now known that physical inactivity is an important risk factor for cardiovascular disease, research into the health effects of physical activity did not start in a formal way until the middle of the twentieth century. The early studies consisted primarily of occupational studies. One of the first of these was conducted in London among bus drivers. It was documented that the bus drivers had higher occurrences of cardiovascular events than conductors. Bus drivers sat all day, but conductors collected fares and were constantly moving around and climbing to the upper levels of the double-decked buses to collect fares. The early studies on physical activity and heart disease were based on occupational groups, and very little was known about the general population. Because it was believed that heart disease was not a problem for women, most early studies focused on men.

Several studies and consensus reports were published in the early 1990s, and it soon became clear that physical activity was a critical component of a healthy lifestyle and its benefits could be felt among children and adults throughout the life span (Pate et al., 1995). By 1996, with the publication of the first Surgeon General's Report on Physical Activity and Health, physical inactivity was viewed as an important a risk factor for cardiovascular disease (leading cause of death) as high blood pressure or high cholesterol (U.S. DHHS, 1996). Consequences of physical inactivity over time include inability to maintain a healthy weight, reduced cardiorespiratory fitness, reduced insulin resistance (leading to diabetes), muscle degeneration, and functional decline.

How Much Physical Activity Is Enough?

The minimal amount of physical activity needed to achieve health benefits is 20 minutes of high intensity activity (such as running) at least 3 times a week. For lower intensity activity (such as walking), the minimal level needed is 30 minutes at least 5 days a week. Any activity over these amounts increases the health benefits, but in previous guidelines there was no mention of combining moderate and vigorous activity counts.

Because of the importance of physical activity and the changing status of the measurement of physical activity, a consensus conference was held in 2008 to update physical activity guidelines (US DHHS, 2008). Based on these updated guidelines, adults should receive approximately 75 minutes per week of high (vigorous) intensity physical activity, or 180 minutes per week of lower (moderate) intensity physical activity, or a combination of both. The consensus group also acknowledged the importance of muscle strengthening activities. Details are shown in Table 11-9.

Epidemiology of Physical Activity

As with any other risk factor, it is important to know the prevalence, or who has the risk factor. Using data from the National Health Interview Survey, Figure 11-8 shows the prevalence of aerobic activity among U.S. adults from 1998-2009. As can be seen, there has been an increase in the overall prevalence of physical activity from 40% in 1998 to 47% in 2009 (Carlson et al., 2010). All numbers are age-adjusted to the 2000 population. Even though these percentages are moving in the right direction, in 2009, 20% of adults were not active enough to achieve health benefits, and 33% of adults reported no physical activity at all.

Adults

Overall, men report more activity than women, younger people report more activity than older people, and whites report more activity than other racial/ethnic groups that are similar. Education is a strong correlate of physical activity, with increases in each category of education. In Figures 11-9, 11-10, and 11-11, the data are shown for each of these

TABLE 11-9 Recommended Levels of Physical Activity Based on the 2008 Physical Activity Guidelines Project

Aerobic Activities

If you choose activities at a moderate level, do at least 2 hours and 30 minutes a week (180 minutes).

If you choose vigorous activities, do at least 1 hour and 15 minutes a week (75 minutes).

1. Slowly build up the amount of time you do physical activities. The more time you spend, the more health benefits you gain. Aim for twice the recommended levels shown for moderate or vigorous activities.

2. Do at least 10 minutes at a time.

3. You can combine moderate and vigorous activities.

Muscle-Strengthening Activities

Do these at least 2 days a week.

1. Exercises for each muscle group should be repeated 8 to 12 times per session.

2. Include all the major muscle groups such as legs, hips, back, chest, stomach, shoulders, and arms.

Based on: http://www.health.gov/PAGuidelines/factSheetAdults.aspx

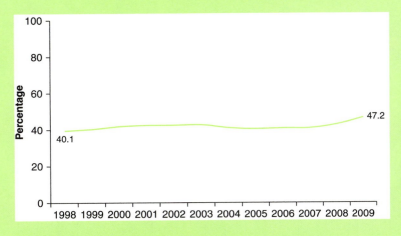

FIGURE 11-8 Trends in Meeting 2008 Aerobic Physical Activity Guidelines among U.S. Adults, 1998–2009
Based on: http://www.cdc.gov/nchs/ppt/nchs2010/06_Schoenborn.pdf

Continues

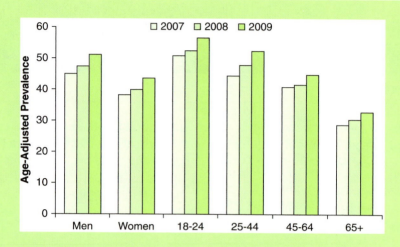

FIGURE 11-9 Trends in Meeting 2008 Aerobic Physical Activity Guidelines among U.S. Adults, by Sex and Age, 2007–2009
Based on: http://www.cdc.gov/nchs/ppt/nchs2010/06_Schoenborn.pdf

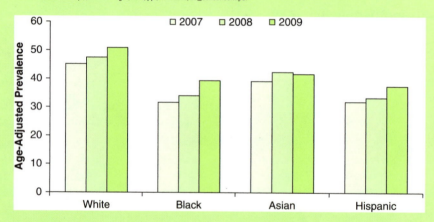

FIGURE 11-10 Trends in Meeting 2008 Aerobic Physical Activity Guidelines among U.S. Adults, by Race/Ethnicity, 2007–2009
Based on: http://www.cdc.gov/nchs/ppt/nchs2010/06_Schoenborn.pdf

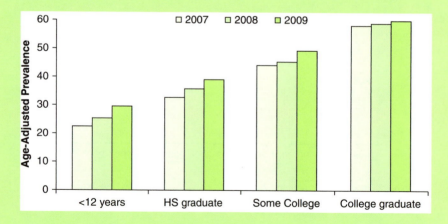

FIGURE 11-11 Trends in Meeting 2008 Aerobic Physical Activity Guidelines among U.S. Adults, by Education, 2007–2009
Based on: http://www.cdc.gov/nchs/ppt/nchs2010/06_Schoenborn.pdf

demographic groups over a three-year period (2007–2009) using the 2008 guidelines for aerobic physical activity. These demographic trends have been consistent for the years 2007–2009 in spite of slight increases in total physical activity. All figures are age-adjusted to the 2000 population.

Youth

The recommended amount of physical activity for children and adolescents is 60 minutes per day (US DHHS, 2008). Participation in physical activity declines as people age. According to data from the Centers for Disease Control and Prevention (http://www.cdc.gov/), 18% of high school students had participated in at least 60 minutes per day of physical activity on each of the 7 days before the survey. The percentage of high school students who attended physical education classes daily decreased from 42% in 1991 to 33% in 2009. In 2009, 47% of 9th grade students, but only 22% of 12th grade students, attended physical education class daily.

   Encouraging youth to become active should occur in schools and home settings. Unfortunately, with budget cuts in the early 1990s, one of the school programs cut was physical education. Sometimes even when physical education classes are present in a curriculum, the lack of coaches or equipment means the class may include listening to health messages, rather than being physically active. Because of this, many school children must obtain all of their activity after school or by participating in organized sports. Consequences of physical inactivity during adolescence can include inability to control weight. Physically inactive adolescents are on track to becoming physically inactive adults.

Going Forward

The need to be physically active has been slowly engineered out of daily life for most Americans. Jobs that once required physical movement are now done by machines (examples include warehouse work, manufacturing, what else?). Safety issues prevent walking in neighborhoods, especially after dark, and are reasons that parents drive children to school rather than letting them walk or bike. Time spent outside of work and school is often used to pursue sedentary activities (for example: using computers, watching television, handheld games, others?). As a result of these lifestyle changes most people have to create ways to be active and incorporate those strategies into their busy lives. Solutions to increasing physical activity prevalence can be most effective if they are based on individual behaviors, along with supportive environmental and policy changes.

Individual Behavior Change

Behavior change is difficult to achieve. Some short-term success (one year) in increasing levels of physical activity has been found with behavioral therapies that include goal setting and monitoring. Although many people know the value of being physically active, it is easy to find barriers or reasons that prevent physical activity. The barriers often cited can include things such as lack of time, motivation, safe venues, equipment, and childcare. These can be categorized as physical barriers (access to equipment and safe venues) or psychological (motivation) or biological (injuries or other limitations) or scheduling (lack of time or childcare). Because behavioral strategies need to be targeted to the individual, it is sometimes important to use a "stages of change" approach. In this model, individuals are categorized as to their readiness to make positive changes. This involves assessing where a person is on a continuum from not wanting to think about changing physical activity behaviors to wanting to make changes but needing help in removing personal barriers or deciding how to start.

Continues

Impact of Environmental/Policy Changes

Many of the barriers people cite as impeding physical activity changes involve access issues. Because of this, a strong environmental and policy approach may be required to effect change in this behavior. Examples of environmental interventions could include designing cities such that neighborhoods are walkable (sidewalks, streetlights) and are mixed-use (stores and services interspersed with living units), with public transportation that is available and affordable. Examples of policy changes that have been successful in removing barriers to physical activity include worksite policies that provide exercise facilities on-site and dedicated time to exercise, and policies that keep school playgrounds open after school hours for community use.

Review Questions

1. The most common type of heart disease in the United States is:
   a. Atherosclerosis
   b. Angina
   c. Coronary heart disease
   d. Rheumatic heart disease

2. **True or False** Men are more likely than women to have coronary heart disease because estrogen is protective.

3. The two ethnic groups at greatest risk for cardiovascular and cerebrovascular diseases are: (Circle two.)
   a. Hispanic Americans
   b. African Americans
   c. Asian Americans
   d. Caucasians

4. The "good cholesterol" is _____. (HDL or LDL)

5. **True or False** Atherosclerosis is an underlying process involved in the majority of cases of both stroke and coronary artery disease.

6. List three prevention strategies for cardiovascular disease and stroke.

   1. _____
   2. _____
   3. _____

7. Which of the following statements regarding stroke is NOT true?

   a. The two types of stroke are hemorrhagic and ischemic.
   b. The risk factors for stroke are the same as those for cardiovascular disease.
   c. The incidence of stroke is higher in men than women.
   d. Stroke is the fourth leading cause of death in the United States.

8. **True or False** The Framingham Heart Study begun in 1948 has been responsible for identifying the major risk factors that contributed to heart disease.

9. **True or False** High blood pressure is not only a cardiovascular disease in itself, but it is also a risk factor for other CVD and stroke.

10. The recommendations for physical activity for adults is:

    a. 2 1/2 hours of moderate activity per week
    b. 1 hour and 15 minutes of vigorous activity per week
    c. Muscle strengthening 2 days a week
    d. Both a and b
    e. All of the above

11. **For Deeper Thought** Design a study that would assess the presence of risk factors for cardiovascular disease among your classmates. Determine the type of study, how you would collect the information needed, what data you would want to collect, and what rates/ratios you would use to assess your data. Use the Framingham Heart Study and the Nurse's Health Study as resources.

Website Resources

American Heart Association: http://www.heart.org

American Heart Association/American Stroke Association: http://www.strokeassociation.org

American Heart Association; Go Red for Women: http://www.goredforwomen.org

American Heart Association: Heart Disease and Stroke Statistics—2011 Update: http://circ.ahajournals.org

Centers for Disease Control and Protection: http://cdc.gov

Framingham Heart Study: http://www.framinghamheartstudy.org

NHIS Physical Activity Information Website: http://www.cdc.gov

National Heart Lung and Blood Institute: http://www.nhlbi.nih.gov

National Institute of Neurological Disorders and Stroke (NINDS), National Institute of Health: http://www.ninds.nih.gov

United States Department of Agriculture (USDA) (modified February 22, 2011); My Pyramid: http://www.mypyramid.gov

For CPR (Cardiopulmonary Resuscitation) training:

Online CPR Training through the American Heart Association: http://www.onlineaha.org/ OR to find a class near you: http://www.heart.org

References

Ainsworth, B. E., Haskell, W. L., Herrmann, S. D., Meckes, N., Bassett, D. R. Jr, Tudor-Locke, C., Greer, J. L., Vezina, J., Whitt-Glover, M. C., & Leon, A. S. (2011). Compendium of Physical Activities: A second update of codes and MET values. *Medicine and Science in Sports and Exercise, 43*(8) ,1575–1581.

American Heart Association. Heart Disease and Stroke Statistics—2011 Update: A Report from the American Heart Association published in *Circulation, 123,* e18-e209 online (December 15, 2010). Retrieved from http://circ.ahajournals.org/cgi/reprint/CIR.0b013e3182009701

American Heart Association. (n.d.). Statistical Fact Sheet, 2010 Update—Populations. Retrieved from http://www.americanheart.org/presenter.jhtml?identifier=2011

American Heart Association. (updated March 3, 2011). Understand Your Risk for Congenital Heart Defects. Retrieved from http://www.heart.org/HEARTORG/Conditions/CongenitalHeartDefects/UnderstandYourRiskforCongenitalHeartDefects/Understand-Your-Risk-for-Congenital-Heart-Defects_UCM_001219_Article.jsp

American Heart Association. (updated January 20, 2011). Peripheral Artery Disease. Retrieved from http://www.heart.org/HEARTORG/Conditions/More/PeripheralArteryDisease/About-Peripheral-Artery-Disease-PAD_UCM_301301_Article.jsp

American Heart Association. (updated March 14, 2011). Smoke-Free Living: Benefits & Milestones. Retrieved from http://www.heart.org/HEARTORG/GettingHealthy/QuitSmoking/QuittingSmoking/Smoke-free-Living-Benefits-Milestones_UCM_322711_Article.jsp

Carlson, S. A., Fulton, J. E., Schoenborn, C. A., & Loustalot, F. (2010, October).Trend and prevalence estimates based on the 2008 Physical Activity Guidelines for Americans. *American Journal of Preventative Medicine, 39*(4), 305–313.

Centers for Disease Control and Prevention. (updated January 28, 2010). Stroke: Stroke Facts. Retrieved from http://www.cdc.gov/stroke/facts.htm

Centers for Disease Control and Prevention. (updated February 9, 2010). Cholesterol—Facts. Retrieved from http://www.cdc.gov/cholesterol/facts.htm

Framingham Heart Study. (updated January 11, 2011). About the Framingham Heart Study. Retrieved from http://www.framinghamheartstudy.org/about/index.html

Framingham Heart Study. (updated January 11, 2011). History of the Framingham Heart Study. Retrieved from http://www.framinghamheartstudy.org/about/history.html

Framingham Heart Study. (updated January 11, 2011). Research Milestones. Retrieved from http://www.framinghamheartstudy.org/about/milestones.html

Medline Plus. (updated March 28, 2011). Blood Pressure. Retrieved from http://www.nlm.nih.gov/medlineplus/ency/article/003398.htm

National Heart Lung and Blood Institute. (Fiscal Year 2009). NHLBI Factbook, Section 4. Disease Statistics. Retrieved from http://www.nhlbi.nih.gov/about/factbook/chapter4.htm

Pate, R. R., Pratt, M., Blair, S. N., Haskell, W. L., Macera, C. A., Bouchard, C., Buchner, D., Ettinger, W., Heath, G. W., King, A. C., Kriska, A., Leon, A. S., Marcus, B. H., Morris, J., Paffenbarger, R., Patrick, K., Pollock, M. L., Rippe, J. M., Sallis, J., & Wilmore, J. H. (1995). Physical activity and public health: A recommendation from the Centers for Disease Control and Prevention and American College of Sports Medicine. *Journal of the American Medical Association, 273*, 402–407.

U.S. Department of Health and Human Services. (1996). *Physical activity and health: A report of the Surgeon General.* Atlanta, GA: U.S. Department of Health and Human Services. Centers for Disease Control and Prevention, National Center for Chronic Disease Prevention and Health Promotion.

U.S. Department of Health and Human Services. (2008). *Physical activity guidelines for Americans.* Retrieved from http://www.health.gov/paguidelines/guidelines/summary.aspx

World Health Organization. (September 2011). Media Centre—Cardiovascular Diseases, Fact Sheet N317. Retrieved from http://www.who.int/mediacentre/factsheets/fs317/en/index.html

Chapter 12

CANCER

Learning Objectives

Upon completion of this chapter, you should be able to:

1. Discuss two primary differences between cancer cells and normal cells.
2. List three external risk factors associated with cancer.
3. Give two examples of vaccines that are being used to prevent cancer.
4. Name the five most commonly occurring cancers (in men and women combined).
5. Name the three most deadly cancers in men and the three most deadly cancers in women.

Key Terms

adenocarcinoma

alternative therapy

basal cell carcinoma

benign

bone marrow stem cell transplants

BRAC1 and BRAC2 genes

cancer

carcinogen

carcinoma

chemotherapy

complementary therapy

electronic cigarettes (e-cigarettes)

genotyping

grading

hormone therapy

immunotherapy

leukemia

lymphoma

malignant

melanoma

metastasis

mutation

neoplasm

neuroblastoma

non-melanomatous skin cancers/carcinomas

oncogenesis

Papanicolaou smear (Pap smear)

primary tumor

prognosis

prostate-specific
antigen (PSA)

radiation therapy

sarcoma

squamous cell
carcinoma

staging

survival rate

tumor

Chapter Outline

INTRODUCTION

What do Jackie Kennedy Onassis (former First Lady), Lance Armstrong (Tour de France bicyclist/champion), Colin Powell (former Secretary of State), and Bob Marley (former Reggae singer) all have in common? Yes, of course. They all have or had cancer.

cancer: cells characterized by uncontrolled growth and the ability to spread to other parts of the body

The term "*cancer*" refers to a group of diseases with a similar underlying process. Cancer is not one disease; there have been over 100 different types of cancer identified. For most people, the word has a negative connotation and many presume cancer = death. This is not always true. Each type of cancer has its own risks, treatments, and prognosis. The commonality of all cancers is that cancer cells are *abnormal cells that divide without control* and are *able to invade other tissues.*

Risk factors are known for some of the more common cancers that may allow for early detection. For example, if she has a family history of breast cancer, a woman would be at a higher risk of developing breast cancer. Genetic testing and earlier mammograms can been used to screen for this type of cancer. Potential for prevention exists for some cancers such as avoiding unprotected sun exposure to prevent skin cancer. Some cancers occur without identified reasons and are more difficult to prevent. Some cancers with known risk factors occur in absence of the risk factor. For example, it is not unknown for lung cancer to appear in someone who has never smoked tobacco. Host resistance may also play a role, particularly in the situation where some with a risk factor do not get the disease whereas others without that risk factor do. It is important to realize that the etiology of cancer is multifactorial and that cancer is a complex disease.

Cancer is the second leading cause of death in the United States, and therefore, interventions to prevent cancer, or to identify it early in its course, would lead to improved longevity and decreased health care costs.

Historical Notes 12·1

Early Pioneers of Cancer Epidemiology

Scientific advances during the Renaissance in Europe led to the early understanding of the human anatomy. Around 1761, Giovanni Morgagni of Italy began to do routine autopsies to associate a person's illness before death to the anatomical findings after death. Shortly thereafter, a Scottish surgeon, John Hunter, began to advocate for surgical removal of certain tumors before death if it had not spread to local tissues and if it was "moveable." Anesthesia, developed a century later, allowed for improved surgical techniques and removal of cancerous tumors. In the nineteenth century, Rudolf Virchow, the father of cellular pathology, correlated the microscopic findings of cancer tissues to the disease with the aid of a microscope. The surgeons now had more information regarding the tumors they were removing— what type it was and if it was completely removed.

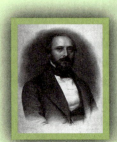

Rudolf Virchow
Courtesy of Wikipedia
Commons: http://
en.wikipedia.org/wiki/
File:Rudolf_Virchow.jpg

The discovery of DNA (an inherited material that contains genetic instructions) by Watson and Crick in the mid-1900s was a major scientific advancement for the understanding of cancer. Once they deciphered the genetic code, physicians could more completely understand the damage caused by mutations. In the 1970s, oncogenes and tumor suppressor genes were discovered, both of which have major roles in directing the growth of cancer cells.

Cancer epidemiology as a field followed three major findings of the eighteenth century. The first finding occurred in 1713 when an Italian physician, Bernardino Ramazzini, recognized that nuns had no cases of cervical cancer but had a high incidence of breast cancer and questioned whether their celibate lifestyle was responsible. The second discovery was that of scrotal cancer in chimney sweeps by Percival Pott in England in 1775. This was the first identification of an occupational exposure (soot collecting in the genital area) as a risk factor for a specific cancer. The third event was when another Londoner, John Hill, became the first to recognize the dangers of tobacco and wrote a book about it in 1761. (What took us so long to listen?)

THE SCOPE OF THE PROBLEM

The statistics presented here are based on data collected by the Surveillance, Epidemiology, and End Results (SEER) Program of the National Cancer Institute for the years from 1975–2008. The SEER Cancer Statistics Review takes these data and provides a report that is published annually and contains the most recent cancer incidence, mortality, survival, prevalence, and lifetime risk statistics. The most recent review includes data from the years 1975–2008. In addition, the National Cancer Institute, with collaboration from the American Cancer Society, the Centers for Disease Control and Prevention, and the North American Association of Central Cancer Registries, uses SEER data to provide annual updates on cancer occurrence trends in the United States. For further information on how these data are collected and reported, refer to the Website Resources at the end of the chapter.

Unless otherwise specified, data presented in this chapter do NOT include **non-melanomatous skin cancers** because these cancers are considered relatively benign

non-melanomatous skin cancers/carcinomas: the more common skin cancers that include basal cell carcinomas and squamous cell carcinomas but not the more invasive melanoma

compared to the invasive cancers and because their extraordinarily high incidence rates would skew the general data. Because of the sheer numbers and potential for prevention, they will be included in the discussion on specific types of cancers later in this chapter.

Lifetime Risk

In the United States, almost 1 in 2 persons (40.77% of men and women) will be diagnosed with cancer at some point in his or her lifetime. This risk will vary based on the site of the primary cancer and the person's gender and race/ethnicity. Men have a lifetime risk slightly higher than women. Looking at lifetime probability of developing cancer by ethnicity, whites have the highest risk, and American Indians and Alaskan Natives have the lowest risk. See Table 12-1 for specific details. Data based on the primary site of several different cancers can be found in Table 12-2.

Ethnicity and gender will also have an impact on lifetime risk of these specific types of cancer. Look around your classroom. How many students are in the class? How many males and how many females? Now look again at Table 12-2. Using this information, calculate how many of you will get cancer of any type or how many will get a specific type. Surprising how common it is!

TABLE 12-1 Lifetime Risk of Being Diagnosed with Cancer by Race/Ethnicity and Gender, 2005-2008

(Percentage)

All Sites	All Races	Whites	Blacks	Asians/Pacific Islanders	American Indians/ Alaskan Natives	Hispanics
Both Sexes	41.21	41.56	37.24	35.65	27.74	36.97
Males	44.85	44.77	41.59	38.19	27.60	40.20
Females	38.08	38.83	33.43	33.67	28.12	34.69

Based on: National Cancer Institute; Lifetime Risk (Percent) of Being Diagnosed with Cancer by Site and Race/Ethnicity, Both Sexes, 17 SEER Areas, 2005–2008; Lifetime Risk (Percent) of Being Diagnosed with Cancer by Site and Race/Ethnicity, Males, 17 SEER Areas, 2005–2008; Lifetime Risk (Percent) of Being Diagnosed with Cancer by Site and Race/Ethnicity, Females, 17 SEER Areas, 2005–2008: http://seer.cancer.gov/csr/1975_2008/results_merged/topic_lifetime_risk.pdf

TABLE 12-2 Lifetime Probability of Developing Cancer by Site, 2006-2008

Site	Risk of Developing	
	Men	**Women**
All Sites	1 in 2	1 in 3
Bladder	1 in 26	1 in 87
Brain/CNS	1 in 147	1 in 189
Breast	1 in 769	1 in 8
Cervix	–	1 in 147
Colorectal	1 in 19	1 in 20
Lung/Bronchus	1 in 13	1 in 16
Melanoma of the skin	1 in 41	1 in 64
Non-Hodgkin lymphoma	1 in 43	1 in 52
Ovary	–	1 in 71
Pancreas	1 in 69	1 in 69
Prostate	1 in 6	–
Testicles	1 in 270	–
Uterine	–	1 in 38

Based on: Data from American Cancer Society—Learn about Cancer, Lifetime Risk of Developing or Dying from Cancer based on SEER data 2006–2008: http://www.cancer.org/Cancer/CancerBasics/lifetime-probability-of-developing-or-dying-from-cancer

Prevalence

On January 1, 2008, the prevalence of all types of cancer was estimated at 11,957,599—or about 4% of the U.S. population. This included persons who currently have, or previously had, a diagnosis of cancer of any site. The prevalence of cancer varies with each type and is dependent on both the incidence of the specific type of cancer and the expected survival time after diagnosis. Therefore, a cancer like lung cancer, which is the second most common cancer, will have a lower prevalence than less common cancers because the survival time is shorter. Factors associated with the prevalence of cancer include:

- *Age:* As would be expected, in general, the prevalence of cancer increases with age. This is dependent on the type of cancer, however; for example, acute lymphocytic leukemia is much more prevalent in the younger years than older years. In January 2008, only 1.9% of all persons with cancer were children aged 0–19 years.

- *Gender:* Based on 2008 data, the prevalence of all types of cancer was slightly higher among women than men. There were 5,505,862 cases among men (46% of total cases) and 6,451,737 (54%) cases among women. Incidence in 2012 was expected to be slightly higher in men (848,170 new cases) versus women (790,740 new cases).

- *Ethnicity:* Prevalence varies among the different ethnicities based on the type of cancer. For example, prostate cancer is far more common in African American men than it is among men of any other ethnicity or race. In general, looking at all sites, Caucasians have a prevalence of cancer about 10 times higher than that of blacks.

Prevalence for the same cancer type may change over the years. This is usually the result of an increase in survival time because of more effective treatment. Every year more and more people survive their cancer because of improved therapies used to treat their disease.

Incidence

The age-adjusted incidence rate for persons diagnosed with cancer between the years 2004–2008 was 464.4 per 100,000 per year. Based on data reported in *Cancer Facts & Figures 2012* published by the American Cancer Society, an estimated 1,638,910 persons in the United States will be diagnosed with some type of cancer in 2012. Of these, 848,170 cases would be expected among men (51.8%) and 790,740 among

TABLE 12-3 Age-Adjusted Incidence Rates by Race and Gender, 2004-2008

Race/Ethnicity	Male	Female
All Races	541.0 per 100,000 men	411.6 per 100,000 women
White	543.6 per 100,000 men	423.0 per 100,000 women
Black	626.1 per 100,000 men	400.9 per 100,000 women
Asian/Pacific Islander	347.7 per 100,000 men	297.0 per 100,000 women
American Indian/Alaska Native	338.0 per 100,000 men	309.0 per 100,000 women
Hispanic	407.3 per 100,000 men	324.4 per 100,000 women

Based on: National Cancer Institute, Surveillance Epidemiology and End Results (SEER); SEER Stat Fact Sheets: All Sites, Incidence and Mortality: http://seer.cancer.gov/statfacts/html/all.html

women (48.2%). The median age for diagnosis of cancer of all sites is 66 years of age, with incidence ranging from 1.1% in persons less than 20 years of age to a peak of 24.7% in those aged 65–74 years. As shown in Table 12-3, by ethnicity and gender, black men have the highest incidence, and Asian/Pacific Islander women have the lowest.

Incidence not only varies by gender or race, but also by the site of the **primary tumor**, or where the cancerous growth originates. For the years 2004–2008, cancers of the prostate, lung, and colorectal sites, in this order, had the most new cases among men of all ethnicities except for Hispanic men who had more colorectal cancer than lung cancer. Breast cancer was the number 1 cancer diagnosed in women of all ethnicities. Lung cancer was number 2 and colorectal cancer was number 3 among all women except those of Asian/Pacific Islander and Hispanic ethnicity for whom these two cancers were reversed.

The *Annual Report to the Nation on the Status of Cancer, 1975–2008* reported trends in the incidence of cancers of different sites among both genders of various races. For the years 2003–2007, there were significant declines in overall incidence rates of lung and colorectal cancer in both men and women, whereas melanomas and pancreatic cancer showed an increase. In men, prostate cancer showed no significant change in either direction; and in women, breast cancer showed a decline in new cases.

> **primary tumor:** the tumor growing in the original site of the cancer

Death Rates

Cancer is the second leading cause of death in the United States. The age-adjusted death rate for the years 2004–2008 was 181.3 per 100,000 men and women per year. As can be seen by Table 12-4, these rates are highest for black men and women and lowest for Asian/Pacific Islander men and women.

TABLE 12-4 Age-Adjusted Death Rates by Race and Gender, 2004-2008

Race/Ethnicity	Male	Female
All Races	223.0 per 100,000 men	153.2 per 100,000 women
White	220.0 per 100,000 men	152.8 per 100,000 women
Black	295.3 per 100,000 men	177.7 per 100,000 women
Asian/Pacific Islander	134.7 per 100,000 men	94.1 per 100,000 women
American Indian/Alaska Native	190.0 per 100,000 men	138.4 per 100,000 women
Hispanic	149.1 per 100,000 men	101.5 per 100,000 women

Based on: National Cancer Institute, Surveillance Epidemiology and End Results (SEER); SEER Stat Fact Sheets: All Sites, Incidence and Mortality: http://seer.cancer.gov/statfacts/html/all.html#incidence-mortality

The cancers with the highest death rates (in order of highest frequency) among men are lung, prostate, and colorectal in all races except Asian/Pacific Islanders for whom liver cancer is the second most deadly cancer. In women, the highest death rates (in order of highest frequency) occur for lung, breast, and colorectal cancers for all women except Hispanic women who have their highest death rates for breast cancer.

According to the *Annual Report to the Nation on the Status of Cancer, 1975–2008*, the trends from 1999–2008 showed a decrease in cancer mortality in both genders across all races/ethnicities except American Indian and Alaskan Native men and women. All men had a decrease in deaths from lung, prostate, and colorectal cancers, except for American Indians and Alaskan Natives in whom the rates remained unchanged. In women, whites, blacks, and Hispanics had a decrease in mortality from breast and colorectal cancer. Women of all ethnicities had decreases in lung cancer deaths.

Financial Costs

Total direct medical costs for cancer in 2010 were $102.8 billion; this includes all expenditures related to the medical care for the disease. The costs for lost productivity as a result of the illness were $20.9 billion, and the costs resulting from lost productivity because of premature death were $140.1 billion.

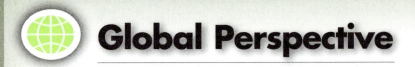

Global Perspective

Cancer: A Leading Cause of Death Worldwide

As in the United States, cancer is a leading cause of death worldwide and is responsible for about 13% of all deaths overall and 21% of noncommunicable disease mortalities. About one-third of cancers are considered to be preventable with tobacco use a major risk factor. Infectious agents are another recognizable cause of cancer and are responsible for about twice the number cases of cancer in the low- and middle-income countries as in the more developed countries. Over two-thirds of cancer deaths occur in the low- and middle-income countries. The top five cancers worldwide are lung (1.4 million deaths), stomach (740,000 deaths), liver (700,000 deaths), colorectal (610,000 deaths), and breast (460,000 deaths). Deaths from cancer are increasing and expected to reach 11 million by 2030. The International Agency for Research on Cancer, an agency of the WHO, collaborates with other United Nations groups in areas of cancer prevention and control worldwide. World Cancer Day is celebrated annually on February 4.

This leads to a total cost of $263.8 billion for cancer in 2010, according to the National Institutes of Health! As you will see later in this chapter, there are lifestyle changes that can be instituted to prevent some cancers. Given the rising health care costs, these measures would have major impact on the national health care budget.

BASIC PHYSIOLOGY AND PATHOPHYSIOLOGY

neoplasm: new growth that may be benign or cancerous

tumor: mass of cells or growth; may be benign or malignant

benign: noncancerous

malignant: cancerous

metastasis: distant spread of cancer cells away from the primary tumor

Cancer is characterized by *uncontrolled growth and the ability to invade other tissues*. In the following sections, the basic process of the change from normal cell to cancerous cell is discussed. There are some basic terms that must be understood when discussing cancers. A **neoplasm** is a new growth, and a **tumor** is a swelling or growth of a tissue. Both of these may be **benign** (noncancerous) or **malignant** (cancerous). **Metastasis** is the spread of disease to a nonadjacent organ and is an example of cancer's ability to invade other tissues.

Basic Pathophysiology of Cancer

The exact cause of cancer is still not fully understood. **Oncogenesis** is the process of malignant transformation of the normal cell. There are likely some parts of the pathway of oncogenesis that are common to all types of cancer, but the process is different for different types of cancer.

The effects that are common to all cancers include an initial **mutation** or change/damage to the cell's DNA and, later, uncontrolled growth of this changed cell. Cancer cells behave differently than normal cells. Instead of dying and being replaced by new normal cells, these abnormal cells continue to grow and divide to produce more abnormal cells. One of the reasons for this is that they lack contact inhibition and therefore do not know when to stop reproducing. These cancer cells are able to spread through the blood and lymph systems and invade other tissues (*metastasis*). This is also partially because of their inability to stick to other cells so that they break off and spread more easily. These two characteristics, *uncontrolled growth* and the *ability to invade other tissues*, are what make cancer cells different from normal cells. Malignant cells also lose the specialized function of the tissues from which they originate. For example, cancerous tumors that originate in the lung no longer perform in the process of respiration.

oncogenesis: process of malignant transformation leading to the formation of a cancer

mutation: change in the normal DNA of a cell

carcinogen: a substance that causes cancer or helps it to grow

Mutations passed on genetically account for only 5%–15% of all cancer cases. More frequently, mutations occur spontaneously as a person ages or is exposed to carcinogens. **Carcinogens** are substances that may be the cause of these mutations leading to a specific cancer. Some examples of the more common and well-studied carcinogens that cause mutations include smoking, radiation exposure, chemical carcinogens such as benzene, and infectious agents like viruses.

Classifications

Cancers are generally named according to the body organ they initially affect, referred to as the "primary tumor," and the type of cells that are affected. Once a cancer is diagnosed, it is classified by the changes in its genes (**genotyping**), the cell (**grading**), and its degree of invasion of local and distant tissues (**staging**). **Prognosis**, or expected outcome, is dependent on these factors, as is the specific treatment plan for that cancer. Having an understanding of these classifications is important in epidemiology to ensure that studies compare like entities.

By Body Organ Origin

Cancer maintains the name of the body organ of origin or primary tumor and does not change once it metastasizes to other organs or tissues. For example, if a cancer starts in the lung, it is considered lung cancer. If it metastasizes to the bone, it does not become known as bone cancer; it is still lung cancer. The distant metastatic tumor retains the same cell types as the primary tumor.

By Cell Type

Cancer is usually named according to the type of cell or tissue from which it originates. **Carcinomas**, which arise from epithelial cells, account for about 85% of all cancers; whereas **sarcomas**, which originate in connective tissues such as bone, tendon, or cartilage, account for only 2%. **Adenocarcinoma** is a term used to describe cancers that start in gland cells (cells that normally secrete a substance). **Melanomas** occur in skin cells that contain melanin (the substance that gives the skin its color) and, although quite rare in the past, are rapidly increasing in frequency because of people's increased sun exposure. **Neuroblastomas** occur in immature cells of the nervous system, primarily in children. **Leukemia** affects white blood cells and is one cancer that primarily manifests in the liquid state of blood; whereas **lymphomas** are solid tumors that arise in the lymphatic system.

Genotyping

Identifying genes or mutations within the cells of a malignant tumor that are characteristic for that specific tumor is called "genotyping." These unique genes are tumor markers and may allow for targeted therapy directed against that specific cancer.

Grading

The grading of a tumor is based on how much the cancer cell's structure deviates from a normal cell's structure when viewed under a microscope. There are different methods used for different cancer types, but all systems grade the cells by determining how great that deviation from normal is, usually on a scale of 1-4 ("1" being least deviation to "4" being most deviation). Those cancer cells with minimal difference from their normal cell counterpart are considered low grade, whereas those with greater differences are considered higher grades.

genotyping: detection of abnormalities in the genes of cancer cells

grading: a classification used to differentiate how much a cancer cell varies from a normal cell

staging: the process of finding out whether cancer has spread and if so, how far

prognosis: the expected outcome of the disease; outlook for chance of survival

carcinoma: cancer that arises in the epithelial cells

sarcoma: a malignant tumor growing from connective tissues, such as cartilage, fat, muscle, or bone

adenocarcinoma: cancer that starts in gland cells (cells that normally secrete a substance)

melanoma: cancer that arises in the pigmented cells (melanocytes) of the skin

neuroblastoma: malignancy arising from the immature cells of the nervous system

leukemia: cancer of the white blood cells

lymphoma: cancer of the lymphatic system

Staging

Staging is based on several factors that may be present at the time of diagnosis:

1. The size of the tumor,

2. The extent of the tumor (e.g., spread to adjacent lymph nodes), and

3. Any distant spread of the tumor or metastasis.

The location of the primary tumor, the cell type, and the tumor grade also impact the staging. Cancers of the blood, such as leukemia, do not have a clear staging system. The determination of a tumor's stage is performed using various specialized tests such as the physical exam, imaging studies like CT (computed tomography) scanning, or MRI (magnetic resonance imaging), laboratory tests, and results of tissue pathology reports from biopsies taken. The stage of a cancer does not change, even if the cancer progresses. A tumor that comes back or spreads is still referred to by the stage it was given at the time of diagnosis and initial staging.

Treatments

Cancer therapy has come a long way over the last 20 years. Death rates for cancer have declined since 1991 and this is in part because of improved therapeutic methods and combinations of treatments, as well as improved preventive interventions. In the past, treatments would attack and destroy the normal cells and organs as easily as the cancer cells, but therapies have improved remarkably over the past several years. The most common therapies include: surgery, chemotherapy, and radiation, or any combination of the three.

Surgery

Surgery is the oldest form of cancer treatment, and most people with cancer have some form of surgery. It can (1) provide tissue for diagnosis, (2) remove or debulk a tumor, and (3) determine if and how far a tumor has spread for staging the cancer. Surgery may be preventative in some cases. A mastectomy (surgical removal of a breast) is an example of possible preventive surgery when done in a woman at a particularly high risk for breast cancer. In tumors that have not metastasized to distant areas, surgery may provide the best chance of cure. There are also special surgical techniques that can be used, including those that use lasers, electrical currents, and cold probes. Modern surgical techniques are more targeted and cause less normal tissue destruction than they did in the past.

Chemotherapy

chemotherapy: treatment of cancer with drugs

Chemotherapy is the use of drugs to kill cancer cells. The goal is to target the effects of the drug only on the rapidly dividing and growing cancer cells and minimize the effects on any normal cells. Chemotherapy is frequently used in conjunction with surgery. It has the advantage of targeting distant metastatic cells or cancer cells that are not visible but may still be local to the primary tumor. Most chemotherapy is given as a combination of agents in which each agent targets a different function or process of the cancer cell. Studies to improve the activity of chemotherapeutic agents and to minimize the adverse side effects of the drugs are ongoing.

Radiation Therapy

Radiation therapy is the use of radiation to treat localized tumors. This therapy is tightly targeted to the tumor to minimize effects to the surrounding tissues. Radiation can be administered to the tumor externally via specialized machines or internally via radioactive seeds or pellets inserted directly into the tumor. Radiation therapy is frequently used to shrink the tumor prior to surgery, but this therapy may also be given after the surgery to kill any remaining cancer cells.

Other Therapies

Hormone therapy is frequently used in combination with the other therapies in the treatment of breast and prostate cancers. **Immunotherapy** uses biologic agents that mimic the body's natural signals. Monoclonal antibodies targeted against specific antigens in the cancer cells are now being used against some tumors, and more work is being done to identify tumor-specific antigens for other cancers. **Bone marrow stem cell transplants** to restore blood-forming cells are frequently used to treat leukemias (cancers of the white blood cells) and lymphomas (cancers of the lymphatic system).

Complementary/Alternative Medicine (CAM)

CAM is used by 25–50% of the general population of cancer patients. **Complementary therapy** is treatment taken along with the standard prescribed treatments, and its aim is to relieve cancer symptoms (but not cure the cancer), treat side effects of the conventional therapy, or promote a healthier body. This is frequently in the form of diets or vitamins or minerals. It is important to note that in some cases, these treatments may actually block or interfere with the conventional treatments and should always be disclosed to the primary physician. **Alternative therapy** is a substitute for mainstream treatment that is meant to achieve a cure. Frequently, there is no scientifically recognized proof of a positive effect from alternative agents. Often the terms "complementary" and "alternative" are used and treated as interchanging terms, but they are different.

Prognosis

As previously mentioned, cancer is not one disease, but many different diseases. As such, the prognosis for cancer varies with the type of cancer, from the more benign non-melanomatous skin cancers to the more aggressive lung cancers. The prognosis for cancer is generally expressed as a 5-year **survival rate**, which is the percentage of cancer patients who are alive five years after their diagnosis. This rate varies by cancer type and stage at time of diagnosis. A limitation of the survival rate is that it does not distinguish between someone who is cured

radiation therapy: treatment with high-energy rays to kill cancer cells and shrink tumors; may be external radiation from a machine or internal from radioactive materials placed directly in the tumor

hormone therapy: use of hormones to treat cancers such as prostate and breast

immunotherapy: treatment designed to boost the cancer patient's own immune system to help fight off the cancer

bone marrow stem cell transplant: a treatment that restores blood-forming stem cells destroyed during chemotherapy or radiation therapy

complementary therapy: treatment taken along with the standard prescribed treatments; not meant as a cure

alternative therapy: used as a substitute for mainstream treatment and is meant to achieve a cure

survival rate: the percentage of people still alive within a certain period of time after diagnosis or treatment; a 5-year survival rate is usually used in cancers versus someone who has relapsed or is still in treatment. In addition, because of the length of time required for the initial data collection and then the 5-year period for survival, this rate does not reflect recent advances in diagnosis or treatment.

During 1975–1977, the overall 5-year survival rate for all types of cancer (adjusted for age, sex, and race) was 50%. By 1999–2005, newly diagnosed cancer cases had a 5-year survival rate of 68% among both males and females. This increase in survival is the result of improved diagnosis and treatment, as well as more widespread preventive measures.

TYPES OF CANCER

In this section, a few of the more common, and more deadly, cancers will be discussed. After these, a few additional cancers that have relevance to young adults will be discussed.

Five Most Common Occurring Cancers

The most commonly occurring cancer is the non-melanomatous skin cancer. Although not included in most statistics because of its sheer numbers and relatively benign nature (it is not considered an invasive cancer), it will be discussed here because of its sheer numbers and its potential for prevention.

Cancer in the lung and bronchus is the second most common cancer when considering men and women combined, although more cases of prostate cancer occur in men and more cases of breast cancer occur in women. Colorectal cancer rounds out the top five most common cancers in the United States. See Table 12-5 for a summary.

TABLE 12-5 Five Most Common Cancers (Number of Estimated New Cases in 2012)	
Skin:	> 3.5 million
Lung/Bronchus:	226,160
Prostate:	241,740
Breast:	229,060
Colorectal:	143,460

Based on: Data obtained from the American Cancer Society: *Cancer Facts & Figures, 2012*: http://www.cancer.org/Research/CancerFactsFigures/index

For males, the top three sites in incidence for *invasive* cancers, therefore, are prostate, lung/bronchus, and colorectal. For women, the top three sites in incidence for *invasive* cancers are breast, lung/bronchus, and colorectal. Figures 12-1 and 12-2 show the trends in incidence of various invasive cancers occurring in men and in women. All age-adjusted incidence and death rates listed for the specific cancers are based on 2003–2007 SEER data.

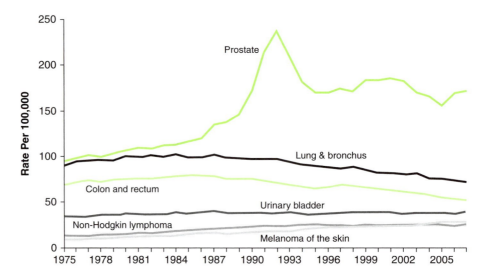

FIGURE 12-1 Cancer Incidence Rates* among Males, U.S., 1975–2007
*Age-adjusted to the 2000 U.S. standard population and adjusted for delays in reporting.

Source: Surveillance, Epidemiology, and End Results Program, Delay-adjusted Incidence database: SEER Incidence Delay-adjusted Rates, 9 Registries, 1975–2007, National Cancer Institute, 2010.

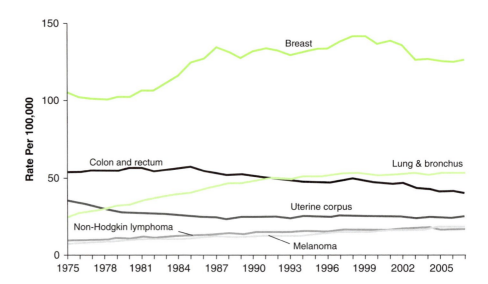

FIGURE 12-2 Cancer Incidence Rates* among Women, U.S., 1975–2007
*Age-adjusted to the 2000 U.S. standard population and adjusted for delays in reporting.

Source: Surveillance, Epidemiology, and End Results Program, Delay-adjusted Incidence database: SEER Incidence Delay-adjusted Rates, 9 Registries, 1975–2007, National Cancer Institute, 2010.

Skin Cancer

There are two major types of skin cancer—the non-melanomatous skin cancers and the melanomas. The non-melanomatous are the more benign and consist primarily of the **basal cell carcinoma** and the **squamous cell carcinoma**. The basal cell cancer starts in the base layer of the epidermis (outer layer) of the skin. Squamous cell cancers start in the flat cells on the surface of the epidermis. Melanomas start in the pigmented cells (melanocytes) that reside in the basal layer of the epidermis. See Figure 12-3 for the anatomy of the skin to further understand the origin of these skin cancers.

Non-melanomatous skin carcinoma (Figure 12-4) is the most commonly occurring cancer. There are estimated to be over 3.5 million new cases diagnosed in the United States each year. Even though these cancers are considered to be relatively benign and are highly curable, there are up to 3,000 deaths (< 0.1% case fatality rate) as a result of basal cell or squamous cell carcinomas. Skin cancers appear most frequently on the sun-exposed skin but can occur anywhere.

The major risk factor is exposure to ultraviolet (UV) light over a lifetime, whether it is from the sun, tanning booths, or sunlamps. Persons with fair skin, light-colored eyes, and red or blonde hair are at particularly higher risk with UV exposure. Other factors that increase risk for skin cancer include immunosuppressive drugs or disease, arsenic exposure, family history of skin cancer, or a personal history of previous skin cancer.

Diagnosis is made by examination of tissue removed by surgical biopsy under a microscope. Frequently, the entire lesion is removed by biopsy and the cancer is

basal cell carcinoma:
a type of non-melanomatous skin cancer that arises in the base layer of cells of the epidermis

squamous cell carcinoma:
a type of non-melanomatous skin cancer that arises from the surface layer of cells of the epidermis

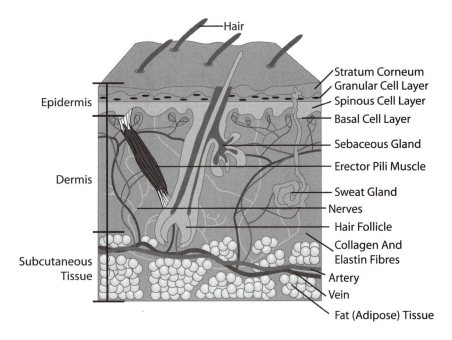

FIGURE 12-3 Anatomy of the Skin
© Anita Potter/www.Shutterstock.com

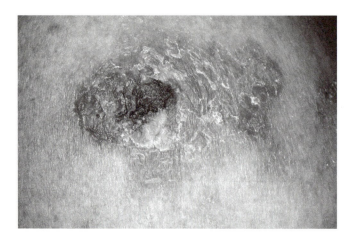

FIGURE 12-4 Non-melanomatous Carcinoma
Courtesy of the Dermatology Branch of the National Cancer Institute (NCI)—Visuals Online: http://visualsonline.cancer.gov/details.cfm?imageid=1947

cured; if not, further surgical removal may be necessary. Topical immunotherapy is an alternative treatment for skin cancers or pre-cancerous lesions. Prognosis and survival for these non-melanomatous skin carcinomas are excellent.

Melanomas are included in the invasive cancers because, unlike basal cell and squamous cell carcinomas, melanomas are more aggressive and cause more deaths. Fortunately, these skin cancers occur much less frequently than their more benign counterparts, but the rates of incidence are increasing in the United States. See Figure 12-5 for a typical melanoma.

In 2012, there will be about 76,250 new cases of melanoma with 9,180 resultant deaths (12.0% case fatality rate). The age-adjusted incidence rate based on 2004–2008 SEER data was 20.8 per 100,000 per year. The risk factors for melanoma are the same as those listed for non-melanomatous carcinomas. A protective factor is black or deeply pigmented skin. Additional risks factors include abnormal

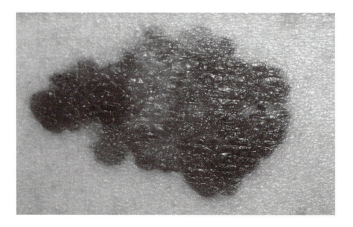

FIGURE 12-5 Seen is Melanoma, with Coloring of Different Shades of Brown, Black, or Tan. Part of the ABCDs for Detection of Melanoma
Courtesy of the National Cancer Institute (NCI)—Visuals Online: http://visualsonline.cancer.gov/details.cfm?imageid=2364

looking moles or more than 50 moles on the body and severe and blistering sunburns. The ABCD's of melanomatous changes in a mole consist of:

Asymmetry,

Border irregularity,

Color change, and

Diameter >6 mm.

Diagnosis is made after the lesion, or part of it, is removed surgically for a biopsy. Staging studies are done that include investigating nearby lymph nodes because melanoma frequently spread via lymph nodes to other parts of the body. Treatment depends on the extent of the original lesion and the presence or absence of spread and may consist of surgery, chemotherapy, radiation therapy, immunotherapy, or a combination of these methods. Ongoing monitoring for future lesions is important. The overall 5-year survival rate for melanoma is 91%; for a localized lesion, it is 98%; with regional spread, it is 62%; and for distant spread, it is 15%. The age-adjusted death rate is 2.7 per 100,000 per year based on data collected from 2004–2008 in the United States.

What famous person died at a young age from melanoma? Bob Marley! (Although darker skin is protective, this is not absolute.)

Cancer of the Lung and Bronchus

Lung cancer accounts for the most cancer-related deaths among both men and women. The incidence and death rates have been declining over the past several decades because of the decrease in the number of male smokers. In the past, it was primarily a disease of men; but in 1987, it overtook breast cancer in women as the most common deadly cancer. In 2012, there will be an anticipated 226,160 new cases of all lung cancers with 116,470 (51.5%) occurring in men and 109,690 (48.5%) occurring in women. The age-adjusted incidence rate is 62.0 per 100,000 per year. The mortality rate in men has decreased much more than it has in women, but still more men die from this cancer than women. In 2012, 160,340 persons with lung cancer will die: 87,750 men and 72,590 women. This will lead to a case fatality rate of 70.9% overall with 75.3% in men and 66.2% in women. Lung cancer frequently starts in the cells lining the airways. See Figure 12-6 for basic lung anatomy and Figure 12-7 for a picture of a lung with cancer. There are two major types of cancer based on what the cells look like under the microscope.

Smoking, by far, is the leading risk factor for cancer. Eighty-seven percent of all lung cancer deaths are associated with a history of smoking. This is discussed in depth in "A Closer Look: Risk Factors—Tobacco" at the end of this chapter. Other well-documented risk factors include exposure to various agents such as radon gas, asbestos fibers, uranium, vinyl chloride, and other chemicals. Air pollution and diesel exhaust are thought to increase a person's risk for lung cancer as is arsenic in drinking water. Persons who have had previous radiation to the chest, usually as a treatment for a prior cancer, are at higher risk; and family history also plays a role in increasing one's likelihood of developing cancer of the lungs.

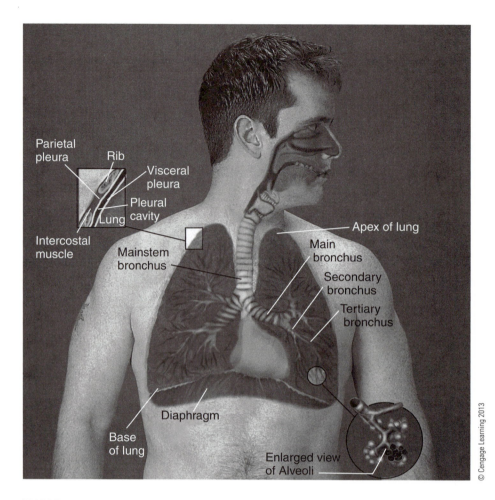

Parietal pleura
Rib
Visceral pleura
Pleural cavity
Lung
Intercostal muscle
Mainstem bronchus
Apex of lung
Main bronchus
Secondary bronchus
Tertiary bronchus
Diaphragm
Base of lung
Enlarged view of Alveoli

© Cengage Learning 2013

FIGURE 12-6 Lung Anatomy

There is currently no screening test available to detect early lung cancer. There has been some promise in preliminary studies that have looked at a special type of CT scan, the spiral CT, as a screening tool for those persons at high risk, but this is not a current recommendation. When symptoms present, diagnosis is usually made by chest X-ray or CT scan and biopsy of the tumor tissue to determine the cancer type.

Treatment may include surgery, chemotherapy, radiation therapy, targeted therapy, or a combination of therapies. Because most lung cancer is diagnosed only after there is distant spread, the overall 5-year survival rate is only 15.6%. One-year survival has increased from 35% in 1975–1979 to 43% in 2003–2006 because of improvements in surgical techniques and combination therapies. Survival varies based on the stage and type of the cancer with local disease having a 5-year survival rate of about 52%, although it only accounts for 15% of all lung cancers. Advanced non-small cell cancers have a 5-year survival rate of less than 1%. The age-adjusted death rate is 51.6 per 100,000 per year.

Persons who have had lung cancer include the creator of Mickey Mouse (Walt Disney), a baseball icon and husband of Marilyn Monroe (Joe DiMaggio), and the wife of Christopher Reeve ("Superman"), Dana Reeve.

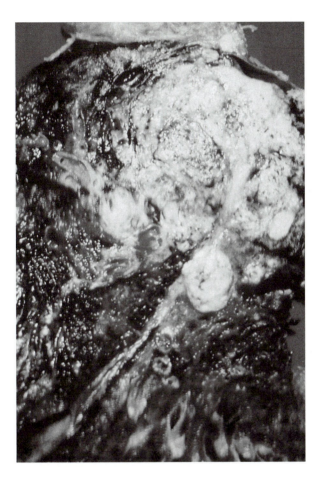

FIGURE 12-7 Cross Section of a Human Lung with Cancer. This Individual was a Smoker as Indicated by the Black Area; the White Area Represents the Cancer
Courtesy of the National Cancer Institute (NCI)—Visuals Online: http://visualsonline.cancer.gov/details.cfm?imageid=2348

Prostate Cancer

The prostate is an organ of the male reproductive system about the size of a walnut that lies below the bladder and in front of the rectum. Its purpose is to make part of the seminal fluid. See Figure 12-8 to understand the relationship of the prostate gland to male anatomy. Because lung cancer occurs in both men and women, it has more cases per year overall; but prostate cancer is the most common *invasive* cancer in men, regardless of race or ethnicity, with 1 in 6 men affected. In 2012, there will be an expected 241,740 new cases, or 152.6 new cases per 100,000 men, and 28,170 deaths (case fatality rate of 11.7%). It is the second leading cause of cancer deaths. Incidence rates peaked in 1992–1993 and then declined sharply from 1992–1995. Since that time, incidence has leveled off.

There have been several risk factors identified for prostate cancer. Age greater than 65 years old is one of the strongest associations because cancer of the prostate is rare among men younger than 45 years of age. Race is another well-documented risk factor as prostate cancer occurs significantly more frequently among black men than among white men and men of Hispanic origin. Death rates have decreased more rapidly for black men than for white men since the early 1990s, but black men still

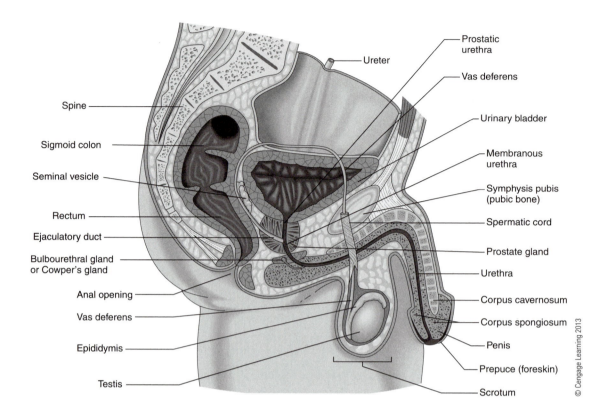

Spine

Sigmoid colon

Seminal vesicle

Rectum

Ejaculatory duct

Bulbourethral gland
or Cowper's gland

Anal opening

Vas deferens

Epididymis

Testis

Ureter

Prostatic
urethra

Vas deferens

Urinary bladder

Membranous
urethra

Symphysis pubis
(pubic bone)

Spermatic cord

Prostate gland

Urethra

Corpus cavernosum

Corpus spongiosum

Penis

Prepuce (foreskin)

Scrotum

© Cengage Learning 2013

FIGURE 12-8 The Male Reproductive System

have twice the risk of death from prostate cancer. Family history of prostate cancer in a father, brother, or son raises a man's risk for developing the same. Other factors that have not been proven but are under investigation include consumption of red meat, obesity, and smoking.

Current recommendations for screening vary by provider. In the past, it was recommended that males have screening examinations every year beginning at age 50. For men at higher risk, screening would begin at age 45. Screening is done by (1) digital rectal examinations (DRE), which is done when the provider feels the prostate gland through the rectum, and by (2) measuring **prostate-specific antigen (PSA)** via a blood sample. Prostate-specific antigen is normally produced by the prostate at a low level, but this level may rise significantly when cancer is present in the gland. Screening with PSA levels has allowed for earlier detection of prostate cancer. Because the progression of this cancer may be very slow, this has led to some procedures and surgeries in which the benefits may not have outweighed the risks of complications. It is for this reason that providers may differ in their recommendations for screening with PSA. All will generally discuss the risks and benefits of having this screening test done in men when they reach the age of 50 and at intervals thereafter.

Diagnosis is usually made with examination of the cells under the microscope after a biopsy or sample of the gland has been removed and processed. Grading the tumor is done with a method called the "Gleason score," which gives information on how likely the tumor is to spread. Treatment can include "watchful waiting,"

prostate-specific antigen (PSA): normally produced by the prostate at a low level, but this level may raise significantly when cancer is present in the gland; used as a screening test for prostate cancer

which is monitoring the cancer with routine DRE and PSA tests and treating only if the tumor shows signs of progressing. Other modalities for treatment depend on the tumor–specific grading and staging and may involve external or internal radiation, hormone therapy, and/or surgery. Approximately 80% of cancer is found when it is still localized to the prostate gland, and the 5-year survival rate for these tumors is almost 100%. This is also true of tumors that have only had regional spread as well. Once the tumor has metastasized to distant parts of the body, the 5-year survival rate drops to about 30%. The age-adjusted death rate for prostate is 24.4 per 100,000 men per year.

Can you name any famous person who has or has had prostate cancer? (*Hints:* a former Army general and Secretary of State, the former president of South Africa, the former manager of the New York Yankees, the mayor of New York City on September 11, 2001, to name only a few!)

Breast Cancer

Sheryl Crow (singer), Betty Ford (former First Lady), and Chief Justice Sandra Day-O'Connor (Supreme Court justice) are all women who have had breast cancer. There are/were many more famous, and not famous, women who have had this disease. Richard Roundtree, the star of the movie *Shaft*, also had breast cancer, which shows that this disease, although primarily one of women, can occur in men as well.

Breast cancer is the most common cancer in women, excluding the non-melanomatous skin cancers. The lifetime chance for a woman to develop breast cancer is a little less than 1 in 8. It is estimated that 226,870 women will be diagnosed with breast cancer in 2012. An additional 63,300 cases of carcinoma in situ (noninvasive), the earliest form of breast cancer, are expected to be diagnosed among women. Although thought of as only a women's disease, 2,190 men are expected to develop breast cancer in 2012. After increasing rapidly for several decades, incidence has been decreasing during the past decade about 2% per year in women over 50 years of age thought to be primarily because of a decrease in the use of hormones to treat menopause.

Breast cancer is the second leading cause of cancer deaths in women, surpassed only by lung cancer. Based on SEER data from 2004–2008, the age-adjusted incidence rate is 124.0 per 100,000 women, and the age-adjusted death rate was 23.5 per 100,000 women. In 2012, there will be 39,920 deaths in total (case fatality rate of 17.4%) expected, with 410 of those deaths in men (case fatality rate of 18.7%) and 39,510 deaths in women (case fatality rate of 17.4%).

Breast cancer can occur in two different forms based on what part of the breast the cancer arises. See Figure 12-9 for the anatomy of the normal female breast. Ductal cancer develops from the lactiferous ducts that are the tubes that bring milk to the nipple during the breastfeeding of an infant. Lobular cancer begins in the glands that make breast milk. Both cancers are treated generally the same way.

There are multiple well-studied risk factors for breast cancer, but the strongest risk factor is gender. In addition, age plays an important role with few women under 45 years of age getting the disease and 2 out of 3 cases occurring among women over the age of 55.

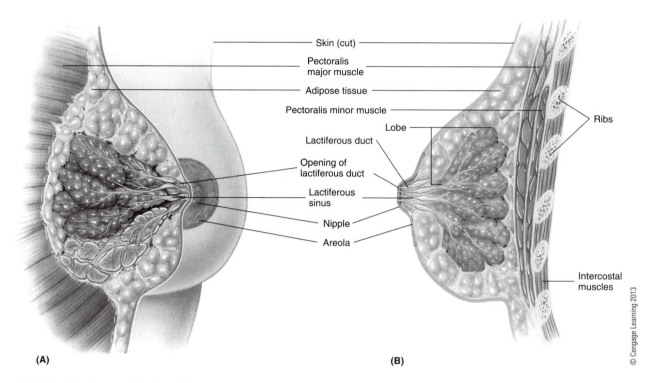

Skin (cut)
Pectoralis
major muscle
Adipose tissue
Pectoralis minor muscle
Lobe
Lactiferous duct
Opening of
lactiferous duct
Lactiferous
sinus
Nipple
Areola
Ribs
Intercostal
muscles

(A)   (B)

© Cengage Learning 2013

FIGURE 12-9 Anatomy of the Female Breast

Genetic factors are thought to be present in about 5–10% of cases with the most common being the mutations known as **BRCA1** and **BRCA2**. The risk for someone who has inherited these mutations to later develop cancer may be as high as 80% and when this occurs, it tends to occur in younger women and in both breasts. Family history unrelated to a specific gene occurring in a mother, sister, or daughter doubles the risk of breast cancer. If a woman has already had cancer in one breast, she has a 3–4-fold increased risk of developing a new cancer in the other breast (considered a second primary cancer rather than a recurrence of the first cancer).

Race is an interesting risk factor because white women are more likely to develop breast cancer, but black women are more likely to have more aggressive tumors and to die from the cancer. Women who started their menstrual cycles early (before age 12) or went through menopause later in life (after age 55), or had their first baby after age 30, or no children at all, are thought to have had longer exposures to estrogen and progesterone and a higher risk of breast cancer. In this same manner, hormonal treatment of menopausal symptoms has been found to increase the risk for breast cancer. Since this association was identified, the use of estrogen replacement therapy for menopause has markedly decreased and so have new cases of breast cancer.

BRCA1 and BRCA2: genes that when mutated or damaged put a woman at higher risk for breast or ovarian cancer and possibly men at higher risk for prostate cancer

Screenings with self breast exams, although they only have a small role in discovering lumps early, can begin in a woman's 20s–30s. Clinical exams by a health care provider also have limitations but are recommended every three years for women in their 20s–30s and yearly after the age of 40. The current recommendations for screening mammograms are for every woman from age 40 on to have the test done

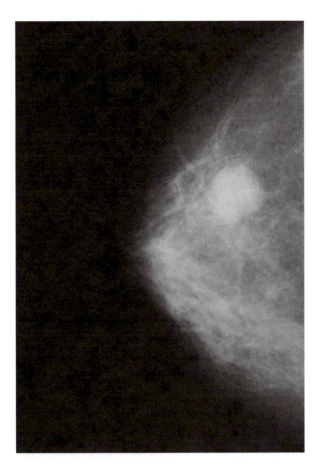

FIGURE 12-10 Shown is a Mammogram of a Fatty Breast with an Obvious Cancer
© Doctor Kan/www.Shutterstock.com

annually. Mammograms, found to be the best method to find tumors early, can detect 80–90% of cancers in women without signs or symptoms of a palpable mass. Note the abnormal mammogram in Figure 12-10. Additionally, women with a strong family history of breast cancer may be offered genetic testing to assess their risk and determine preventive measures. MRIs are also being used to screen high-risk women. Once a tumor has been found, a needle can be inserted into the tumor to obtain a biopsy for study under the microscope.

Treatment for breast cancer includes surgery, ranging from lumpectomy (removing only the tumor) to total radical mastectomy (removing all breast tissue, underlying chest muscles, and local lymph nodes). Additional treatments include chemotherapy, radiation therapy, hormone therapy, and targeted therapy, or a combination of therapies. The specific course of treatment used is based on the stage of the tumor at the time of diagnosis. Survival rate is also dependent on the stage of disease at diagnosis. Fortunately, for those with breast cancer, about 60% of tumors are found when they are still localized, and the 5-year survival rate for these tumors is 98%. Regional spread to local lymph nodes decreases this rate to 84%, and metastatic spread to other parts of the body lowers it further to 23%.

Colorectal Cancer

What do a U.S. president (Ronald Reagan), an actress (Farrah Fawcett), a British media personality (Sharon Osbourne), and the creator of *Peanuts* (Charles Schultz) have in common? Cancer of the colon or rectum.

Colon and rectal cancers are usually of the same cell types with the same beginnings and risk factors and so are grouped together. The colon is synonymous with the "large intestine" and consists of about five feet of muscular intestine in the digestive tract. The rectum is the last six inches of the digestive system before the exit out of the body (anus). (See Figure 12-11.) The colon absorbs water from the digested food matter and serves as a storage place for the waste product.

Colon cancer usually starts in a previously benign polyp (small growth) or in an area of dysplasia (abnormal cells usually found in areas of inflammation) from diseases like ulcerative colitis. Once the cancer cells break through the wall of the colon, they can spread to distant parts of the body via the blood or lymph system. There are several types of colorectal cancers, but 95% are tumors called "adenocarcinomas" that start in the mucous-forming cells that line the colon.

Colorectal cancer is the third most common occurring invasive cancer when men and women are considered separately. Both incidence rates and death rates have been decreasing over the past 20 years because of improved screening and earlier detection and improved treatment. There will be an anticipated 103,170 new cases of colon cancer and 40,290 new cases of rectal cancer in 2012. These will occur about equally between men and women with women having a few more cases of colon cancer and men having a few more cases of rectal cancer. By sheer numbers, colorectal cancer is the second most deadly cancer in men and women combined, or third if men and women are considered separately. The age-adjusted incidence rate is 47.2 per 100,000 men and women per year. In 2012, there will be approximately

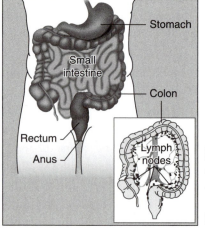

© Cengage Learning 2013

FIGURE 12-11 A Diagram of Digestive Organs, Including the Large and Small Intestine, and Accessory Organs Involved in the Process of Digestion

51,690 deaths (case fatality rate of 36.0%) with 26,470 deaths in men (case fatality rate of 36.1%) and 25,220 deaths in females (case fatality rate of 36.0%).

Most persons who develop colorectal tumors are generally over the age of 50. A personal past history of polyps or a family history of colon cancer are significant risk factors. There are several inherited disorders that are associated with colon cancer, but the most common are hereditary non-polyposis colon cancer and familial adenomatous polyposis. Inflammatory conditions such as ulcerative colitis and Crohn's disease lead to dysplasia and a higher risk of cancer. Race and ethnicity play a role in this disease as blacks and Ashkenazi Jews have increased risks over other groups. Lifestyle factors that increase a person's risk for developing this tumor include excessive alcohol consumption, smoking, obesity, and diets high in red meat or processed meats. Diets high in fiber, vegetables, and fruit seem to decrease the risk. Of special note is the known association between anal cancers and human papillomavirus infections (similar to the association of HPV with cervical cancer).

Successful, proven screening tools are available for colorectal cancer, but they are vastly underused. It is estimated that over 18,000 deaths per year from colorectal cancer could be prevented with properly used screening methods. The current recommendations for screening for colorectal cancer include: (1) using high-sensitivity fecal occult blood tests (FOBT) every year and/or (2) direct visualization of the colon with colonoscopy every 10 years, or (3) flexible sigmoidoscopy (visualization of just the last part of the colon and rectum) every 5 years. Screening is recommended for those persons aged 50–75. A "virtual" colonoscopy done with a CT scan is currently being studied for use as a screening method. If blood in the stool is detected on FOBT, visualization by colonoscopy would be recommended. This is the basis for diagnosis, and a sample of abnormal appearing tissue or a polyp would be sent as a biopsy for examination under a microscope.

Treatment is dependent on the location of the tumor, extent of disease, and stage at the time of diagnosis. Surgery, chemotherapy, biological therapy, radiation therapy, or a combination of these modalities may be used. Five-year survival rates vary according to stage of disease from 90% if still confined to the primary site (localized), to 69% if there is spread to regional lymph nodes, and to 12% if there is metastatic disease. The age-adjusted death rate for colorectal cancer is 17.1 per 100,000 men and women per year.

Check It Out

Risk assessment tools for breast cancer, colorectal cancer, and melanoma can be found online at http://www.cancer.gov

Five Most Deadly Cancers

As can be seen by comparing Table 12-5 and Table 12-6, four of the most common cancers that occur in men and women of the United States are also four of the most deadly. Only skin cancers are not included in this second category. They are replaced by cancer of the pancreas. Figures 12-12 and 12-13 show the trends in deaths from several types of cancers since 1930.

TABLE 12-6 Five Most Deadly Cancers (Estimated Number of Deaths in 2012)	
Lung/Bronchus:	160,340
Colorectal:	51,690
Breast:	39,920
Pancreas:	37,390
Prostate:	28,170

Based on: Data obtained from the American Cancer Society: *Cancer Facts & Figures, 2012:* http://www.cancer.org/Research/CancerFactsFigures/index

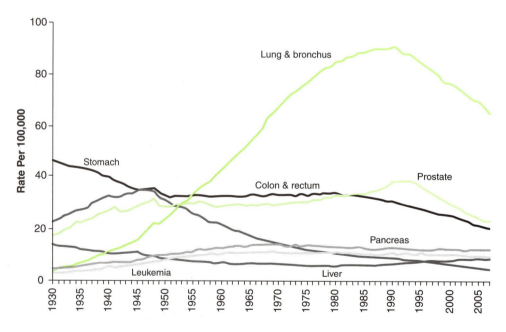

FIGURE 12-12 Cancer Death Rates* among Men, U.S., 1930-2007
*Age-adjusted to the 2000 U.S. standard population.

Source: U.S. Mortality Data 1960-2007, U.S. Mortality Volumes 1930–1959. National Center for Health Statistics, Centers for Disease Control and Prevention.

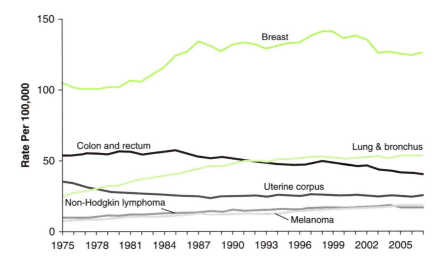

FIGURE 12-13 Cancer Incidence Rates* among Women, U.S., 1930–2007
*Age-adjusted to the 2000 U.S. standard population and adjusted for delays in reporting.

Source: Surveillance, Epidemiology, and End Results Program, Delay-adjusted Incidence database: SEER Incidence Delay-adjusted rates, 9 Registries, 1975–2007, National Cancer Institute, 2010.

Pancreatic Cancer

Patrick Swayze (actor), Steve Jobs (Apple CEO), and Ruth Bader Ginsburg (Supreme Court Justice) have all battled with this deadly cancer.

The pancreas is an organ of the digestive tract that lies behind the stomach in the abdomen. (See Figure 13–1 in Chapter 13: Diabetes Mellitus.) It has two primary functions: (1) exocrine, to produce and release enzymes that help with digestion, and (2) endocrine, to produce and release hormones that control blood sugars. The endocrine function is discussed further in Chapter 13, Diabetes Mellitus. The exocrine cells are the source of the majority of the cases of pancreatic cancer. About 95% of these tumors arise from the ducts in the pancreas and are adenocarcinoma in type. There are other cancers that start in exocrine cells and some rare cancers that arise from endocrine cells, but cancer of the pancreas is treated based more on its stage rather than the cell type.

Pancreatic cancer is the tenth most common cancer occurring in both men and in women (counted separately), yet is the fourth most common cause of cancer deaths in both genders. In 2012, 43,920 new cases of this tumor are expected with fairly equal incidence in men (50.3% of cases) and women (49.7% of cases). The age-adjusted incidence rate based on SEER data from 2004–2008 is 12.0 cases per 100,000 men and women. Based on this same data, the age-adjusted mortality rate is 10.8 deaths per 100,000 men and women. For 2012, there will be 37,390 expected deaths from pancreatic cancer (85.1% case fatality rate), again occurring relatively equally between men (85.3% case fatality rate) and women (84.9% case fatality rate). As can be determined by these case fatality rates, it is a highly fatal disease.

Smoking is the strongest risk factor for pancreatic cancer with the risk increased 2–3 times over that of nonsmokers. This is a dose-dependent association in that heavy smokers are more likely than casual smokers to get the disease. Almost 90%

of persons with this disease are diagnosed after the age of 55 years, and the majority of those are over 65 years of age. Chronic pancreatitis (inflammation of the pancreas usually resulting from either infection or trauma) is also recognized as a risk factor for later development of malignant changes. Other well-studied risk factors include obesity, family history of this cancer, and diabetes. Some factors currently under study include diets high in animal fats and excessive alcohol consumption. As with any cancer, many persons who are diagnosed with this tumor have no known risk factors. Previous concerns about an association between coffee or caffeine use and pancreatic cancer have not been confirmed by scientific studies.

There are currently no available screening tests for pancreatic cancer. The pancreas is located deeper in the abdomen, and therefore, it is unusual for symptoms to develop before the disease has spread to other organs. It is because of these two reasons there is a high mortality rate for this disease. An imaging study such as a CT scan is required for diagnosis.

Surgery is the primary treatment and is done either to remove the whole tumor, in the rare cases that it is found early, or for palliative treatment to relieve severe symptoms associated with the disease. Other modalities used are dependent on the spread of the disease and include radiation therapy, chemotherapy, and targeted therapy. Survival is dismal with this cancer. Even when it is found early and still localized to the primary site, the 5-year survival rate is only 21.5%. If there is spread to the regional lymph nodes, this rate drops to 8.7%; and when there is distant spread, it drops even further to 1.8%.

Other Important Cancers

The cancers discussed in this section were chosen because they may occur in the age group of the typical college-aged student, unlike those previously discussed that tend to occur in the older person, or because they may be of particular interest to students.

Testicular Cancer

Testicular cancer occurs primarily between the ages of 20–54 years. It is the most common cancer in men 15–34 years of age. There are several types of testicular tumors, but over 90% develop in the germ cells (cells that produce sperm) of the testicles. The age-adjusted incidence rate for testicular cancer is 5.5 per 100,000 men per year. In the United States in 2012, there will be an estimated 8,590 new cases and 360 deaths (case fatality rate of 4.2%) from this disease. The incidence has been increasing over recent years worldwide and in the United States. Not a frequent cancer (<1% of cancers in men), testicular cancer is considered an easily treated and highly curable cancer.

The most strongly associated risk factor is that of a young man having a testicle that did not fully descend into the scrotum by one year of age. Early surgical correction of this condition may have a protective effect. In addition, this is primarily a cancer of white men, though it is not understood why. A personal history of a

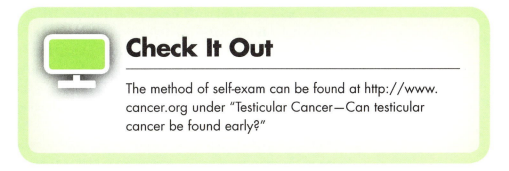

Check It Out

The method of self-exam can be found at http://www.cancer.org under "Testicular Cancer—Can testicular cancer be found early?"

previous testicular tumor or family history in a father or brother increases the risk slightly. Most tumors present as a palpable lump in the testicle. In the past, testicular self-exams were recommended as young men hit puberty to improve early detection. There is currently not enough scientific evidence to determine that this decreases the risk of dying from testicular cancer. Some physicians may still recommend self-exams in young men at higher risk of developing the disease. Five-year survival rates for all testicular tumors are excellent with a 99% survival if localized, 96% survival if there is only regional spread, and 72% survival even with distant metastasis. The age-adjusted death rate is 0.2 per 100,000 men per year.

Cervical Cancer

The cervix of a woman lies at the junction of the uterus and vagina (see Figure 12-14). Cervical cancer occurs in women primarily between the ages of 30–50, although 20% of cases will occur in women over 65 years old. Hispanic and black women have much higher incidence rates than do women of other ethnicities. The age-adjusted incidence rate for invasive cervical cancer is 8.1 cases per 100,000 women per year. There will be an estimated 12,170 new cases of invasive disease in 2012 with 4,220 deaths (34.7% case fatality rate). In situ (localized to the surface) cancer

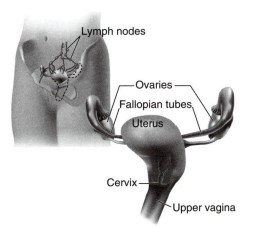

FIGURE 12-14 Female Anatomy
Courtesy of the National Cancer Institute (NCI)—Visuals Online: http://visualsonline.cancer.gov/details.cfm?imageid=4350

of the cervix occurs about 4 times more frequently than the invasive type. The age-adjusted death rate is 2.4 per 100,000 women per year. Fortunately, 48% of these cancers are confined locally at presentation and have a 5-year survival rate of 91%; 36% present with regional spread only and have a survival rate of 57%; whereas only 12% present with distal spread and have a survival rate of only 17%. Routine use of the HPV vaccine will be expected to have a major impact on decreasing the incidence and death rates of cervical cancer.

Although cervical cancer is not one of the more common cancers in women, it is one of the most preventable. From 1952–1992, deaths from this cancer decreased by 70% because of increased screening, and rates continue to decrease about 3% per year. Much has been published recently because of the association of human papillomavirus (HPV) and cervical cancer. The vaccine against this virus recently introduced will serve as a further preventive measure. Other known risk factors include immunosuppression, smoking (twice the risk), birth control pills (twice the risk), delivery of three or more children, less than 17-years-old with first pregnancy (twice the risk), history of maternal use of diethylstilbestrol during pregnancy (used during the years 1940–1971), and family history of cervical cancer (2–3 times the risk).

Screening is done with a **Papanicolaou smear (Pap smear)**, which is when cells from the surface of the cervix are collected and then viewed under the microscope for evidence of early malignant changes (dysplasia). Because the process of a normal cervical cell changing to a premalignant cell and then to a cancerous cell occurs slowly, routine Pap smears give medical personnel the ability to detect changes early and thus prevent progression to cancer. The current recommendations from the American Cancer Society is for a woman to have her first Pap smear at the age of 21 years or within 3 years of becoming sexually active, and this is repeated annually until the age of 30. At that point, if three prior screens have been negative, the frequency can decrease to every 2–3 years.

Lymphomas

Lymphomas are cancers that originate in the lymph cells and tissues of the body. There are two main types: Hodgkin lymphoma and non-Hodgkin lymphoma. Each of these main types has several subtypes. Most all lymphomas present the same way with painless, swollen lymph nodes, fever, unexplained weight loss, chest pain, and night sweats. See Figure 12-15 for the anatomy of the lymphatic system.

Hodgkin lymphoma usually begins in the lymph nodes of the neck and chest, although it can start in any lymph node of the body. The most common variant of this disease occurs primarily in younger adults in their 20s, although it can occur at a younger or older age. The age-adjusted incidence rate for Hodgkin disease is 2.8 per 100,000 men and women per year. In 2012, there will be about 9,060 new cases with 4,960 (55%) occurring in males and 4,100 (45%) occurring in females. There were 1,190 deaths from this tumor (case fatality rate 13.5%) with 670 in males (case fatality rate 15.8%) and 520 in females (case fatality rate 12.7%).

The most well-known risk for this tumor is a past history of infection with Epstein-Barr virus (EBV), the virus that causes mononucleosis, but it is also associated with infection with the human immunodeficiency virus (HIV). It is seen more

Papanicolaou smear (Pap smear): cells from the surface of the cervix are collected and viewed under the microscope for evidence of early malignant changes

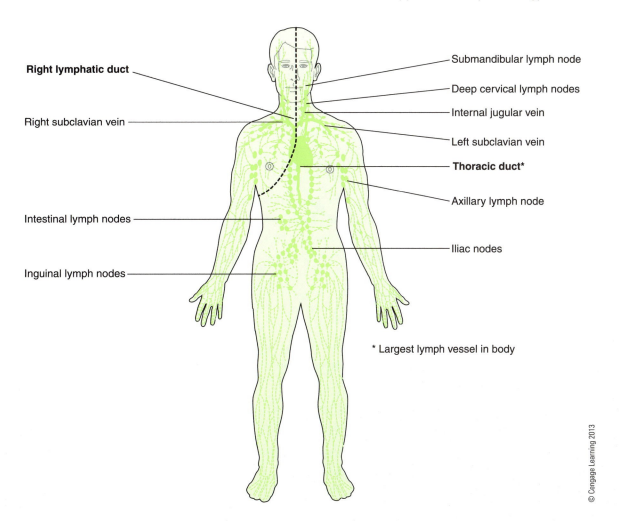

Right lymphatic duct

Right subclavian vein

Intestinal lymph nodes

Inguinal lymph nodes

Submandibular lymph node

Deep cervical lymph nodes

Internal jugular vein

Left subclavian vein

Thoracic duct*

Axillary lymph node

Iliac nodes

* Largest lymph vessel in body

© Cengage Learning 2013

FIGURE 12-15 The Lymphatic System

commonly in persons from the United States, Canada, and Northern Europe, as well as persons of a higher socioeconomic status, but these associations have not been explained. A sibling of a person with Hodgkin disease is at higher risk for developing the same tumor, but this is still uncommon. The overall 5-year survival rate is 85% with rates up to greater than 90% in localized disease. The age-adjusted death rate is 0.4 per 100,000 per year.

Non-Hodgkin lymphoma (NHL) has many different subtypes and may start in any part of the lymph system. The age-adjusted incidence rate for non-Hodgkin lymphoma is 19.8 per 100,000 men and women per year. There will be an estimated 70,130 new cases of NHL in 2012 with 18,940 deaths from the disease (case fatality rate 27.0%). The risk of this disease increases with age with most cases occurring in persons over the age of 60; only about 800 cases per year occur in children up to 19 years of age. It tends to occur more frequently in whites than any other race or ethnicity and in males slightly more than females. It has been associated with immune system disorders, as well as with certain infectious agents such as Epstein-Barr virus (cause of infectious mononucleosis) and HIV. Radiation exposure, either environmentally or as treatment for disease, increases the risk of development of NHL. Five-year survival rates are based on the specific subtype of disease, spread of the disease, and certain other prognostic indicators such as laboratory study results. Overall, the 5-year survival rate for NHL is 67%, much lower than that of Hodgkin lymphoma. The age-adjusted death rate is 6.7 per 100,000 per year.

RISK FACTORS AND PREVENTION

Risk factors have been mentioned as they related to the specific cancers discussed. In this section, some of the common risk factors for cancer are reviewed. Some of them are lifestyle behaviors that can be modified and, therefore, have potential for intervention, whereas others are nonmodifiable.

Risk Factors

- *Age:* The strongest risk factor for developing cancer is nonmodifiable; it is growing older. Seventy-seven percent of all cancers occur in persons over the age of 55 years.

- *Genetics:* A known genetic mutation is only associated with about 5% of all cancers. This may be slightly higher in some cancers and lower in others.

- *Exposure to carcinogens:* Examples of these substances include asbestos, benzene, vinyl chloride and others. The most studied carcinogen is tobacco smoking, which is discussed in more detail in "A Closer Look" at the end of this chapter. Some exposures are easily prevented such as quitting tobacco products or removing asbestos. Others may be more difficult to modify, such as some occupational exposures.

- *Ultraviolet light radiation:* Unprotected exposure to ultraviolet light is one of the most easily modified risk factors. Exposures include the sun, tanning booths, and sun lamps, which are so popular these days with young adults.

- *Ionizing radiation:* This includes diagnostic radiologic imaging, radiation therapy for other cancers, and radon exposure. More recent extensive studies have found no association between nonionizing radiation exposure from cell phone use and brain cancers. This had been a concern in the past, and the potential for this association continues to be investigated.

- *Infectious agents:* Current evidence suggests that 20% of cancers may be caused by infectious agents. This has resulted in the development of vaccines against some of these agents specifically to prevent the later complication of cancer. Well-studied infectious diseases that have potential for later development of cancer include (1) HIV as a precursor to lymphomas and potentially others, (2) HHV-8 and its link to Kaposi's sarcoma and non-Hodgkin lymphoma, (3) EBV (the cause of infectious mononucleosis) and non-Hodgkin lymphoma and nasopharyngeal carcinoma, (4) hepatitis B and C infections associated with liver cancer, and (5) *H. pylori* and stomach cancer. Human papillomavirus (HPV) is the cause of sexually transmitted anogenital warts and has been found to be the cause of anogenital cancers. This association is most notable with cervical cancer, but is also linked to cancer of the penis, oral cavity, anus, vagina, and vulva. Identifying other infectious agents and potentially preventing their associated cancers is an area of intense research.

Prevention

The major focus of prevention is aimed at the modifiable risk factors. Lifestyle changes are the primary focus for breaking the progression to cancer. Smoking is the most preventable cause of invasive cancer and is discussed in detail in "A Closer Look" at the end of this chapter. Given the large number of skin cancers, avoiding unprotected exposure to UV light whether it is in the form of the sun, tanning booths, or sunlamps is another target for protection. Preventive measures would include avoidance of exposure during peak sunlight hours from 10 a.m.-4 p.m. and use of sunscreen effective against both UVA and UVB light. The SPF (sun protection factor) of a sunscreen denotes protection against UVB sunlight only and a minimal SPF of 30 is recommended. Dietary changes that have been associated with prevention of cancer include avoiding excessive alcohol consumption and eating foods low in fat and high in fiber. Avoidance of exposure to known carcinogens when possible will also have an impact on the incidence of cancers.

Routine screening, when available, may not prevent cancers but will help to identify them earlier when treatment may be more successful. This would include routine visits to a physician for skin exams, full physical exams, and screening procedures when indicated, as well as self-screening exams. Vaccines that have been developed against certain infectious agents associated with later cancer development may be the future of prevention and are already playing a role.

As scientists continue to identify the genetic changes identified with familial heritable cancers, they are able to develop genetic testing that can be used to monitor high-risk persons and allow preventive measures when available. Genetic testing may also allow for earlier diagnosis that, for most invasive cancers, leads to an improved prognosis. Identifying genetic changes found in different cancer types may also lead to development of targeted treatments against the cancer cells that are present.

THE FUTURE

In 2005, the National Cancer Institute and the National Human Genome Research Institute began the Cancer Genome Atlas. This is a large-scale effort to identify the genomic changes associated with the development of the various cancers. The initial tumors studied were lung cancer, ovarian cancer, and glioblastoma, a brain cancer. There are more planned for in future years. This information may later be

Check It Out

To see more about the Cancer Genome Atlas, go to http://cancergenome.nih.gov/.

used for screening in high-risk patients, for diagnosis, and for studying different targeted treatments.

In addition to the genomic studies, ongoing research into drug development aims to find medications that will target the malignant cells and limit their effects on the normal cells, thereby minimizing severe side effects. Another major focus of investigations is the relationship between certain infectious agents and later development of cancers. We have already started the prevention of these cancers with the use of vaccines against hepatitis B and human papillomavirus.

Summary

Cancer is not one disease, but many, dependent on the origin of the mutated cells. Because of this, the incidence, prevalence, lifetime risk, and mortality rates vary greatly. The characteristic finding in all cancers is *uncontrolled growth* of cells and the *ability to invade other tissues*. Cancers can be classified by their tissue and organ of origin, by how much the cancer cells differ from their normal counterparts (grading), by the DNA changes in the malignant cells (genotyping), and by how much the cancer has spread (staging). Non-melanomatous skin cancers are by far the most commonly occurring cancers, but because of their benign nature, they are not considered *invasive* cancers. By sheer numbers, the five most commonly occurring cancers are skin, lung, prostate, breast, and colorectal. Looking only at invasive cancers, the three most common cancers in men are prostate, lung, and colorectal. In women, they are breast, lung, and colorectal. The five most deadly cancers are lung, colorectal, breast, pancreas, and prostate. This chapter discussed these cancers in some detail. Lymphomas, cervical, and testicular cancers were also discussed because of their importance to the college-age student.

Cancer is the second most common cause of death in the United States. By identifying risk factors that can be modified, the incidence of a specific cancer may be reduced and health care costs contained. Two common cancers that prevention can have a major impact on are skin cancers, which can be reduced by reducing unprotected sun exposure, and lung cancer, which can be reduced by smoking cessation.

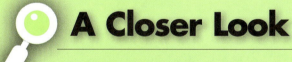

A Closer Look

Risk Factors—Tobacco

Smoking is the most preventable cause of death in the United States. It is responsible for more deaths than motor vehicle accidents, AIDS, suicides, murders, alcohol, and illicit drugs, combined. The average smoker will die 13–14 years earlier than the nonsmoker. In 2006, users spent $89.4 billion on tobacco products. Of these costs, $83.6 billion was spent on cigarettes, $3.2 billion on cigars, and $2.6 billion on smokeless tobacco products. Direct health care costs associated with tobacco that year were $96 billion. Another $97 billion was associated with indirect costs such as those resulting from lost productivity. Therefore, tobacco-related costs for the year 2006 were $282.4 billion!

Types of Exposure

Cigarettes, cigars, and pipe tobacco are all made from dried tobacco leaves. See Figure 12-16. Some have substances added for flavor or other reasons. There are more than

Continues

4,000 substances, including ammonia, tar, and carbon monoxide, in tobacco. Over 60 of these substances are known to be carcinogens. There are several forms of tobacco use, but it is important to know that all forms of tobacco use are dangerous to a person's health. The "tar" in cigarettes is the sticky brown residue that contains the toxins and carcinogens. It accumulates in the lungs and paralyzes the cilia (hair-like projections on the surface of the cells that propel mucus and debris out of the lungs), leading to lung diseases and cancer. The inhaled toxins increase as the cigarette burns down, such that the last puff may have up to twice the amount as the first puff. Filters initially developed to decrease the amount of tar absorbed by the lungs have been found not to work as efficiently as they were designed. In addition, the low-tar cigarettes are not any safer than regular cigarettes. Smokers tend to compensate by taking deeper inhalations, larger puffs, and more frequent puffs.

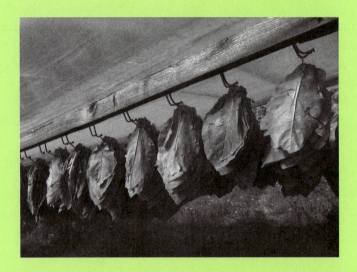

FIGURE 12-16 Tobacco Leaves Hanging to Dry
©ollirg/www.Shutterstock.com

Nicotine is a substance common to all types of tobacco products and has been identified as the substance that is addictive. It does not cause cancer. The U.S. Surgeon General reported that nicotine was the addictive substance to the public initially in 1988. That is still true today. The level of nicotine absorbed into the bloodstream depends on the type of tobacco product used, the numbers of puffs, how deep the tobacco is inhaled, and other factors.

Cigarettes

Cigarettes are made of different blends of tobacco, frequently with additives, and then wrapped in porous paper. They tend to contain about 1 gram of tobacco. Cigarette smoking accounts for the majority of tobacco use in the United States and, therefore, for the majority of smoking-related disease and cancer. See Figure 12-17 for trends in cigarette smoking in the United States.

The Family Smoking Prevention and Tobacco Control Act signed by President Obama gives control over tobacco products to the Federal Drug Administration (FDA). It requires that the manufacturers report all ingredients used in their cigarettes and bans the use of the terms, "mild" or "light," which suggest a lower-risk alternative.

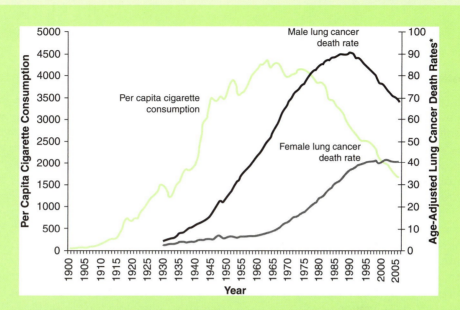

FIGURE 12-17 Tobacco Use and Death Rates in the United States, 1900–2006
*Age-adjusted to 2000 U.S. standard population.

Source: Death rates: U.S. Mortality Data, 1960-2006, U.S. Mortality Volumes, 1930–1959, National Center for Health Statistics, Centers for Disease Control and Prevention, 2009. Cigarette consumption: U.S. Department of Agriculture, 1900–2007.

Secondhand Smoke

Secondhand smoke consists of the sidestream smoke that comes from the burning cigarette, as well as the smoke exhaled by the smoker. Sidestream smoke passes easily through the porous paper that wraps the tobacco of a cigarette and contains more cancer-causing substances than the exhaled smoke. Both of these smokes contain toxins and carcinogens and put those who are exposed to them at risk for the same diseases and lung cancer as the smoker.

Cigars

The tobacco leaves for cigars are aged for about a year and then fermented. One large cigar can contain as much tobacco as an entire package of cigarettes, and it is wrapped in a tobacco leaf with no filter. Cigars are usually not inhaled completely, so that there is slower absorption in the lungs, but the absorption in the saliva is very significant. In addition, the sidestream smoke contains the same toxins and carcinogens as cigarettes.

Smokeless Tobacco

Smokeless tobacco is defined as tobacco that is not burned. All smokeless tobacco products contain nicotine, toxins, and carcinogens. Two examples are *chewing tobacco*, which is loose leaves or plugs of tobacco that are chewed or placed between the cheek and the gum, and *snuff*, which is finely ground tobacco in cans or pouches that can be moist or dry and also is placed between the gum and cheek. In both cases, nicotine and the other substances are absorbed easily through the mucous membranes of the oral cavity. One of the most harmful chemicals in smokeless tobacco is nitrosamines, which are known carcinogens. Although not associated with lung cancer like the smoked tobacco products, these products are strongly

Continues

associated with cancers of the oral cavity and esophagus, as well as gum disease and destruction of the teeth and boney sockets around them.

E-cigarettes

Around for several years now, **electronic cigarettes (e-cigarettes)** may resemble an actual cigarette but use an atomizer to heat a solution in a cartridge using a battery as the power supply. The solution contains nicotine (known to be the addictive substance in cigarettes), various flavorings, and other substances that may or may not have health risks. Nicotine levels may vary in these products, and other substances that have been found include diethylene glycol (a chemical found in antifreeze) and nitrosamines (known carcinogens).

There are those who promote the potential benefits of e-cigarettes, including the delivery of nicotine without the other carcinogens and chemicals of regular cigarettes and the absence of secondhand smoke. In addition, because they look and feel like their real counterparts and the level of nicotine contained can be varied, they are potential aides in smoking cessation. On the other hand, there is currently no scientific data regarding their general safety or their efficacy in helping smokers quit. There are concerns that the contents of the cartridges used have not been standardized. Whether children may use them and be led into smoking real cigarettes also needs investigation. Although e-cigarettes were previously unregulated, a recent federal ruling allows the FDA oversight of marketing and labeling, monitoring of the substances contained in the cartridges, and restriction of sales to those persons over 18 years of age. Studies looking at potential risks and benefits are ongoing.

Others

Manufacturers have found ways to supply tobacco in other forms that may be more attractive to users. Some examples include clove cigarettes from Indonesia and fruit-flavored cigarettes from India. A new social event popular on college campuses involves smoking flavored tobacco through a water pipe or hookah. It is mistakenly thought that the water filters out the toxins of the tobacco, but this smoke actually contains more toxins than others. In addition, infectious diseases have been known to be transmitted by hookahs because users share the mouthpiece.

Health Consequences

All forms of tobacco use increase the risk for health problems. Cigarette smoking is the most common use of tobacco and, therefore, is responsible for a higher occurrence of the sequelae. Damage from tobacco use is dose-dependent. That is, the more a person smokes or uses smokeless tobacco products and the longer they use tobacco in any form, the higher risk they have for developing some kind of health problem. The major medical consequences of tobacco use include cancer, cardiovascular disease, chronic respiratory diseases, and early death. There are other health issues related to tobacco that may be specific to a particular demographic such as pregnant women or infants.

electronic cigarettes (e-cigarettes): resemble actual cigarettes but use an atomizer to heat a solution containing nicotine and other substances

Cancer

Smoking is a major leading preventable cause of cancer and cancer deaths in the United States. A man who smokes is 23 times more likely to develop lung cancer than a male nonsmoker, and a female smoker is 13 times more likely to develop lung cancer than a female nonsmoker. Smoking is responsible for 90% of lung cancer deaths in men and 80% of lung cancer deaths in women.

Although lung cancer is the most well-known and studied cancer related to cigarette smoking, smokers are also at higher risk for cancer of the larynx, oral cavity (mouth), esophagus, stomach, pancreas, kidney, bladder, and cervix. Cigars are associated with cancers of the mouth, larynx, esophagus, pancreas, and lung. Smokeless tobacco use is associated primarily with cancer of the oral cavity, but also with cancer of the esophagus, stomach, and pancreas.

Cardiovascular Disease and Stroke

Smokers are 2–4 times more likely to develop coronary heart disease and up to 6 times more likely to have a heart attack than nonsmokers. They are also 2–4 times more likely to suffer from a stroke. Cigar smokers are less likely to have these complications, but they still have a higher risk than nonsmokers. The same is true for smokeless tobacco users. Other cardiovascular diseases that occur more frequently in smokers include atherosclerosis, peripheral vascular disease, and aortic aneurysms.

Chronic Respiratory Diseases

Chronic obstructive pulmonary disease (COPD), also known as "emphysema," is strongly associated with smoking, and 90% of deaths from this chronic respiratory disease are seen in smokers. Bronchitis is more common in smokers; and when a smoker gets pneumonia, he or she usually has a more severe course. Asthma is also worse in smokers, and asthma exacerbations or flares are seen commonly in children exposed to secondhand smoke.

Deaths

There are about 443,000 deaths per year in the United States attributable directly to smoking. This is greater than the mortality from HIV, alcohol, motor vehicle accidents, suicide, and murder, all combined! Of these deaths, 46,000 occur in nonsmokers who live with smokers. Male smokers die about 13.2 years early, and women smokers lose about 14.5 years of life as compared to their nonsmoking counterparts. See Figure 12-18.

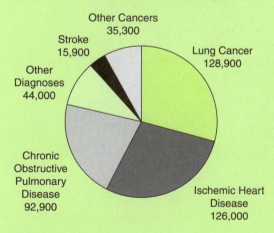

About 443,000 U.S. Deaths Attributable Each Year to Cigarette Smoking*

Other Cancers 35,300
Stroke 15,900
Other Diagnoses 44,000
Lung Cancer 128,900
Chronic Obstructive Pulmonary Disease 92,900
Ischemic Heart Disease 126,000

FIGURE 12-18 Deaths Attributable to Smoking
*Average annual number of deaths, 2000–2004.

Source: *MMWR* 2008; 57(45): 1226–1228.

Courtesy of Centers for Disease Control and Prevention: http://www.cdc.gov/
tobacco/data_statistics/tables/health/attrdeaths/index.htm

Continues

Other

Smokers are at higher risk for miscellaneous conditions such as gum disease, bone thinning, and stomach ulcers. Bone loss around the teeth and tooth loss are frequently seen in smokeless tobacco users. Children of smokers are at increased risk for ear infections, lung infections, and asthma; and because of these risks, children who are exposed have more hospitalizations as compared to children of nonsmokers.

Treatment

The U.S. Surgeon General's report in 1990 stated that once someone quits smoking, the beneficial effects start right away. See Figure 12-19. The report also states that ex-smokers live longer and lower their risk of lung cancer, heart attacks and strokes, and chronic lung disease. If smokers quit in their 30s, they avoid most of the risks associated with smoking. Even when quitting after 50 years old, an ex-smoker will live longer. The risk of delivering a baby with low birth weight can be prevented if a pregnant woman quits smoking before or during the first 3–4 months of her pregnancy.

The Centers for Disease Control reports there are more than 46 million smokers in the United States. About 70% of these smokers report that they would like to quit smoking, and about 40%

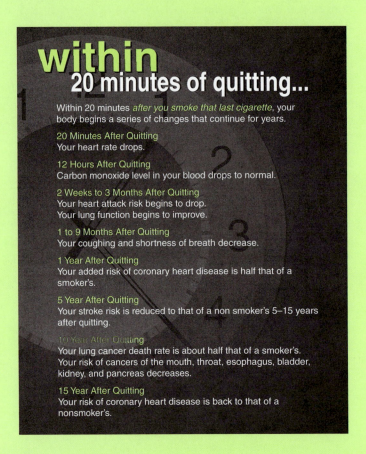

FIGURE 12-19 After Quitting…

Courtesy of Centers for Disease Control and Prevention: http://www.cdc.gov/tobacco/data_statistics/sgr/2004/posters/20mins/index.htm

of smokers will try to quit each year. Because of the strongly addictive nature of the nicotine contained in tobacco, only 4–7% of smokers will succeed in stopping without help. Most cessation programs recommend using a nicotine replacement method. Several forms are available to purchase without a prescription such as the nicotine gum, lozenges, and patches. Nicotine inhalers and nasal spray that require a doctor's prescription are also available. It is important for smokers to remember that they cannot use these nicotine replacements therapies and continue to smoke. The nicotine toxicity can be dangerous. Medications in the form of pills are available to ease the withdrawal from nicotine, but these also require a prescription. There are several websites listed at the end of this chapter that focus on helping a smoker quit successfully.

Epidemiology of Tobacco Use

The prevalence of smoking among adults in the United States dropped from 24.7% of the population in 1997 to 20.6% in 2009. This downward trend has leveled out over the past couple of years. By gender, 23.5% of men are smokers and 17.9% of women are smokers. By age, about 20% of high school students smoke, 24% of persons aged 25–44 smoke, and only 9.5% of persons over the age of 65 years smoke. (Is this because most smokers die by this age or because they have become wiser and quit?) Whites, African Americans, and Native Americans/Alaskan Natives smoke much more than their Hispanic and Asian American counterparts.

Cigar smokers used to be middle-aged and older men, but now younger men and teenagers have taken up the habit. Cigars have lower taxes than cigarettes and therefore may be easier to afford for younger people. In 2009, 27% of twelfth-grade boys and 10% of twelfth-grade girls reportedly had smoked cigars. The largest group of smokeless tobacco users is Major League baseball players. In 2003, one in three players chewed tobacco!

Review Questions

1. Number the following cancers in order of incidence with the most common first:

<u>In Men:</u>

_____ Colorectal

_____ Lung

_____ Prostate

_____ Testicular

_____ Skin (non-melanomatous)

<u>In Women:</u>

_____ Breast

_____ Skin (non-melanoma)

_____ Colorectal

_____ Lung

_____ Cervical

2. The cancer that causes the most cancer-related deaths among men and women is

_____.

3. **True or False** Cancer is characterized by the uncontrolled growth and spread of abnormal cells.

4. Five-year survival rates:

    a. Describe the percent of cancer patients who are alive after five years
    b. Does not distinguish between those who are cured, those who are still in treatment, or those who have relapsed
    c. Does not reflect recent advances in diagnosis and treatment
    d. All of the above

5. Name two risk factors for skin cancer (either melanomas or non-melanomatous):

    1._____
    2._____

6. The ethnicity of males at highest risk for prostate cancer is:

    a. Caucasians
    b. Hispanic Americans
    c. African Americans
    d. Asian Americans

7. BRCA1 and BRCA2 are genes associated with:

    a. Lung
    b. Breast
    c. Colorectal
    d. Pancreatic

8. The major source of data and statistics regarding cancers comes from the _____ Program of the National Cancer Institute.

    a. Annual Report to the Nation on the Status of Cancer
    b. Surveillance, Epidemiology, and End Results (SEER)
    c. North American Association of Central Cancer Registries
    d. American Cancer Society

9. **True or False** Prevalence of a specific cancer type is dependent on the incidence of the cancer and the survival time.

10. In the United States, almost one in _____ persons will be diagnosed with cancer at some point during his or her lifetime.

11. **For Deeper Thought** Choose one of the following topics and come up with a "campaign" that could be used on your college campus to address the issues. Choose the information you would use to present your case to your fellow students—e.g., would statistics be helpful, consequences, difficulty in behavior modification, etc.

    - Why a fellow student should stop smoking
    - Why a fellow student should never start smoking
    - Why fellow students should not use tanning booths, sunlamps
    - Why it is important to get the HPV vaccine now (while a student)

Website Resources

American Cancer Society: http://www.cancer.org

American Heart Association: htpp://www.americanheart.org

American Lung Association: http://www.lungusa.org

Centers for Disease Control and Prevention: http://www.cdc.gov

Centers for Disease Control and Prevention: National Program of Cancer Registries, United States Cancer Statistics (USCS): http://apps.nccd.cdc.gov/uscs/index.aspx

National Cancer Institute: http://www.cancer.gov

National Library of Medicine: http://www.nlm.nih.gov

Surveillance Epidemiology and End Results: http://seer.cancer.gov

U.S. Preventive Services Task Force: http://www.ahrq.gov/clinic/prevenix.htm

World Health Organization: http://www.who.int

Smoking Cessation Resources:

    American Lung Association: http://www.lungusa.org

    Smokefree.gov: http://www.smokefree.gov

    Centers for Disease Control: http://www.cdc.gov/tobacco

    American Heart Association: http://www.americanheart.org

References

American Cancer Society. (2011). Cancer Facts and Figures. Retrieved from http://www.cancer.org/Research/CancerFactsFigures/CancerFactsFigures/cancer-facts-figures-2011

American Cancer Society. (2012). Cancer Facts and Figures. Retrieved from http://www.cancer.org/Research/CancerFactsFigures/CancerFactsFigures/cancer-facts-figures-2012

Buzzle.com. (n.d.). Famous People with Lung Cancer. Retrieved from http://www.buzzle.com/articles/famous-people-with-lung-cancer.html

Centers for Disease Control and Prevention. (updated October 24, 2011). FastStats—Death and Mortality. Retrieved from http://www.cdc.gov/nchs/fastats/deaths.htm

Centers for Disease Control and Prevention. (updated March 21, 2011). Smoking and Tobacco Use. Retrieved from http://www.cdc.gov/tobacco/index.htm

Joe DiMaggio. (n.d.). The Life Story. Retrieved from http://www.joedimaggio.com/LifeStory.php?n=&n=1&lspg=6

National Cancer Institute. (2010). Surveillance Epidemiology and End Results—SEER Stat Fact Sheets: All Sites. Retrieved from http://seer.cancer.gov/statfacts/html/all.html#incidence-mortality

National Comprehensive Cancer Network. (2010). Cancer Staging Guide. Retrieved from http://www.nccn.com/understanding-cancer/cancer-staging.html

U. S. Preventive Services Task Force. (October 2008). Screening for Colorectal Cancer. Retrieved from http://www.uspreventiveservicestaskforce.org/uspstf08/colocancer/colors.htm

Wiley Online Library. (August 15, 1998). Cancer—The Prevalence of Complementary/Alternative Medicine in Cancer. Retrieved from http://onlinelibrary.wiley.com/doi/10.1002/(SICI)1097-0142(19980815)83:4%3C777::AID-CNCR22%3E3.0.CO;2-O/full

World Health Organization. (February 2011). Health Topics—Cancer. Retrieved from http://www.who.int/mediacentre/factsheets/fs297/en/index.html

Chapter 13

DIABETES MELLITUS

Learning Objectives

Upon completion of this chapter, you should be able to:

1. Define diabetes and the function of insulin.
2. Describe the prevalence of diabetes as it occurs among different age groups, genders, and ethnic groups.
3. Define prediabetes and explain the findings of the Diabetes Prevention Plan (DPP).
4. Explain the difference between Type 1, Type 2, and gestational diabetes, including the underlying cause and prevalence in the United States.
5. List the risk factors for each type of diabetes and describe their association to any preventive measures.

Key Terms

acanthosis nigricans

autoimmune

beta cell

diabetes mellitus

endocrine

gestational diabetes mellitus

glucose

glycosuria

hyperglycemia

hypoglycemia

impaired fasting glucose

impaired glucose tolerance

insulin

insulin resistance

islets of Langerhans

metabolic

metabolic syndrome

pancreas

polycystic ovary syndrome (PCOS)

polydipsia

polyphagia

polyuria

prediabetes

Type 1 diabetes mellitus

Type 2 diabetes mellitus

Chapter Outline

INTRODUCTION

diabetes mellitus: group of disorders characterized by high blood sugar resulting in polyuria

endocrine: system of glands that produce hormones that regulate functions of the body

insulin resistance: state in which the pancreas produces insulin but the body cells do not respond to it as they should to allow for glucose uptake

metabolic: relating to the breakdown of food and use for energy

glucose: sugar used by cells for energy for cellular processes

What do Mike Huckabee (politician), Randy Jackson (*American Idol* judge), Bobby Clarke (NHL—Philadelphia Flyers), and Arthur Ashe (ex–tennis pro) all have (or had) in common? Yes, they all have diabetes!

Diabetes mellitus is an **endocrine** disorder that is *characterized by high blood sugar*. This disease is caused by inadequate production of insulin, lack of response to the insulin that is produced, also known as **insulin resistance**, or both. It is also sometimes referred to as a **metabolic** disease because it affects the way our body uses digested food for energy and growth. You may have heard your grandmother call it "sugar in the blood," but this is not entirely accurate because we all have sugar (**glucose**) in our blood. The problem in people with diabetes is that they have too much sugar in the blood. Why this occurs will be explained in a later section. Different types of diabetes have different causes but may share risk factors that either precipitate the disease or worsen the disease.

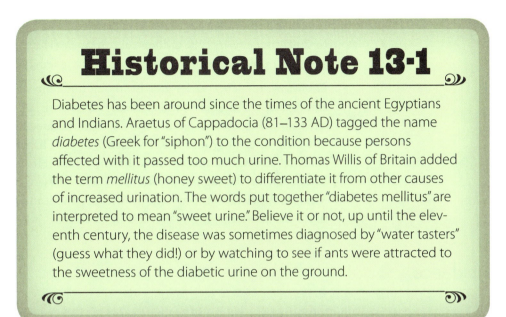

Historical Note 13-1

Diabetes has been around since the times of the ancient Egyptians and Indians. Araetus of Cappadocia (81–133 AD) tagged the name *diabetes* (Greek for "siphon") to the condition because persons affected with it passed too much urine. Thomas Willis of Britain added the term *mellitus* (honey sweet) to differentiate it from other causes of increased urination. The words put together "diabetes mellitus" are interpreted to mean "sweet urine." Believe it or not, up until the eleventh century, the disease was sometimes diagnosed by "water tasters" (guess what they did!) or by watching to see if ants were attracted to the sweetness of the diabetic urine on the ground.

THE SCOPE OF THE PROBLEM

The statistics presented here are based on information published by the Centers for Disease Control and Prevention (CDC) in the 2007 National Diabetes Fact Sheet. This fact sheet, the most current available, uses various databases, studies, and surveys to derive its estimates. See the website referring to this fact sheet listed at the end of this chapter for further information.

Prevalence

The total reported prevalence of all types of diabetes in the U. S. population (2007) was 23.6 million people affected, or 7.8% of the U.S. population. This included 17.9 million diagnosed with the disease and the estimated 5.7 million undiagnosed. (For an explanation of how "undiagnosed" cases were inferred, see the reference at the end of this chapter for the 2007 National Diabetes Fact Sheet.) Prevalence varies based on age, gender, and ethnicity.

- *Age:* Prevalence for diabetes in the United States varies according to age. In persons less than 20 years old, there were 186,300 cases (0.2% of the population in this age group). In persons more than 20 years old, there were 23.5 million cases (10.7% of the population in this age group); but in the subgroup of those persons more than 60 years old, there were 12.2 million cases (23.1% of the population in this age group). Although the total numbers of cases in those 20 years of age and older are the highest, the percentage is highest in the subgroup of persons over 60 years old, putting this age category in higher risk.

- *Gender:* The prevalence of diabetes is about equal in adult men and adult women. In 2007, there were 12.0 million cases in men (11.2% of the male population) and 11.5 million cases in women (10.2% of the female population).

- *Ethnicity:* Prevalence varies greatly among different ethnic groups. It is highest among Native Americans and Alaskan natives with 16.5% of those populations affected. There is even variation in this group based on the geographic region in which different groups live. Prevalence in the Hispanic population is 10.4%, and this also varies among the different ethnic Hispanic groups with Puerto Ricans having the highest prevalence, Cubans having the least prevalence, and Mexican Americans in between. In African Americans, the prevalence is 11.8%. In Asian Americans, it is 7.5%, and in Caucasians it is 6.6%.

Incidence

In 2007, there were 1.6 million new cases of diabetes diagnosed in the U.S. population (5.3 new cases per 1,000 persons in the U.S. population). By age, there were 281,000 new cases in persons 20–39 years old (2.2 new cases per 1,000 persons of that age); 819,808 new cases in persons aged 40–59 (10.7 new cases per 1,000 persons of that age); and 536,000 new cases in persons over 69 years old (14.2 new cases per 1,000 persons of that age). Among those less than 20 years old in 2002–2003, there were 15,000 new cases (18 new cases per 100,000 persons of that age) of Type 1 disease and 3,700 new cases (4.4 new cases per 100,000 persons of that age) of Type 2 disease. Caucasian youth had the highest incidence of new onset Type 1 disease, which was greater than the incidence of Type 2 diabetes in this group. Asian Americans and Pacific Islanders, as well as Native Americans and Alaskan natives, had a higher incidence of Type 2 disease across all age groups as compared to Type 1 disease. African Americans and Hispanics had similar incidences of Type 1 and Type 2 disease.

The incidence of Type 2 disease among adolescents has been steadily increasing in the United States and worldwide and is trending along with the rise in obesity among youth. Type 2 diabetes, which two decades ago occurred only rarely in children (hence the previous name of "adult onset" diabetes), now accounts for 50% of all new cases of diabetes in youth aged 10–19 years. The potential impact of this on the health care delivery system is enormous.

Death Rates

Diabetes mellitus was the seventh leading cause of death in the United States in 2007. The number of deaths actually may be underreported because of poor documentation on death certificates. Only approximately 35–40% of death certificates of known diabetics had diabetes listed on the death certificate even as an underlying disease. The risk of death overall is two times that of persons the same age but without diabetes. Heart disease and stroke account for the majority of deaths in persons with diabetes.

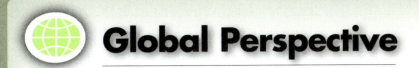

Global Perspective

The World Health Organization (WHO) reports that 346 million people worldwide have diabetes mellitus. In 2008, 9% of the world's population over the age of 25 years had elevated blood sugars. In 2004, 3.4 million persons died from complications of elevated blood sugars with 80% of those deaths occurring in the lower- and middle-income countries. The top three countries in diabetes prevalence include (in decreasing order) India, China, and the United States. Prevalence in both developed and developing countries is expected to rise significantly to 2030 across all age groups (20–44 years, 45–64 years, 65+ years), except for the 20–44 years group from the developed countries. The WHO Global Strategy on diet, physical activity, and health supports the WHO'S diabetes work. WHO also collaborates with the International Diabetes Federation to celebrate the World Diabetes Day each year on November 14.

Financial Costs

Direct medical costs for diabetes for the year 2007 in the United States were $116 billion. Indirect costs for work loss, disability, and early death were $58 billion, leading to the total cost of $174 billion per year! The health care costs incurred for someone with diabetes are about 2.3 times the health care costs for someone without diabetes. According to Huang et al. in a December 2009 article in *Diabetes Care*, produced by the American Diabetes Association, the number of people with diagnosed and undiagnosed diabetes will increase from 23.7 million persons in 2009 with a total annual cost of $113 billion to 44.1 million persons in 2034 with an annual cost of $336 billion dollars! Isolating the costs for the older Medicare-eligible population, costs are expected to rise from $45 billion in 2009 to $171 billion in 2034.

BASIC PHYSIOLOGY AND PATHOPHYSIOLOGY

insulin: a hormone produced by the pancreas that is involved in the uptake of glucose by the body's cells to be used for energy

Because its primary symptom is an excess of urine production, diabetes was considered a disorder of the kidneys until 1889 when the pancreas was shown to have a major role in the disease. In 1921, the hormone **insulin**, which is responsible for facilitating the movement of glucose from the bloodstream into the cells for use as energy, was isolated.

Normal Physiology

beta cells: specialized cells, found in the islets of Langerhans regions of the pancreas, that produce insulin

islets of Langerhans: area of the pancreas that is related to its endocrine function, including the production of insulin; comprises only 1–2% of the mass of the pancreas

pancreas: located behind and below the stomach, a body organ that contains the cells that produce insulin

Insulin is a hormone produced by specialized cells, the **beta cells**, in the **islets of Langerhans** of the **pancreas**, an organ that lies just behind and below the stomach. See Figure 13-1 for a view of this anatomy. Release of insulin from the pancreas is stimulated by food eaten during a meal, especially foods containing sugars or carbohydrates. These carbohydrates and sugars are broken down into simple sugars, particularly glucose. This glucose passes into the bloodstream and is delivered to all parts of the body. It is the rise in blood glucose levels after a meal that triggers the release of insulin from the pancreas. Glucose is the primary source of energy for many of the body's cells, and insulin's role is to move the glucose from the bloodstream into the cells for use as energy for the cell's functions. Please refer to Figure 13-2, which shows a normal insulin response to a glucose load in the bloodstream. Insulin also has a role in the use of proteins and fats, as well as in glucose storage, that has an impact on persons with diabetes.

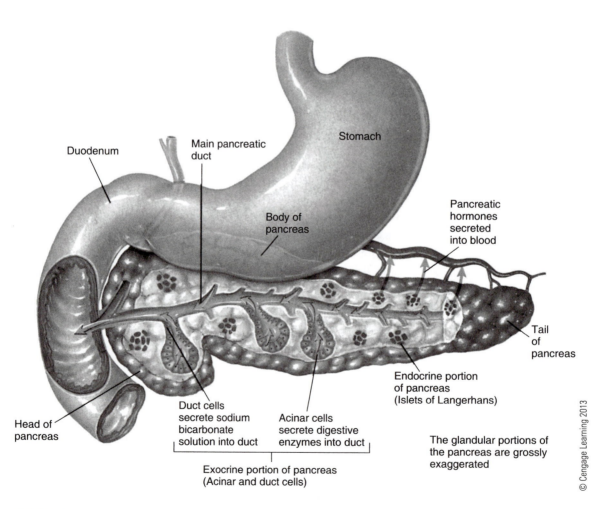

Duodenum

Main pancreatic duct

Stomach

Body of pancreas

Pancreatic hormones secreted into blood

Tail of pancreas

Endocrine portion of pancreas (Islets of Langerhans)

Head of pancreas

Duct cells secrete sodium bicarbonate solution into duct

Acinar cells secrete digestive enzymes into duct

Exocrine portion of pancreas (Acinar and duct cells)

The glandular portions of the pancreas are grossly exaggerated

© Cengage Learning 2013

FIGURE 13–1 Anatomy of Pancreas

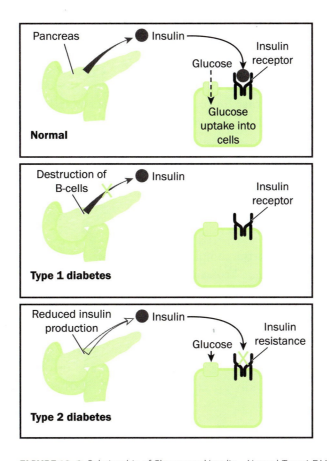

FIGURE 13–2 Relationship of Glucose and Insulin—Normal, Type 1 DM, Type 2 DM
© Blamb/www.Shutterstock.com

Blood sugar levels vary throughout the day over a relatively narrow range. These levels are highest after a meal, return to normal at about two hours after a meal, and are lowest after an overnight fast. When blood glucose levels return to normal, insulin release decreases.

Basic Pathophysiology and Symptoms

If the glucose cannot get into the cells, either because there is no insulin to promote its uptake or because the cells are not responding to the insulin that is present, sugar levels rise in the bloodstream, a condition known as **hyperglycemia**. Cells lose their primary source of energy, even though there is plenty of glucose around, because it cannot get into the cell. As glucose levels rise in the bloodstream, a threshold is met. At this point, the kidneys attempt to excrete the excess glucose by passing it in urine. As levels continue to rise, more and more urine is produced to help get rid of the excess glucose. This condition of excess urine productions is called **polyuria**, which is a primary symptom of diabetes. The urine now has excess glucose in it, a condition called **glycosuria**, and this is one of the ways the disease can be diagnosed. As more and more water is lost as urine production

hyperglycemia: high blood glucose (sugar)

polyuria: excessive urine production

glycosuria: glucose in the urine

increases, excess thirst occurs, **polydipsia**, to replace this loss. Because cells cannot use glucose for energy, the body gives the signal to replenish the source of energy by increased appetite, **polyphagia**. Therefore, the typical symptoms of all types of diabetes include these 3 Ps (polyuria, polydipsia, and polyphagia). Because of the loss of glucose and therefore calories, weight loss and fatigue can occur, most commonly with Type 1. Blurred vision can also occur because when there is excess glucose in the bloodstream, some sugar will deposit in the lenses of the eyes, drawing fluid in with it and distorting the shape of the lenses.

polydipsia: increased thirst
polyphagia: increased hunger

Complications

Besides short-term complications of diabetes such as **hypoglycemia** (low blood sugar) or diabetic ketoacidosis (a complication of high blood sugar), people with diabetes frequently develop serious, long-term complications, usually after years of having the disease. Over time hyperglycemia leads to narrowing of the blood vessels. In addition, insulin resistance itself is associated with atherosclerosis, also known as hardening of the arteries. Most of the long-term complications of diabetes are related to these vascular changes and involve the cardiovascular system, eyes, kidneys, skin, or central nervous system. This vascular damage is progressive over time.

hypoglycemia: low blood glucose (sugar)

Heart Disease and Stroke

There is an increased risk of heart disease and stroke in persons with diabetes. In 2004, 68% of diabetes-related deaths were from heart disease and 16% from stroke in those patients over 65 years of age. Adults with diabetes have heart disease death rates about 2–4 times higher than their counterparts without diabetes. Their risk for stroke is also 2–4 times higher than the general population. High blood pressure is found in 75% of those with diabetes.

Eye Disease (Retinopathy)

Diabetes is the leading cause of new cases of blindness among adults aged 20–74 years. This is a result of the damage in the blood vessels supplying the eyes, specifically the retina. There are 12,000 to 24,000 new cases of blindness per year as a result of diabetic vascular changes.

Kidney Disease

Diabetes is the leading cause of kidney failure in adults and for the need for chronic dialysis. It caused about 44% of the new cases of renal failure in 2004. In 2005, about 180,000 patients with diabetes had end stage kidney failure, requiring chronic dialysis or kidney transplant.

Nervous System Problems (Neuropathy)

About two-thirds of all diabetics have mild to severe nervous system disease such as poor sensation, slowed digestion, carpal tunnel syndrome, erectile dysfunction, weakness of arms or legs, and others. One-third of those have poor sensation in the feet and lower legs, leading to ulcers that can become severe enough to require lower extremity amputations. Two-thirds of all nontraumatic amputations of the lower legs are performed on people with diabetes.

Dental

Severe gum disease is more common in diabetics. This very frequently leads to an increase in tooth loss and resulting decrease in quality of life for persons with diabetes.

Pregnancy

Diabetes occurring before pregnancy or early in the first trimester is associated with major birth defects and a higher incidence of spontaneous abortion (miscarriage). This is in addition to the complications that occur with gestational diabetes that occurs later in pregnancy.

TYPES OF DIABETES MELLITUS

Diabetes mellitus, usually referred to simply as diabetes, is actually a group of common endocrine/metabolic diseases characterized by high blood sugar. There are generally three defined types of diabetes: Type 1, Type 2, and gestational. Each type is distinct but may share risk factors and management methods. Prediabetes is a condition that may occur for years without symptoms before the diagnosis of diabetes is made. Though not really diabetes (YET!), prediabetes may be a precursor and is potentially modifiable.

Prediabetes

prediabetes: state of impaired glucose tolerance, impaired fasting glucose, or both; blood glucose is higher than normal but not in the range for a diagnosis of diabetes

impaired fasting glucose (IFG): fasting glucose level that is above normal (70–100 mg/dL) but not in the range for a diagnosis of diabetes

impaired glucose tolerance (IGT): glucose level taken two hours after a glucose load—either a meal or a liquid glucose solution—(two-hour postprandial level) that is above normal (<140 mg/dL) but not in the range for a diagnosis of diabetes

Prediabetes is a condition in which blood sugar levels are higher than normal, but not high enough for the diagnosis of diabetes. Normal blood sugar levels obtained after an overnight fast (FPG = fasting plasma glucose) would range from 70–100 mg/dL. Another measurement of blood sugar that aids in the diagnosis of diabetes or prediabetes is the two-hour postprandial sugar level (OGTT = oral glucose tolerance test). This is a blood level obtained two hours after a sugar load (usually an oral glucose solution) and is normally less than 140 mg/dL. It would simulate a glucose level that would be obtained two hours after a meal. For a diagnosis of prediabetes, one must have **impaired fasting glucose** (IFG) or **impaired glucose tolerance** (IGT) or both. See Table 13-1.

A U. S. study from 1988–1994 tested 40–74-year-olds not previously identified as having prediabetes or diabetes and found that 33.8% had impaired fasting glucose levels (IFG) and 15.4% had impaired glucose tolerance (IGT); 40.1% of all those tested could be diagnosed with prediabetes. In 2010, the U.S. Department of Health and Human Services estimated that there were 79 million persons in the United States over the age of 20 years with prediabetes.

TABLE 13-1 Common Laboratory Values Used in the Diagnosis of Diabetes

	Fasting Plasma Glucose (mg/dL) (FPG)	2-Hour Postprandial (mg/dL) (OGTT)
Normal	70–100	< 140
Prediabetes	100–125	140–199
Diabetes	≥ 126	≥ 200

© Cengage Learning 2013

Identifying persons with prediabetes is important because they have an increased risk for future development of Type 2 diabetes or development of heart disease or stroke. Prediabetes may exist for years before this progression occurs. A recent study done by the Diabetes Prevention Program (DPP) showed that progression from prediabetes to Type 2 diabetes was not inevitable and could be delayed or even prevented. This study showed increased physical activity of 30 minutes per day for at least 3 days a week and a 5–7% weight loss reduced the risk of developing diabetes by 58% over 3 years. For some people, their blood sugars even returned to normal. Medication use also showed a 31% decrease in risk over 3 years but was most effective in the younger age group (25–40-year-olds) and those who were 50–80 pounds overweight.

Prediabetes is becoming more common in the United States. Those people with prediabetes are likely to develop Type 2 diabetes within 10 years, unless they take steps to prevent or delay it. The Diabetes Prevention Program study showed that lifestyle changes were more effective than medications, making interventions to prevent or delay Type 2 diabetes in persons with prediabetes feasible and cost-effective.

Type 1 Diabetes Mellitus

Anne Rice (*Interview with a Vampire*), Tom Foster (Foster Farms Chicken), Sonia Sotomayor (U.S. Supreme Court Justice), Nick Jonas (Jonas Brothers), Jay Cutler (Denver Broncos), and Halle Berry (actress) all reportedly have Type 1 diabetes mellitus! And all of them have been able to make significant contributions despite their disease.

Type 1 diabetes mellitus was formerly called juvenile onset diabetes (JOD) and insulin-dependent diabetes (IDDM), both describing important aspects of this disease. It accounts for only 5–10% of all cases of diabetes. As the prior name suggests, this type of diabetes is most commonly diagnosed in childhood but may occur in adults as well. In Type 1 diabetes mellitus, there is *no production of insulin*. See Figure 13-2 for an understanding of how this affects blood glucose.

Type 1 diabetes mellitus: disease where no insulin is produced because of an autoimmune response against the beta cells of the pancreas

Genetic factors play a major role in the occurrence of Type 1 diabetes and are likely responsible for the predisposition for acquiring the disease. An environmental trigger, possibly a viral infection or nutritional factor in early childhood or young adulthood, starts a cascade that precipitates the disease. Most Type 1 diabetes is secondary to an **autoimmune** attack on the beta cells of the pancreas. An environmental trigger occurs that causes that person's immune system to attack its own cells, which are recognized as foreign to the body. The ability of the beta cells to produce insulin is then permanently destroyed. This destruction of beta cells usually begins years before symptoms begin. Because the pancreas is no longer able to produce insulin, treatment is with insulin replacement provided by injections, hence the prior name of "insulin-dependent." The goal of therapy is to maintain normal blood sugars and to prevent the short- and long-term complications of the disease. Diet, exercise, and education are also important in management of the disease. There are *no preventive measures*, but better control can be achieved with lifestyle changes when used in conjunction with insulin therapy.

autoimmune: an immune response against one's own cells or tissues

Type 2 Diabetes Mellitus

Well-known persons with Type 2 diabetes include David Wells (pitcher, Major League Baseball), Thomas Edison (inventor), Ernest Hemingway (author), Walt Frazier (former NBA player), and Larry King (television personality). And they, too, have been able to make significant achievements despite their disease.

Type 2 diabetes mellitus was previously called adult-onset diabetes mellitus (AODM) and noninsulin-dependent diabetes mellitus (NIDDM). Again, as the name implies, this condition is more common in the adult population and becomes progressively more common with advancing age. In recent years, however, Type 2 diabetes has been increasing in alarming rates in the adolescent population following the rise in obesity in this age group. This form of diabetes accounts for 90–95% of all cases of diabetes and is a major health problem in the United States.

In Type 2 diabetes, insulin is still produced by the pancreas, at least early in the disease, but the body's cells do not respond to the insulin effectively. See Figure 13-2, which shows this effect on blood glucose. This is most frequently referred to as *insulin resistance* because the cells are resistant to the effects of the insulin. After several years' progression of the disease, the pancreas decreases its production of insulin and this effect is then the same as with Type 1. Presenting symptoms in both types of diabetes, e.g., the 3 Ps, are the same, but onset is more gradual in Type 2.

The genetic link with diabetes is present in both types of diabetes but lifestyle factors, particularly obesity, play a major role in Type 2 disease. The focus of treatment in this type of diabetes is therefore on diet, weight loss and control, and exercise. Oral medications are required in most cases, and insulin may be used in more severe cases that have been present for many years. Because Type 2 diabetes is so common and lifestyle interventions can be so successful, the American Diabetes Association (ADA) recommends routine screening with urine and blood glucose tests beginning at age 45 or before if risk factors exist.

Type 2 diabetes mellitus: disease in which insulin is produced normally, at least initially, but the body's cells do not respond; a state of insulin resistance

Gestational Diabetes Mellitus

Gestational diabetes mellitus occurs in pregnant women who have high blood glucose levels and no history of diabetes prior to pregnancy. It affects about 4% of all pregnant women, usually later in the pregnancy. This form of diabetes is similar to Type 2 in that the glucose intolerance is caused by insulin resistance. After the birth of the baby, the high blood sugars usually resolve. Gestational diabetes does leave the mother with a 20–60% higher risk for developing Type 2 diabetes. The symptoms and treatment are similar to the other types of diabetes. Although it is similar to the insulin resistance of Type 2, gestational diabetes frequently requires insulin injections. The goal is to maintain normal blood sugars throughout the pregnancy.

Even though gestational diabetes is transient, if left untreated, it can lead to complications to the fetus and newborn. The placenta produces hormones that help the fetus grow but inhibit maternal insulin. This leads to high blood sugar levels in the mother. Maternal insulin does not cross through the placenta into the fetus's bloodstream, but the glucose does. This leads to high blood glucose levels in the infant. The fetal pancreas responds by producing its own insulin. The excess glucose in the fetal bloodstream is then stored as fat. Infants of mothers with diabetes tend to have large bodies (macrosomia) and are at higher risk for trauma during delivery. Other potential complications to the newborn include seizures secondary to low blood sugars after birth, congenital malformations, respiratory distress after birth, and jaundice. Like their mothers, these infants are also at an increased risk of developing Type 2 disease later in life.

gestational diabetes mellitus: occurring during pregnancy, gestational diabetes is similar to Type 2 diabetes in that the glucose intolerance is caused by insulin resistance

Other Causes

Less common causes of diabetes include specific genetic conditions (like cystic fibrosis), maturity onset diabetes of youth (MODY), certain surgical procedures, certain drugs (particularly steroids), infections that involve the pancreas (pancreatitis), and malnutrition. Severe stress, e.g., from prolonged intensive care unit hospital stays as a result of major surgical procedures or from severe medical illnesses, is known to respond with hyperglycemia that resolves as the stress resolves but may need to be treated as with the more common types.

RISK FACTORS AND PREVENTION

As with most chronic diseases, there are modifiable and nonmodifiable risk factors associated with the development of diabetes. Knowledge of lifestyle modifications that impact this disease and implementation of these changes on a major scale can have a significant impact on prevention.

Risk Factors: Type 1 Diabetes Mellitus

There are few known risk factors for Type 1 diabetes mellitus. Those that are known include family history or genetics and geography or climate. The incidence of this type of diabetes increases as one travels farther from the equator. It is highest in Finland—about 2 to 3 times higher than that in the United States and 400 times higher than that in Venezuela. It is also more common during winter months than in summer months. Possible risk factors associated with an increased risk of developing Type 1 diabetes also include exposure to a virus, low vitamin D levels, formula-fed infants (rather than breastfed), and early introduction of solid foods to infants. Viruses are thought to be the trigger that stimulates the onset of diabetes in at-risk persons. Viruses currently thought as responsible include the coxsackie virus, Epstein-Barr virus, mumps virus, or cytomegalovirus, all relatively common in early childhood and adolescence.

Risk Factors: Type 2 Diabetes Mellitus

polycystic ovary syndrome (PCOS): excess insulin and insulin resistance resulting in overproduction of testosterone in women

acanthosis nigricans: a skin disorder found commonly in obesity and diabetes; dark, velvety patches found in body creases

Family history of diabetes in a first-degree relative (parent or sibling) and obesity are the strongest risk factors for Type 2 diabetes, and, in fact, obesity is present in 80% of diabetics and is the single best predictor for diabetes. (See "A Closer Look: Risk Factors—Obesity" at the end of this chapter.) Ethnicity plays an important role in diabetes with Hispanic Americans, African Americans, Native Americans, and Asian Americans/Pacific Islanders being at the highest risk. Age greater than 45 years has been a well-documented risk factor in the past, but more recently Type 2 diabetes has become an increasing problem in adolescents primarily related to an increase in obesity in this age group. Because exercise helps maintain a healthy weight, increases the use of glucose, and makes cells more sensitive to the activity of insulin, a sedentary lifestyle (exercise less than 3 times a week) makes a person more likely to develop diabetes. A personal past medical history of gestational diabetes, **polycystic ovary disease**, a skin condition called **acanthosis nigricans**, high blood pressure, cardiovascular disease, and high cholesterol and/or high triglycerides are also associated with a higher risk of developing diabetes.

Risk Factors: Gestational Diabetes Mellitus

Risk factors associated with gestational diabetes include being overweight or obese, a previous history of prediabetes or previous history of gestational diabetes with a prior pregnancy, family history of diabetes, especially on the maternal side, and over 25 years of age at the time of the pregnancy.

Metabolic Syndrome

Identified only about 20 years ago, **metabolic syndrome**, also known as Syndrome X or insulin-resistance syndrome, is actually a group of risk factors that have been associated with an increased risk of cardiovascular diseases and Type 2 diabetes mellitus and are thought to be the result of the metabolic complications of obesity. To be diagnosed with this syndrome, one must have *three or more* of the following findings:

1. Elevated blood pressure (≥130/85 mmHg);

2. Elevated blood sugar (FBS ≥ 100 mg/dL);

3. Elevated triglycerides (≥150 mg/dL);

4. Waist circumference ≥ 40 inches in men or ≥ 35 inches in women, and/or

5. A low HDL (high density lipoprotein) of ≤ 50mg/dL in women or ≤ 40mg/dL in men.

metabolic syndrome: also known as Syndrome X or insulin-resistance syndrome; a group of risk factors that has been associated with an increased risk of cardiovascular diseases and Type 2 diabetes mellitus

These risk factors appear clustered together and are thought to be caused by insulin resistance and obesity. Other risk factors for this medical condition include aging, genetics, hormone changes, and lack of physical activity. The consequences of metabolic syndrome are related to the increased risk for atherosclerosis, coronary artery disease, heart attack, stroke, peripheral vascular disease, liver disease, and Type 2 diabetes. According to the American Heart Association, it is estimated to involve about 20–25% of the U.S. population. Mexican Americans have a higher incidence than whites or blacks. Mexican American and black women have a higher incidence than their male counterparts, but it occurs almost equally in white men and women. Worldwide it is found to occur with high incidence among south Asians. Metabolic syndrome is the focus of ongoing research into cardiovascular disease and diabetes.

Prevention

There is no prevention measure currently available for Type 1 diabetes. There is a blood test that detects antibodies against islet cells that can be given to those at risk to help ascertain their present risk. A balanced diet low in fats and concentrated sugars, weight management, and physical activity can all help in better management of the disease and prevention or at least delay of some of the complications.

Maintaining a healthy weight and observing an exercise schedule are the best preventive measures for Type 2 diabetes. A recent study done through Johns Hopkins University found that 75% of obese adults with Type 2 diabetes were able to

Check It Out

To assess your own current risk for diabetes mellitus, go to http://www.diabetes.org. Click on "Diabetes Basics" and then on "Risk Test."

discontinue their medication after stomach reducing surgery, and 85% of those patients were still off their medication after two years. The federally funded study, Diabetes Prevention Program (DPP), showed that persons with prediabetes could prevent or delay the onset of Type 2 disease simply by losing 5–7% of their total body weight and exercising 30 minutes at least 3 times a week. They found similar positive results with the use of certain medications, but the effects were not as frequent as those with weight loss and exercise alone. Screening is recommended for overweight adults who have other risk factors and for persons over 45 years of age. This is repeated every three years for monitoring. For obese children and adolescents who have other risk factors, screening is recommended every two years.

Maintaining a healthy weight, control of blood pressure, control of cholesterol and triglycerides, yearly evaluations by a kidney doctor (nephrologist) and eye doctor (ophthalmologist), proper foot care, and routine visits to a primary physician will all help in better management of Type 2 disease and prevention or delay of its complications.

THE FUTURE

Research into the "cure" for diabetes has many challenges. If looking at pancreas transplantation or even transplantation of the islet cells alone, researchers must contend with the phenomena of rejection of the foreign organ or cells. Although there are medications available now to assist with preventing rejection, they are not without significant side effects that must be contended with for life. When transplanting cells alone, finding the adequate numbers of cells needed to transplant to function as needed and keeping those transplanted cells alive can be a difficult task. Progress is being made in these areas though.

Other areas under investigation include artificial pancreas development and genetic manipulation. One genetic focus is in using non-beta cells to produce insulin for use in persons with Type 1 diabetes mellitus.

Summary

Diabetes mellitus is a group of common endocrine/metabolic diseases characterized by *high blood sugar*. The disease and its complications have a significant impact on the health of the U.S. population and on our health care costs. At least in part, there are identifiable risk factors that may be modified or, in some cases, even allow for prevention or delay of some cases of the disease. These public health measures may allow for decreased morbidity, mortality, and medical costs. This chapter discusses diabetes mellitus—the different types and causes, the scope of the problem, associated risk factors, focusing on obesity—and preventive measures.

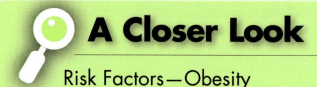 **A Closer Look**

Risk Factors—Obesity

Definition

Both "overweight" and "obesity" are terms used to describe weights that range above those considered healthy for a given height. *Body mass index (BMI)* is the measure used to define overweight and obesity. For adults, a BMI between 25 and 29.9 is considered *overweight*. A BMI of 30 or over is considered *obese*.

Measuring the exact amount of a person's body fat is not easy. The most accurate measures are to weigh a person underwater or in a chamber that uses air displacement to measure body volume or to use a special X-ray test. These methods are not practical for the average person and are done only in research centers with special equipment. Another simpler measure to estimate body fat is to use a caliper to measure fat just below the skin at several areas of the body. Weight-for-height tables were used in the past, but these tables do not distinguish between excess body fat and muscle.

Body mass index correlates with body fat but is not a direct measure of body fat. BMI is calculated by dividing a person's weight in pounds by height in inches squared and multiplied by 703 ($BMI = Weight/Height^2 \times 703$). See Table 13-2. This formula also has its limitations in that some persons such as athletes would be identified as overweight even though they are not. In children and adolescents, BMI is calculated to account for differences in gender and in body fat found at different ages. These figures are recorded as "BMI for age."

 Check It Out

To assess your own body mass index, go to http://www.nhlbisupport.com/bmi

Another predictor of obesity is an individual's waist circumference. Women typically collect their fat around the hips and buttocks, giving them a "pear shape." Men collect fat around their abdomen, giving them an "apple shape." Abdominal fat (apple shape) is predictive of obesity-related diseases. Women with a waist measurement of more than 35 inches and men with a waist measurement of more than 40 inches may have more health risks than people with lower waist measurements because of their body fat distribution.

Causes and Consequences

There are several factors that play a role in obesity. Body weight is a result of genes, metabolism, and behavior. Environment, culture, and socioeconomic status also play a role. Behavior and environment are the greatest area for prevention and treatment. There are only a few medical disorders that contribute to obesity—for example, hypothyroidism, polycystic ovary syndrome, Cushing's syndrome.

The easiest way to interpret weight management is to think about weight control. Weight control is dependent on caloric balance. That is, to maintain a certain weight, calories taken in the body in the form of food and drink must equal calories expended in the form of body functions and physical activity. If one is gaining weight, calories taken in are greater than calories expended. If one is losing weight, calories taken in are less than calories expended. Genetics play a role in making one susceptible to personal weight gain.

The consequences of obesity include a decreased life expectancy and higher risk for certain diseases. These medical conditions include diabetes, high blood pressure, arthritis, cardiovascular disease, stroke, gallbladder disease and stones, gastroesophageal reflux, gout, some pulmonary problems, and some forms of cancer. Much of this morbidity can be prevented or controlled by maintaining a healthy body weight.

Treatment

Treatment is strongly recommended for those persons with a family history of diabetes and other medical conditions, as well as for those who already have those diseases. In addition, those with waist circumferences above normal should also be encouraged to lose weight.

The mainstay of weight loss is diet and increased physical activity. A weight loss as simple as 5–10% can play a significant role in minimizing the risk for associated disorders. Moderate physical activity of 30 minutes, 5 times a week also has positive health benefits.

Epidemiology

Data from the Behavioral Risk Factor Surveillance System (BRFSS) showed that 35.7% of adults in the United States were obese, 35.5% of men and 35.8% of women. Obesity prevalence was highest for black women, followed by black men. It increased with age. There was a geographical difference with the South having the highest prevalence and the West having the lowest. Data from the 2009–2010 NHANES estimated that 16.9% of children aged 2–19 years were obese.

A recent study published in the *Journal of the American Medical Association* (JAMA) suggests that although the prevalence of obesity in U.S. adults is still high, new data show the rate of increase may be slowing. Figure 13-3 shows this trend of increasing obesity among different age groups.

Continues

TABLE 13-2 Body Mass Index

BMI	NORMAL						OVERWEIGHT					OBESE										EXTREME OBESITY		
Height (Feet-Inches)	19	20	21	22	23	24	25	26	27	28	29	30	31	32	33	34	35	36	37	38	39	40	41	42
	Weight (Pounds)																							
4'10"	91	96	100	105	110	115	119	124	129	134	138	143	148	153	158	162	167	172	177	181	186	191	196	201
4'11"	94	99	104	109	114	119	124	128	133	138	143	148	153	158	163	168	173	178	183	188	193	198	203	208
5'00"	97	102	107	112	118	123	128	133	138	143	148	153	158	163	168	174	179	184	189	194	199	204	209	215
5'01"	100	106	111	116	122	127	132	137	143	148	153	158	164	169	174	180	185	190	195	201	206	211	217	222
5'02"	104	109	115	120	126	131	136	142	147	153	158	164	169	175	180	186	191	196	202	207	213	218	224	229
5'03"	107	112	118	124	130	135	141	146	152	158	163	169	174	180	186	191	197	203	208	214	220	225	231	237
5'04"	110	116	122	128	134	140	145	151	157	163	169	175	180	186	191	197	204	209	215	221	227	232	238	244
5'05"	114	120	126	132	138	144	150	156	162	168	174	180	186	192	198	204	210	216	222	228	234	240	246	252
5'06"	118	124	130	136	142	148	155	161	167	173	179	186	192	198	204	210	216	223	229	235	241	247	253	260
5'07"	121	127	134	140	146	153	159	166	172	178	185	191	198	204	211	217	223	230	236	242	249	255	261	268
5'08"	125	131	138	144	151	158	164	171	177	184	190	197	204	210	216	223	230	236	243	249	256	262	269	276
5'09"	128	135	142	149	155	162	169	176	182	189	196	203	210	216	223	230	236	243	250	257	263	270	277	284
5'10"	132	139	146	153	160	167	174	181	188	195	202	209	216	222	229	236	243	250	257	264	271	278	285	292
5'11"	136	143	150	157	165	172	179	186	193	200	208	215	222	229	236	243	250	257	265	272	279	286	293	301
6'00"	140	147	154	162	169	177	184	191	199	206	213	221	228	235	242	250	258	265	272	279	287	294	302	309
6'01"	144	151	159	166	174	182	189	197	204	212	219	227	235	242	250	257	265	275	280	288	295	302	310	318
6'02"	148	155	163	171	179	186	194	202	210	218	225	233	241	249	256	264	272	280	287	295	303	311	319	326
6'03"	152	160	168	176	184	192	200	208	216	224	232	240	248	256	264	272	279	287	295	303	311	319	327	335
6'04"	156	164	172	180	189	197	205	213	221	230	238	246	254	263	271	279	287	295	304	312	320	328	336	344

Adapted from: George Bray, Pennington Biomedical Research Centre, *Clinical Guidelines on the Identification, Evaluation, and Treatment of Overweight and Obesity in Adults; The Evidence Report*, National Institutes of Health, National Heart, Lung, and Blood Institute, September 1998.

Source: National Heart, Lung. Blood Institute. http://www.nhlbi.nih.gov/guidelines/obesity/bmi_tbl.pdf

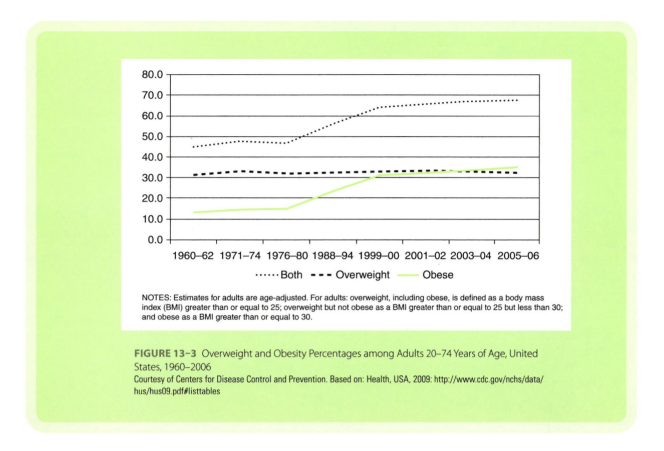

NOTES: Estimates for adults are age-adjusted. For adults: overweight, including obese, is defined as a body mass index (BMI) greater than or equal to 25; overweight but not obese as a BMI greater than or equal to 25 but less than 30; and obese as a BMI greater than or equal to 30.

FIGURE 13-3 Overweight and Obesity Percentages among Adults 20–74 Years of Age, United States, 1960–2006
Courtesy of Centers for Disease Control and Prevention. Based on: Health, USA, 2009: http://www.cdc.gov/nchs/data/hus/hus09.pdf#listtables

Review Questions

1. Diabetes is characterized by (defined by) _____.

2. Insulin resistance is the cause of _____ (Type 1 OR Type 2) diabetes, and a lack of insulin production is the primary defect in _____ (Type 1 OR Type 2) diabetes.

3. Briefly discuss the findings of the study by the Diabetes Prevention Program (DPP) regarding the progression of prediabetes to Type 2 diabetes.

4. Define the metabolic syndrome and list the five criteria used to determine its presence.

5. **True or False** Type I diabetes can be prevented by maintaining normal BMI/body weight and regular exercise.

6. Gestational diabetes is diabetes that occurs during:

    a. Childhood
    b. Older age
    c. Obesity
    d. Pregnancy

7. **True or False** Males are more likely to develop diabetes than women.

8. Arrange the following ethnic groups in order of increasing prevalence of Type 2 diabetes: Caucasians, African Americans, Native Americans/Alaskan natives, Hispanics, Asian Americans/Pacific Islanders

    1._____
    2._____
    3._____
    4._____
    5._____

9. The two most strongly associated risk factors for Type 2 diabetes include:

    a. Family history
    b. Age
    c. Ethnicity
    d. Obesity

10. Discuss the incidence of Type 2 diabetes in youth aged 10–19 years as it relates to the current trend, associated risk factors, and ethnic preference.

11. **For Deeper Thought** Briefly discuss how you would design a study to determine if there is an association between being obese and developing Type 2 diabetes. Include the study type/design, population of importance/where you would collect your data, five variables that might be important to include, and defined outcome.

Website Resources

American Diabetes Association: http://www.diabetes.org

National Diabetes Information Clearinghouse: http://www.diabetes.niddk.nih.gov

Centers for Disease Control and Prevention: http://www.cdc.gov

WebMD Diabetes Health Center: http://diabetes.webmd.com

National Library of Medicine: http://www.nlm.nih.gov

The Obesity Society: http://www.obesity.org

World Health Organization: http://www.who.int/en

For country and regional facts on diabetes worldwide, go to: http://www.who.int/diabetes/actionnow/en/mapdiabprev.pdf OR http://www.who.int/diabetes/facts/world_figures/en

References

American Diabetes Association. (n.d.). Diabetes Basics—Gestational. Retrieved from www.diabetes.org/diabetes-basics/gestational

American Diabetes Association. (August 17, 2010). News and Research—Study: Surgery May Reduce [Diabetes Patients'] Need for Drugs. Retrieved from www.diabetes.org/news-research/news/diabetes-in-the-news/study-surgery-may-reduce.html

American Heart Association. (July 11, 2011). About Metabolic Syndrome. Retrieved from http://www.heart.org/HEARTORG/Conditions/More/MetabolicSyndrome/About-Metabolic-Syndrome_UCM_301920_Article.jsp

Centers for Disease Control and Prevention. (updated June 4, 2010). Diabetes Public Health Resource, 2007 National Diabetes Fact Sheet. Retrieved from http://www.cdc.gov/diabetes/pubs/estimates07.htm

Centers for Disease Control and Prevention. (June 28, 2010). FastStats—Deaths and Mortalities. Retrieved from http://www.cdc.gov/nchs/fastats/deaths.htm

Centers for Disease Control and Prevention. (August 4, 2010). Overweight and Obesity—Data and Statistics. Retrieved from http://www.cdc.gov/obesity/data/index.html

dLife for Your Diabetes Life! (updated May 25, 2010). Inspiration and Expert Advice: Famous People. Retrieved from http://www.dlife.com/diabetes/information/inspiration_expert_advice/famous_people

Huang E. S., Basu, A., O'Grady, M., & Capretta, J. C. (2009). Projecting the future diabetes population size and related costs for the U.S. *Diabetes Care, 32*(12), 2225–2229. Retrieved from http://www.ncbi.nlm.nih.gov/pmc/articles/PMC2782981

Mayo Clinic. (updated July 8, 2010). Type 1 Diabetes—Risk Factors. Retrieved from http://www.mayoclinic.com/health/type-1-diabetes/DS00329/DSECTION=risk-factors

National Diabetes Information Clearinghouse. (June 2008). National Diabetes Statistics, 2007. Retrieved from http://www.diabetes.niddk.nih.gov/dm/pubs/statistics/index.htm

National Heart, Lung, and Blood Institute. (n.d.). Metabolic Syndrome—Who Is at Risk for Metabolic Syndrome. Retrieved from http://www.nhlbi.nih.gov/health/dci/Diseases/ms/ms_whoisatrisk.html

The Obesity Society. (n.d.). Obesity Statistics—Obesity in U.S. Adults: 2007. Retrieved from http://www.obesity.org/statistics

World Health Organization. (n.d.). Health Topics—Diabetes. Retrieved from http://www.who.int/topics/diabetes_mellitus/en

Chapter 14

REPRODUCTIVE HEALTH

Learning Objectives

Upon completion of this chapter, you should be able to:

1. List at least three reproductive health problems.
2. Describe at least three of the most common birth defects.
3. Identify health benefits and risks associated with certain types of contraception.
4. Describe how common lifestyle behaviors may adversely affect human reproduction.
5. Identify reproductive risks associated with maternal age.
6. Describe the association between obesity and reproductive health.

Key Terms

abortion	chorionic villus sampling	fecundity
amniocentesis	conception	fertility
anovulatory	contraception	fertilization
assisted reproductive technology (ART)	corpus luteum	fetal alcohol syndrome (FAS)
birth defects	environmental tobacco smoke (ETS)	fetal death
caesarean section (C-section)	estrogen	folic acid
		gestation

infant mortality

infertility

low birth weight

maternal mortality

menarche

menses

miscarriage

neonatal mortality

neural tube defects

ovulation

ovulatory cycles

precocious puberty

preterm

progesterone

reproductive health

spontaneous abortion
  or miscarriage

stillbirth

sudden infant death
  syndrome (SIDS)

teenage abortion rate

teenage birth rate

teenage pregnancy

teratogenic

testosterone

trimester

very low birth weight

viable

zygote

Chapter Outline

Introduction
The Scope of the Problem
Basic Physiology and Pathophysiology
  Normal Physiology
  Reproductive Pathophysiology
Types of Reproductive Health Problems
  Infertility
  Infertility Treatments
  Contraception
  Abortion and Miscarriage
  Cesarean or C-section
  Multiple Births
  Neonatal Complications
  Maternal Mortality
Risk Factors and Prevention
  Risk Factors
  Prevention
  Issues in Conducting Research
The Future
Summary
A Closer Look: Teenage Pregnancy
Review Questions
Website Resources
References

INTRODUCTION

conception: the joining of an egg and sperm; interchangeable with "fertilization"

reproductive health: encompasses physical, mental, and social well-being in all matters relating to the reproductive system

infertility: inability to conceive after 12 consecutive months

abortion: refers to any termination of pregnancy, but most often applies to intentional termination of pregnancy

miscarriage: the spontaneous end of a pregnancy at a stage where the embryo or fetus is incapable of surviving, generally defined in humans at prior to 20 weeks of gestation

The broad field of reproductive epidemiology includes the study of diseases and conditions of the male and female reproductive system that affect **conception**, as well as pregnancy outcomes. **Reproductive health** encompasses physical, mental, and social well-being in all matters relating to the reproductive system processes and, therefore, includes information and access to safe, effective, and acceptable methods of family planning. Reproductive health is an important problem worldwide and a major focus of the World Health Organization (WHO), the coordinating authority for health within the United Nations system of 193 member countries. This chapter will cover discussion on male and female reproductive issues, including **infertility** (defined as the inability to conceive after 12 consecutive months), **abortion** (used here as the intentional termination of pregnancy), and **miscarriage** (the unintentional termination of pregnancy), as well as health effects of the mother and child during and after delivery. This chapter also covers risk factors from a variety of perspectives, including nutritional, infections, behavioral/lifestyle, environmental/occupational, and personal characteristics. A discussion of prevention will conclude this chapter. These reproductive health problems are particularly important because they affect young, otherwise healthy persons and because the consequences of these problems extend to the entire family.

THE SCOPE OF THE PROBLEM

infant mortality: an infant death during the first year after live birth

maternal mortality: death of a woman while pregnant or within 42 days of termination of pregnancy from any cause related to or aggravated by the pregnancy

Reproductive problems are complex and occur frequently, making it difficult to summarize the overall field in terms of basic epidemiology. Unlike other health conditions, reproductive problems can affect the mother, father, infant, and the entire family. These problems occur worldwide. According to the World Health Organization, in 2004, reproductive and sexual ill-health accounted for 20% of the global burden of ill-health for women and 14% for men. The most serious of reproductive health problems are those that result in death of the child (**infant mortality**) or mother (**maternal mortality**). The health status of a country is often measured by the country's rates of infant and/or maternal mortality. Furthermore, these deaths of infants or young women contribute to a lower estimate of life expectancy for the population.

The burden of reproductive problems can be measured in both direct costs (those associated with office visits, medical procedures, and prescriptions) and indirect costs (those associated with other measures such as loss of income or caregiving costs). For example, a child born weighing less than 2,500 grams may have high *direct* medical costs associated with prolonged hospital care and specialized equipment, but the *indirect* costs associated with the child's slow learning and developmental problems may mean that the child's future earning potential is limited. These indirect costs have a societal burden that is difficult to quantify. In this chapter, we will focus on the most common problems resulting in death or lifelong disability or disrupted lives. Specific data on prevalence, trends, and financial impact (when available) will be provided for each reproductive health problem.

BASIC PHYSIOLOGY AND PATHOPHYSIOLOGY

An understanding of the basic processes involved in reproduction is necessary to understand what can go wrong in reproductive health issues. This section will first discuss the "normal" processes involved in male and female reproductive health and then follow with a brief discussion of how various events may alter these processes.

Normal Physiology

"Normal" reproductive health generally refers to those reproductive processes that most males and females experience. There are ranges involved in most of these processes, however, that include the outliers that are still considered "normal."

Puberty

Menarche, the age of onset of menstruation in females, typically occurs around the age of 12 years, but varies by ethnicity and country of origin. Early **menses**, menstrual periods, are typically associated with **anovulatory** cycles or cycles that do not produce an egg and therefore are not capable of resulting in pregnancy. Onset of ovulation is related to the onset of menarche. When menarche occurs before 12 years of age, onset of **ovulatory cycles**, or menstrual cycles that do produce a viable egg capable of being fertilized by a viable sperm and resulting in pregnancy, occur within one year of the first menstrual period in 50% of females. By contrast, in young girls who begin menstruating after the age of 12 years, fully ovulatory cycles *may* not occur until 8–12 years later.

The menstrual cycle in a woman is necessary for reproduction and typically repeats every 28 days. Onset of the cycle is considered to be on the first day of menstrual bleeding. Menstrual bleeding stops after 3–7 days, and a follicle in the ovary that contains an egg begins to develop. Over the next 14 days, **estrogen**, a female hormone produced by the ovary, begins to increase as other hormones come into play. At mid cycle, about day 14, **ovulation** occurs when an egg is released from its follicle and begins its journey through the fallopian tube. The ruptured follicle becomes a **corpus luteum** and begins producing **progesterone**, the hormone responsible for causing the lining of the uterus to prepare for the fertilized egg to implant and begin a pregnancy. If the egg is not fertilized by a sperm within about 24 hours or if a fertilized egg does not implant in the thickened lining of the uterus within two weeks, the cycle begins again with the shedding of the uterine lining (menses).

The onset of sperm production occurs mid-puberty in boys and is associated with a surge of testosterone. **Testosterone** is a male hormone produced primarily in the testes, but a small amount is produced in the ovaries of a female and in the adrenal glands in both sexes. This increase in testosterone is also associated with the male sexual response and development of the male penis, scrotum, and testes. The median age of this stage of pubertal development is 14 years. Sperm are produced in the

menarche: age of onset of menstruation in females

menses: menstrual periods in females, also known as "menstruation"

anovulatory: not accompanied by the release of an egg from the ovary and therefore not capable of resulting in pregnancy

ovulatory cycles: menstrual cycles that produce a viable egg capable of being fertilized by a viable sperm and therefore capable of resulting in pregnancy

estrogen: a female hormone produced by the ovary

ovulation: release of an egg from its follicle in the ovary

corpus luteum: ruptured ovarian follicle after the release of an egg; produces the hormone progesterone

progesterone: the female hormone produced by the ovarian corpus luteum and responsible for causing the lining of the uterus to prepare for the fertilized egg to implant

testosterone: a male hormone produced primarily in the testes; a surge in this hormone is responsible for the onset of puberty in males

testes and carried out of the body in semen during ejaculation. Sperm have flagella, or tails, that move back and forth and propel them up the fallopian tube to reach a newly released egg.

Conception

As previously discussed, during the second week of an ovulatory cycle, the lining of a woman's uterus is stimulated to become a blood-rich layer capable of supporting a fertilized egg, and around day 12–16, ovulation occurs. When intercourse occurs during this ovulation period, about 400 of the 250 million sperm in an ejaculate will make the trip up through the uterus and into the fallopian tube. One sperm may be successful in penetrating the egg, and their DNA will merge. This is conception, also known as **fertilization**. The fertilized egg is now a **zygote** and will begin to divide and grow as it continues to travel through the fallopian tube to eventually embed in the prepared lining of the uterus. During the next 38 weeks or so after fertilization, the uterus will expand to accommodate the growing baby.

Pregnancy

Pregnancy is divided into three **trimesters**, approximately 3 months each, to allow for easier reference to different stages of development. The first trimester is from conception to week 12 of fetal development. About the fourth week, the pregnancy test will become positive and early signs of pregnancy begin. The first prenatal visit to a medical facility is ideally around 8 weeks of **gestation**. At the initial prenatal visits, the pregnant woman is tested for previous exposure to or current infection with several infectious diseases known to have potential deleterious effects on a fetus. By the fifth week of pregnancy, the brain, spinal cord, heart and gastrointestinal tract of the fetus have begun to form. By week 9, all essential organs have started to form. Exposures to environmental hazards, nutritional deficiencies, alcohol, drugs, and infectious diseases have their biggest impact during this trimester.

The second trimester is from 13 to 27 weeks. Prenatal testing with blood tests and ultrasounds may be performed to rule out some of the more common abnormalities such as **neural tube defects** (defects that affect the developing spinal cord or brain), Down syndrome, and other common problems. If indicated by medical history or abnormal findings, an **amniocentesis** (collection of amniotic fluid from the gestational sac, see Figure 14-1) or **chorionic villus sampling** (removing cells from the placenta) may be done to identify genetic or chromosomal disorders in the baby. Fetal movement is usually felt around weeks 16–22.

The third trimester is from 28 weeks through delivery at about 40 weeks. During prenatal visits, blood pressure and urine testing for protein and sugar are monitored to evaluate for the presence of hypertension and gestational diabetes, which can have adverse effects on the developing baby, as well as on the mother. Full-term deliveries occur at 37–42 weeks of pregnancy. Fetal development in the third trimester consists of the final maturation of the organ systems and further growth of the baby in general. Babies born as early as 25 weeks estimated gestational age have well-established potential for viability. As would be expected at this age, the fetal organ systems such as respiratory, cardiac, nervous system, and others are not fully

fertilization: the joining of an egg and sperm; interchangeable with "conception"

zygote: the cell formed by the union of a sperm and an egg that divides and grows into an embryo

trimester: division of a 9-month pregnancy into three periods of 3 months

gestation: the period during which an embryo/fetus develops; also called "pregnancy"

neural tube defects: defects that occur early in pregnancy and affect the developing spinal cord or brain; an example is spina bifida

amniocentesis: procedure that collects a sample of the amniotic fluid that surrounds the developing fetus; fluid is used to perform laboratory tests to detect genetic and other diseases

chorionic villus sampling: procedure that collects a small piece of the placenta from the uterus; used for laboratory testing for genetic and other diseases early in pregnancy

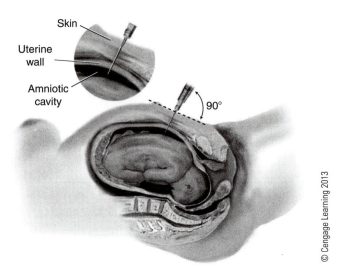

Skin

Uterine wall

Amniotic cavity

90°

© Cengage Learning 2013

FIGURE 14-1 Amniocentesis

developed and put a preterm infant at risk of serious complications. By age 32–34 weeks estimated gestational age, most infants will be born able to breathe on their own but may still have complications related to prematurity.

Delivery

Only about 5% of babies are actually born on their expected date of delivery. Labor is the physical process of uterine contractions that open the cervix to allow the infant passage out of the uterus through the vagina. On occasion, for various medical reasons, the infant cannot pass easily out of the uterus through the vagina, and a surgical procedure known as a **caesarean section (C-section)** removes the infant through an incision in the woman's abdomen and uterus. This procedure may also be indicated when there is fetal distress and delivery via the vaginal canal is not imminent.

After delivery of the infant, the umbilical cord that had been connecting the mother's circulatory system with the baby's is cut. The placenta is delivered shortly thereafter. Pregnancy is now completed. There are continued reproductive health issues that impact health care in the postpartum, or post-delivery, time period in the woman and neonatal (birth to 28 days of life) period of the infant. These can include neonatal and maternal mortalities, postpartum depression in the mother and birth problems in the infant as examples. These health issues will be discussed in more detail later in this chapter.

> **caesarean section (C-section):** refers to a surgical procedure in which one or more incisions are made through a mother's abdomen and uterus to deliver one or more babies

Reproductive Pathophysiology

Reproductive health problems are numerous and varied, and the underlying processes involved in these conditions are as numerous and varied. The problems associated with the conditions discussed in this chapter will be mentioned in the section of that condition, but a brief general discussion follows here.

During Puberty

Early onset of puberty is also known as **precocious puberty**. In girls, this is generally defined as puberty occurring before 8 years of age and in boys, as occurring before 9 years of age. In most cases, this early onset of puberty occurs in the same manner as normal puberty would occur. Usually it occurs as a variant of normal, but in some girls and boys, it is the result of tumors, disease, or even obesity. A Danish study in 2005 reported that the incidence of precocious puberty in girls 0–4 years old was less than 1 per 10,000 and rises to 8 per 100,000 in girls 5–9 years old. In boys less than 10 years old, the incidence is much less at 1–2 per 10,000. The prevalence of precocious puberty was 20–23 girls per 10,000 and fewer than 5 boys per 10,000. A medical evaluation with imaging studies and laboratory testing helps differentiate the cause. This condition is more common in girls than in boys, but an underlying medical cause is more likely in boys who present with precocious puberty. There are also racial differences in that African American girls tend to start puberty earlier than white girls and are more likely to have early puberty than are white girls. Even when early puberty occurs in an otherwise normal child, there can be adverse effects on the child's psychological state or in his or her social behavior. There may also be other health effects such as increasing risks for later chronic diseases or by affecting the child's ultimate height potential.

precocious puberty: defined as puberty occurring before 8 years of age in girls and before 9 years of age in boys

During Conception

Fertility (the ability to produce children) requires the union of a **viable** egg and a viable sperm, travel through the fallopian tube into the lining of the uterus, embedding of the zygote into the lining, and then cell division and growth that can continue without interruption. This process was discussed in the previous section. In the cases of infertility, any step of this process may be affected. The eggs may not be released, the fallopian tubes may be obstructed secondary to previous infections, there may be no sperm or a low number of motile sperm in the male's ejaculate, and the lining of the uterus may not be sufficient to sustain the zygote and its growth. Heritable and genetic disorders from either the maternal DNA or paternal DNA or from the combination of the two may become possible when fertilization occurs. Fertilization of more than one egg by sperms or division of the fertilized egg into more than one embryo results in multiple births.

fertility: the ability to produce children

viable: able to survive

During Pregnancy

If pregnancy results, multiple events may occur that can have adverse effects. Interruptions in the pregnancy can occur electively, by abortion, or unintentionally via miscarriage. Environmental exposures to substances such as paints, tobacco smoke, and other potential **teratogenic** chemicals or substances may have deleterious effects on the developing baby. Thalidomide, a medication used in the past to treat morning sickness, is one of the more known teratogens. It has been identified as causing severe limb defects in the infants born to mothers who took this drug. Nutritional issues also impact the pregnancy and status of the infant. An example of this is folate deficiency, associated with neural tube defects in the fetus, which is

teratogenic: the ability to produce fetal malformations

discussed later in this chapter. Infectious diseases, such as rubella, have long been known for their effects on the developing fetus. HIV infection in the mother that can be passed on to the baby is discussed in "A Closer Look" at the end of Chapter 8, Infectious Diseases. Alcohol freely passes into the fetal circulation, and its use and abuse during pregnancy has been associated with an adverse impact on growth and with psychological and physical problems of the child. Illicit drug use by the pregnant mother can have similar effects. Many of these risky exposures put an infant at risk for **birth defects**, which are faults or imperfections present in a baby at birth.

> **birth defects:** faults or imperfections present in a baby at birth

At Delivery

Preterm (before 37 weeks gestational age) delivery presents multiple complications in the infant, the severity of which are dependent on how early the delivery occurs. Reviewing the events that occur during each trimester as discussed earlier in this section will give an idea of the problems that may arise if an infant is delivered at that particular time. For about two decades prior to 2006, the preterm birth rates had been rising; but since 2006, these rates have been declining. In 2008, the preterm birth rate was 12.3% and had shown a downward trend among white, black, and Hispanic women alike. This decline was noted primarily for preterm infants born at 34–36 weeks of gestation, or the "late preterm births."

Other possible health issues that present during delivery include **low birth weight** (birth weight less than 2,500 grams) and, in the case of infants born to mothers with gestational diabetes, even infants who are large for gestational age (birth weight > 90th percentile for that age) and therefore at risk for birth trauma. Less commonly, delivery may have an outcome of maternal or neonatal death.

> **preterm:** delivery occurring before 37 weeks of gestational age
>
> **low birth weight:** birth weight less than 2,500 grams

TYPES OF REPRODUCTIVE HEALTH PROBLEMS

A reproductive health problem can be defined as anything that interferes with conception, the developing fetus, and birth of a healthy infant. There are many ways in which these processes can be interrupted, and not all of them can be covered in this chapter. Therefore, only the most common or most preventable problems affecting human reproduction will be discussed in this section.

Infertility

Two terms used to measure childbearing are *fertility* (the ability to produce children) and **fecundity** (difficulty conceiving or bringing a pregnancy to term). In this context, "fecundity" refers to the potential production of children, whereas "fertility" refers to the actual production of children. Fertility declines with age, with the most fertile years for women occurring in their 20s. With the advent of oral contraceptives in the 1960s, women had more options regarding family planning, and many women opted to delay childbearing into their late 20s or early 30s, which may lead to difficulty in getting pregnant.

> **fecundity:** difficulty conceiving or bringing a pregnancy to term

Among the reproductive health problems, *infertility*, defined as difficulty or failure to conceive after 12 months of trying, is a condition that affects about 6.1 million Americans, or 10 percent of the reproductive age population (age 15–44), according to the Centers for Disease Control and Prevention. Men and women are equally affected. In the U.S., trends in fertility have been relatively stable over time with a slight decline from 2007 to 2010 (Figure 14-2). Based on data from the 2002 National Survey of Family Growth, the percent of women aged 15–44 with impaired fecundity was 11.8%, whereas the percent of married women aged 15–44 who were infertile was 7.4% (Chandra et al., 2005).

Infertility Treatments

Depending on the reason for infertility, there are many treatment options available ranging from surgery to allow pregnancy to take place to hormone augmentation to allow the pregnancy to carry to full term. However, for those with resistant problems, **assisted reproductive technology (ART)**, which involves fertility treatments in which both egg and sperm are manipulated, can provide an effective treatment. ART procedures are very expensive and involve surgically removing eggs from a woman's ovaries, combining them with sperm in the laboratory, and returning them to the woman's body or donating them to another woman. The costs of ART are prohibitive for most couples. Just one cycle of treatment can cost $12,000, and the national estimate for diagnosing and treating couples with infertility issues is likely to be about $5 billion dollars a year (Staniec & Webb, 2007). Although

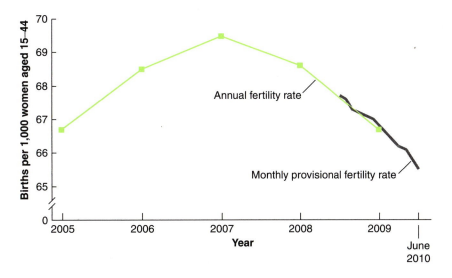

FIGURE 14-2 Fertility Rate: United States, 2005–2009, and Provisional, June 2009–June 2010
Notes: Monthly provisional fertility rates for June 2009–June 2010 are based on 12 months of provisional counts ending with the specified month. The 2009 rate is from preliminary data. Rates for 2005–2008 are from final data.
Source: CDC/NCHS, National Vital Statistics System.
Courtesy of Centers for Disease Control and Prevention/National Center for Health Statistics: http://www.cdc.gov/nchs/data/hestat/births2010/births2010.htm#figure

assisted reproductive technology (ART): all fertility treatments in which both eggs and sperm are manipulated

Historical Note 14·1

The Suleman Octuplets

Nadya Denise Doud-Suleman (born Natalie Denise Suleman on July 11, 1975), mother of 14 children and known as "Octomom" in the media, is an American woman who came to international attention when she gave birth to octuplets in January 2009. The Suleman octuplets are only the second full set of octuplets to be born alive in the United States. One week after their birth, they surpassed the previous worldwide survival rate for a complete set of octuplets by the Chukwu octuplets in 1998. Public reaction turned negative when it was discovered that the single mother already had six other young children and was unemployed and on public assistance programs. She conceived the octuplets and her six older children through in vitro fertilization. The circumstances of the octuplets' high-order multiple births have led to controversy in the field of assisted reproductive technology, as well as to an investigation by the Medical Board of California of the fertility specialist involved. California officials ruled that the doctor involved in implanting the embryos committed "gross negligence" with "repeated negligent acts, for an excessive number of embryo transfers" into Suleman and stripped the fertility specialist of his state medical license.

this process is very expensive, there is a trend for insurance companies to pay for this treatment, which will increase its use and provide more comprehensive and accurate estimates of its cost.

Contraception

To prevent unplanned pregnancies, men and women have a variety of **contraception** (or birth control) methods available that are generally effective if used properly. However, the types of contraception used may have an impact on future fertility problems, some intended and some not intended. For women, contraception choices include surgery (tubal sterilization, removal of the uterus or ovaries), hormones (oral contraceptive pills, injections, or patches), and barrier methods (diaphragm, sponge, female condom, spermicides, and intrauterine device or IUD). Refer to Figure 14-3 A-C. For men, contraception choices include surgery (vasectomy), hormones (injections to suppress sperm development or to make sperm immobile),

contraception: also called "birth control"; refers to any strategy that reduces or eliminates the chance of fertilization

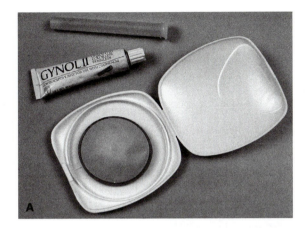

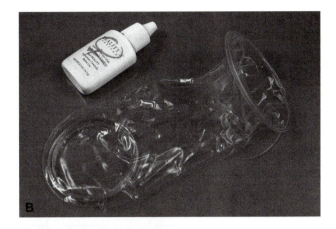

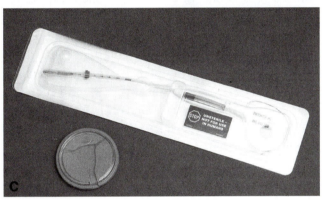

© Cengage Learning 2013

FIGURE 14-3 Female Contraceptive Devices. (A) Diaphragm with Contraceptive Jelly (B) Female Condom (C) Intrauterine Device—IUD

and barrier methods (condom). According to a 2010 report from the Guttmacher Institute, more than 99% of all women aged 15–44 who have ever had sexual intercourse have used at least one contraceptive method. Although there are many types of contraceptives, the most common types, representing 81% of the total, are oral contraceptive pills, tubal sterilization, male condom, and vasectomy.

Abortion and Miscarriage

Although *abortion* means the termination of a pregnancy for any cause, it commonly refers to pregnancies that are ended intentionally, and that is how it is used here. *Miscarriage* or **spontaneous abortion** refers to pregnancies terminated because of medical problems or unintentional conditions. Although data on either type of abortion is difficult to come by, 846,181 legally induced abortions were reported to CDC from 49 reporting areas in 2006, representing a 3% increase from 2005. The abortion rate for 2006 was 16.1 legal-induced abortions per 1,000 women aged 15–44 years. The majority (62.0%) of abortions in 2006 were performed at 8 weeks or less of gestation (MMWR, 2009).

spontaneous abortion: also called "miscarriage"; the loss of a fetus before the 20th week of pregnancy; refers to naturally occurring events, not to medical or surgical abortions

Miscarriage or spontaneous abortion is the most common complication of early pregnancy. It is estimated that between 25–50% of conceptions spontaneously abort. Researchers do not have an exact figure because if this occurs very early on, many women do not know that they were ever pregnant. Among clinically recognized pregnancies less than 20 weeks of gestation, 8 to 20% will end in miscarriage.

Cesarean or C-section

When normal vaginal delivery is difficult or impossible or if doing so would cause distress to the mother or the fetus, the child is often born by cutting through the mother's uterus using a surgical procedure called a "cesarean section" or, more commonly, a "C-section." In 2007, nearly one-third (32%) of all births were cesarean deliveries. From 1996 to 2007, cesarean rates increased for all women, regardless of age, race and origin, or state of residence (Figure 14-4). Cesarean rates also increased for infants of all gestational ages and may be partly related to the increased rate of multiple births because infants in multiple births are much more likely than singletons to be cesarean births. In addition to clinical reasons, nonmedical factors suggested for the widespread and continuing rise of the cesarean rate may include maternal demographic characteristics (e.g., older maternal age), physician practice patterns, and maternal choice.

Although there are often clear clinical indications for a cesarean delivery, the short- and long-term benefits and risks for both mother and infant have been the subject of intense debate for more than 25 years. Cesarean delivery involves major abdominal surgery and is associated with higher rates of surgical complications and maternal re-hospitalization, as well as with complications requiring neonatal intensive care unit admission. In addition to health and safety risks for mothers and newborns, hospital charges for a cesarean delivery are almost double those for a vaginal delivery, imposing significant costs.

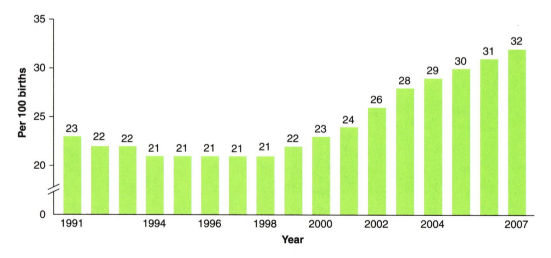

FIGURE 14-4 Cesarean Delivery Rates: United States, 1991–2007
Courtesy of Centers for Disease Control and Prevention/National Vital Statistics Systems Data Brief, No. 35, March 2010: http://www.cdc.gov/nchs/data/databriefs/db35.pdf

Historical Note 14-2

The Cesarean Section (C-section)

The best historical view of the Cesarean section comes from the National Library of Medicine (http://www.nlm.nih.gov/exhibition/cesarean). As described in that source, cesarean surgeries have been reported since ancient times in both Western and non-Western cultures. Yet, the early history of cesarean surgery remains shrouded in myth. The origin of the term "cesarean" is commonly believed to be derived from the surgical birth of Julius Caesar; however, this seems unlikely because at that time, the procedure was performed only when the mother was dead or dying. Caesar's mother, Aurelia, is reputed to have lived to hear of her son's invasion of Britain. Roman law under Caesar decreed that all women who were so fated by childbirth must be cut open; hence, cesarean. Other possible Latin origins include the verb "caedare," meaning to cut, and the term "caesones" that was applied to infants born by postmortem operations. Ultimately, though, it is not known for sure where or when the term "cesarean" was derived.

During its evolution, the cesarean section has changed dramatically from ancient to modern times. The initial purpose of the procedure was to retrieve the infant from a dead or dying mother in the hope of saving the baby's life. It was a measure of last resort, and the operation was not intended to preserve the mother's life. There were, however, sporadic early reports of heroic efforts to save women's lives. Perhaps the first written record of a mother and baby surviving a cesarean section comes from Switzerland in 1500 when Jacob Nufer performed the operation on his wife. After several days in labor and help from 13 midwives, the woman was unable to deliver her baby. Her desperate husband eventually gained permission from the local authorities to attempt a cesarean. The mother lived and subsequently gave birth normally to five children, including twins. The baby born by cesarean lived to be 77 years old. However, because this story was not recorded until 82 years later, historians question its accuracy.

Many of the earliest successful cesarean sections took place in remote rural areas lacking in medical staff and facilities. This meant that cesareans could be undertaken at an earlier stage in failing labor when the mother was not near death and the fetus was less distressed. Under these circumstances, the chances of one or both surviving were greater. These operations were performed on kitchen

Continues

tables and beds, without access to hospital facilities, and this was probably an advantage until the late nineteenth century. Surgery in hospitals was accompanied by infections passed between patients, often by the unclean hands of medical attendants. These factors may help to explain such successes as Jacob Nufer's.

The first successful cesarean section performed in America took place in what was formerly Mason County, Virginia (now Mason County, West Virginia), in 1794. The procedure was performed by Dr. Jesse Bennett on his wife Elizabeth. Both mother and child survived.

Multiple Births

Having two or more fetuses sharing the same uterus can result in many problems because of crowding and lack of sufficient nutrients. Before availability of ART, multiple births were rare. Using ART, several fertilized embryos are implanted at one time to ensure success, and it has become common to see multiple births. Although ART is rarely used, as of 2000, it accounted for 1% of all single births and 18% of multiple births in the United States (Reynolds et al., 2003). The twin birth rate was 32.2 per 1,000 births in 2007, compared to 19.3 per 1,000 births in 1980. The 2007 triplet/+ birth rate was 148.9 per 100,000 births, compared to 37 per 100,000 births in 1980. Although low overall, the triplet/+ birth rate climbed more than 400 percent between 1980 and 1998, but has since generally trended downward (Figure 14-5). Women aged 35 and over are much more likely to have

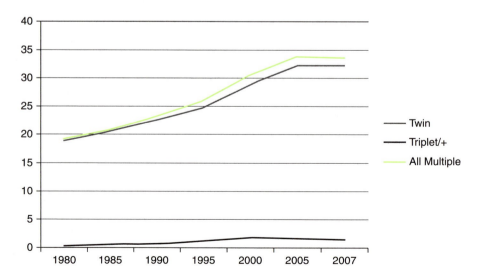

FIGURE 14-5 Twin and Multiple Birth Rates per 1,000 Live Births

Based on data provided by the National Vital Statistics Reports, Volume 58, Number 24, August 9, 2010 (Table 39).

a twin or triplet/+ birth than younger mothers. In 2007, less than 2 percent of teenagers giving birth had a twin birth compared with 5 percent of mothers aged 35–44 and more than 20 percent of mothers aged 45 and older. The range in age-specific triplet/+ rates is even wider; 1 in about 4,500 mothers under age 20 had a triplet/+ birth in 2007, compared with 1 in 70 women aged 45 and older (Martin et al., 2010).

Babies born in twin and triplet/+ deliveries are much more likely to be born too soon and too small and possibly not survive the first year of life. These twin and triplet/+ births are occurring more frequently in older women, thus increasing age-associated risks. Some of the complications of multiple births include spontaneous abortion, early delivery, and low birth weight. More than half of all twins (57%) and nearly all triplets (96%) were low birth weight in 2007 compared with 6 percent of singletons. In 2006, 3% of twins and 7% of triplets died during infancy compared with less than 1% of all single births (Martin et al., 2010).

Neonatal Complications

Even when all goes well with the pregnancy, the infant could have problems during and after delivery. The three most important complications are low birth weight (because of lifelong learning and motor disabilities that may result), birth defects that may affect physical, social, and mental development of the child, and of course, mortality. The top two causes of infant mortality in the United States in 2006 were birth defects and low birth weight/prematurity (Heron et al., 2009).

Low Birth Weight

Although there is considerable variability in the optimal birth weight for infants, it is generally recommended that a term infant weigh at least 2,500 grams (5 pounds, 8 ounces). Although the definition of "low birth weight" is less than 2,500 grams, another measure, **very low birth weight** (defined as less than 1,500 grams or 3 pounds 4 ounces) is also used to characterize risk. Although low birth weight is most frequently encountered in infants who are born prematurely, it can also be seen in infants who are born at term. The problems associated with term infants who are low birth weight but whose organ systems have formed completely may be different than the issues encountered in preterm infants whose organ systems are in a premature state.

In general, in the United States, 8.16% of infants born weighed less than 2,500 grams in 2009, and 1.45% weighed less than 1,500 grams. These infants are at high risk for lifelong problems, including mental and physical development (Hamilton et al., 2010). Although improvements in medical technology have resulted in many low- and very low birth-weight infants surviving, the direct medical and indirect social costs are high. A recent report estimated the average cost of direct medical care for the first year of life of a premature or low birth-weight baby is about $49,000. This compares to the first-year costs of a newborn without complications of $4,551. Newborns with other kinds of complications, such as congenital defects, have first-year medical expenses of $10,273 on average (Russell et al., 2007).

very low birth weight: defined as weighing less than 1,500 grams or 3 pounds 4 ounces at birth

Birth Defects

Birth defects occur in 3% of infants born in the United States and are the leading cause of infant mortality accounting for more than 20% of infant deaths and are the fifth leading cause of years of potential life lost. Although birth defects usually develop during the first three months of pregnancy, some are diagnosed at birth, whereas most are diagnosed during the first year of life or sometimes later. Common birth defects can include those that are easy to detect (cleft lip or palate, clubfoot) and those that are harder to detect (hearing loss, heart defects). Of all birth defects, heart defects occur in 1 out of 100–200 births. This represents 25–35% of all birth defects. Orofacial (cleft palate) and neural tube defects (spina bifida, anencephaly) occur in 1 out of 750–1,000 pregnancies. Other birth defects include genetic defects (Down syndrome and hemophilia) and metabolic disorders (Tay-Sachs, phenylketonuria).

The direct medical costs of treating birth defects (e.g., hospitalizations, surgery) can be substantial because of the lifelong care that may be required. According to a report from the Agency for Healthcare Research and Quality, hospitals spent $2.6 billion in 2004 for the treatment of birth defects, with half of the costs treating congenital heart and circulatory problems. However, indirect costs may include social costs of family caregiving, special educational resources, and personal costs of limited potential income and limited independence, which are much harder to estimate.

Infant Mortality

There are several sub-definitions of mortality rates used when looking at reproductive health issues. A **fetal death** occurs when a fetus of 20 or more weeks of gestation dies before being delivered. When a child is delivered after 20 or more weeks of gestation, but not alive or breathing, it is called a **stillbirth**. When a child dies within 28 days after birth, it is termed **neonatal mortality**. Infants who die within the first year after birth are termed *infant mortality*. Losing a child at this stage of its life is devastating to a family. Because of its impact on population and life expectancy, infant mortality rates are used as one of the indicators of the health of a country.

In 2006, the infant mortality rate in the United States was about 6.7 per 1,000 live births. There was little change in the infant mortality rate from 2000–2006. Although infant mortality rates fell fairly rapidly from 1950 to 1980, then more slowly until 1995, they have declined much more slowly since 1995 (Figure 14-6). The 2006 infant mortality rate was 77% lower than in 1950 as a result of annual declines from 1960–2000 (Health USA, 2009). In 2006, infant mortality rates were highest for mothers in the youngest and oldest age groups. The infant mortality rate for single births to mothers less than 15 years old was 16.7 infant deaths per 1,000 live births, approximately three times the rates for the age groups at lowest risk, those mothers aged 25–39 years, 30–34 years, and 35–39 years (Figure 14-7). The infant mortality rate for single births to mothers aged 45 years and older was 11.46, approximately twice the rate for mothers in the age groups at lowest risk (Mathews, et al, 2010).

fetal death: death prior to completed delivery of a fetus of 20 or more weeks of gestation; also called "stillbirth"

stillbirth: death of a fetus after 20 or more weeks of gestation, prior to completed delivery

neonatal mortality: refers to the death of an infant within the first 28 days after birth

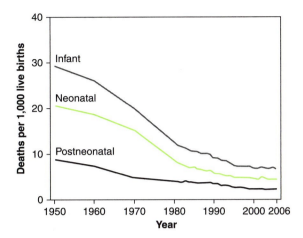

FIGURE 14-6 Infant, Neonatal, and Postneonatal Mortality Rates, U.S., 1940–2007

Source: CDC/NCHS, *Health, United States, 2009*, Figure 17. Data from the National Vital Statistics System.

Courtesy of Centers for Disease Control and Prevention/National Vital Statistics Reports, Volume 58, No. 19, May 2010, Table 7.

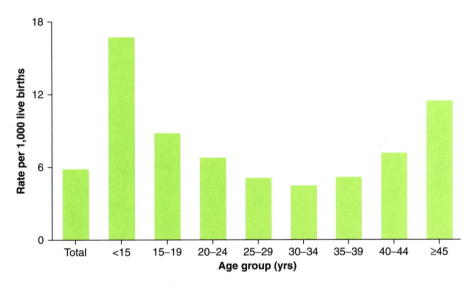

FIGURE 14-7 Infant Mortality Rates* for Single Births, by Age Group of Mother—United States, 2006
*Per 1,000 live births

National Center for Health Statistics. Linked birth/infant death data set, 2006. Available at http://www.cdc.gov/nchs/linked.htm

Although the overall U.S. infant mortality rate was 6.7 per 1,000 live births, this rate varies by racial/ethnic status. In 2006, the highest infant mortality rate was 12.9 deaths per 1,000 live births to black or African American mothers, followed by 8.6 deaths per 1,000 live births among children born to Alaska natives and American Indian mothers. Among the lowest infant mortality rates were 4.5 deaths per 1,000 live births for Asian and Pacific Islanders mothers, 5.4 deaths per 1,000 live births for Hispanic mothers, and 5.6 deaths per 1,000 live births to white mothers.

Internationally, the United States ranked 28th among 32 countries for whom data were available (Health USA, 2009). Countries (or reporting areas) with lower

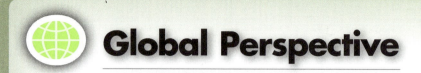

Global Perspective

Reducing the Maternal Mortality Ratio Worldwide

The Millennium Development Goals (MDG) of the United Nations (UN) has identified Goal 5 as improving maternal health with the target of reducing the maternal mortality ratio by three-quarters between 1990 and 2015. According to the 2010 UN report, "the maternal mortality ratio in developing regions in 2008 was 290 maternal deaths per 100,000 live births, representing a 34% decline since 1990." The risk of maternal death in a developing country is 1 in 31; the risk of maternal death in a developing region is 1 in 4,300, according to the UN report. The majority of these deaths (87%) occur in sub-Saharan Africa and southern Asia. The average annual decline in this ratio (2.3%) still falls short of the 5.5% annual decline needed to meet this MDG.

infant mortality rates than that of the U.S. rate of 6.7 per 1,000 live births include: Hong Kong (1.8 per 1,000 live births), Japan (2.6 per 1,000 live births), Norway (3.2 per 1,000 live births), and Sweden (2.8 per 1,000 live births). Those countries with higher rates included Romania (13.9 per 1,000 live births), Russia (10.2 per 1,000 live births), Costa Rica (9.6 per 1,000 live births), and Chile (7.6 per 1,000 live births).

Maternal Mortality

Although maternal mortality is rare in developed countries, it remains a problem in developing countries where 99% of all maternal deaths occur (WHO, 2010). Worldwide about 20% of women die as a result of diseases aggravated by pregnancy, including anemia, malaria, tuberculosis, and HIV/AIDS. In the United States, death of mothers related to childbirth has decreased from 73.7 deaths per 100,000 live births in 1950 to 11.2 deaths per 100,000 live births in 2006 (Health USA, 2009). In developing countries, the rate is much higher; but from 1990 to 2008, the rates of maternal mortality have dropped by one-third. The social effects of this problem affect the family and the newborn child for years to come; so it is a problem that deserves full attention of public health officials.

Note that the rates may have fluctuated over time because of differing definitions of maternal mortality. As of 1994 and the use of the International Classification of Disease (ICD), version 10, the current definition of maternal mortality is "death of

Historical Note 14·3

Philipp Semmelweis

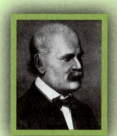

Philipp Semmelweis (July 1, 1818–August 13, 1865), a Hungarian physician, is now known as an early pioneer of antiseptic procedures. Described as the "savior of mothers," Semmelweis discovered that the incidence of childbed fever could be drastically cut by the use of hand disinfection in obstetrical clinics. Childbed fever was common in mid-nineteenth century hospitals and often fatal, with maternal mortality at 10%–35%. Semmelweis postulated the theory of washing with chlorinated lime solutions in 1847 while working in Vienna General Hospital's First Obstetrical Clinic, where doctors' wards had three times the maternal mortality of midwives' wards.

Wikipedia Commons: http://en.wikipedia.org/wiki/File:Ignaz_Semmelweis_1860.jpg

Despite various publications of results where hand washing reduced maternal mortality to below 1%, Semmelweis's observations conflicted with the established scientific and medical opinions of the time, and the medical community rejected his ideas. Some doctors were offended at the suggestion that they should wash their hands, and Semmelweis could offer no acceptable scientific explanation for his findings. Semmelweis's practice earned widespread acceptance only years after his death, when Louis Pasteur confirmed the germ theory. In 1865, Semmelweis was committed to an asylum, where he died of a blood infection at age 47.

a woman while pregnant or within 42 days of termination of pregnancy from any cause related to or aggravated by the pregnancy or its management, but not from accidental or incidental causes" (Hoyert, 2007). Using a standardized definition will make it easier to track changes over time.

RISK FACTORS AND PREVENTION

The most important way to prevent reproductive problems is to identify and modify factors that may cause these problems. Using the epidemiological methods discussed earlier in this text to study this problem, numerous risk factors have been identified. Although some risk factors (such as smoking) are modifiable, others (such as age) are not. To reduce the impact of reproductive problems, the goal is to find modifiable risk factors that can be changed or unmodifiable risk factors that can be avoided.

Risk Factors

From a public health standpoint, it is important to understand what factors or exposures are associated with adverse reproductive outcomes and, if modified, can lead to healthier families. Although there is still more to learn, a number of harmful exposures have been identified. Note that there is a lot of overlap between exposure and suspected outcome as one type of exposure could affect several domains of reproduction (e.g., alcohol use is associated with low birth weight and may also lead to birth defects). As described in the sections that follow and summarized in Table 14-1, these exposures can be grouped into categories that include nutrition, infection, behavior and lifestyle, environmental hazards and occupational hazards, and personal characteristics.

Nutrition

One of the best ways to ensure a healthy child is for the mother to practice good nutritional behaviors. This includes eating a balanced diet that includes sufficient intake of vitamins and minerals needed to support a growing fetus. In developed countries such as the United States, one of the most common nutritional deficiencies is lack of dietary nutrients such as iron, **folic acid** (one of the B vitamins that is a key factor in the making of nucleic acid), and calcium. If these nutrients are not available, the growing fetus taps the mother's stores, if available. The result may be a smaller baby or one with birth defects and brittle teeth, hair, and bones for the mother. In developing countries, malnutrition is a common problem, and this results in lack of many dietary nutrients, particularly iron. After a child is born, breastfeeding is the best way for a child to receive important antibodies that the immature immune system needs. However, breastfeeding requires that the mother have an adequate diet including protein, calcium, and iron. This is a particular problem in developing countries where nutritional support is difficult to obtain or where the mother has other health conditions (e.g., HIV positive) that can be transmitted to the child through breast milk.

Although malnutrition is a problem that affects the developing fetus, overnutrition or obesity, which is common throughout the world, is an equally important problem. Overnutrition is characterized by excessive weight gain. Risks to the mother include development of gestational hypertension, gestational diabetes, miscarriage, difficult delivery, and likelihood of a C-section. Risks of maternal overnutrition to the infant include trauma during delivery, birth defects, stillbirth, and neonatal mortality.

folic acid: one of the B vitamins that is a key factor in preventing neural tube defects

Infection

Infections can present problems for the reproductive system in many ways. Prior to conception, pelvic inflammatory disease can result in tubal damage and lead to infertility. The presence of an infection in the mother can affect a fetus in a number of ways, depending on the stage of development. Most common infections that

TABLE 14-1 General Summary of Risk Factors for Reproductive Health Problems

Exposure	Risk Factor	Major Effect (Outcome)
Nutrition		
• Nutrients	Lack of vitamins, folic acid, calcium, iron	Low birth weight, birth defects (neural tube defects), miscarriage
• Caloric intake	Obesity, malnutrition	Maternal mortality, motor or learning disabilities, infertility (male or female), low birth weight, macrosomia
Infection		
• Sexually transmitted diseases	Gonorrhea, syphilis, HIV, herpes	Birth defects, miscarriage, maternal and infant mortality
• Infectious diseases	Varicella (chickenpox), rubella (German measles)	Birth defects, maternal and infant mortality
• Vaccines	Measles/mumps/rubella (MMR) vaccine	Birth defects, low birth weight
Behavior and Lifestyle	Use of alcohol, tobacco, drugs, medications; lack of exercise	Infertility, low birth weight, sudden infant death syndrome (SIDS), birth defects, fetal alcohol syndrome (FAS), miscarriage
Environmental/ Occupational (men or women)	Lead, PCBs, benzene, pesticides, pollution, ionizing radiation, environmental tobacco smoke	Infertility (male or female), birth defects, low birth weight
Personal Characteristics	Maternal age less than 15 or older than 40	Low birth weight, congenital heart defects, Down syndrome, infant mortality
	Chronic disease (e.g., diabetes or hypertension)	Low birth weight, large for gestational age (diabetes)

occur during pregnancy, such as those of the skin and respiratory tract, cause no serious problems. However, some infections can be passed to the fetus before or during birth and damage the fetus or cause a miscarriage or premature birth. These infections are summarized in Table 14-2.

TABLE 14-2 Infections and Potential Effects

Sexually transmitted diseases that can cause problems include:

Chlamydia	May cause preterm labor and premature rupture of the membranes; also eye inflammation (conjunctivitis) in newborns
Gonorrhea	Can also cause conjunctivitis in newborns
Syphilis	Can be transmitted from a mother to the fetus through the placenta; can cause several birth defects
Human immunodeficiency virus (HIV)	Is transmitted to the fetus in one-fourth of pregnant women who have the infection and are not treated. For some women with HIV infection, a C-section, planned in advance, may further reduce the risk of transmitting HIV to the baby.
Genital herpes	Can be transmitted to the baby during a vaginal delivery. Babies who are infected with herpes can develop a life-threatening brain infection called "herpes encephalitis"; can also damage other internal organs and cause skin and mouth sores, permanent brain damage, or even death.

Infections not transmitted sexually that can cause problems include:

German measles (rubella)	Can cause birth defects, particularly of the heart and inner ear, and cognitive deficiency
Cytomegalovirus	Can cross the placenta and damage the fetus's liver and brain
Listeriosis	Increases the risk of a premature birth, miscarriage, or stillbirth. Newborns may have the infection.
Bacterial infections of the vagina	May lead to preterm labor or premature rupture of the amniotic membranes containing the fetus; can be transmitted to newborn
Chronic viral hepatitis	Increases the risk of miscarriage and premature birth; may cause chronic hepatitis in the newborn
Chickenpox (varicella)	Increases the risk of a miscarriage; may damage the eyes of the fetus or cause defects of the limbs, blindness, or mental retardation. The fetus's head may be smaller than normal.
Toxoplasmosis	May cause a miscarriage, death of the fetus, serious birth defects

Behavior/Lifestyle

There are many lifestyle choices that can affect the developing fetus. One of the more important is smoking, which can affect the size of the developing embryo and lead to stunted growth and motor problems. Smoking around infants has been shown to be associated with breathing problems and is a suspected risk factor of **sudden infant death syndrome (SIDS)**, a condition in which an infant stops breathing and dies during sleep.

Alcohol consumption is another problem that can have major effects on a developing embryo. Children born to mothers who drank alcohol during pregnancy are at risk to have a condition known as **fetal alcohol syndrome (FAS)**. The defect could be in the form of characteristic physical changes of the face and head, social problems because of behavioral deficits, or learning disabilities. This syndrome can be obvious at delivery if physical problems are apparent, but mild cases are often not diagnosed until the child is ready for school. Because of the difficulty in diagnosing this disorder, it is difficult to obtain accurate statistics on its prevalence; however, it is 100% preventable if women who may become pregnant refrain from drinking alcohol. Based on current knowledge, CDC recommends that there is no safe level of alcohol consumption during pregnancy (http://www.cdc.gov/ncbddd/fasd/facts.html).

Many over-the-counter (OTC) drugs that are generally safe for adults may cause problems for a developing fetus. A notable example of this is thalidomide, a drug used in the late 1950s as a sedative. If taken during pregnancy, the drug affected the development of the limbs, resulting in children born with deformed or absent arms or legs. Although it is best to avoid all drugs (prescription or over-the-counter) during pregnancy, that may not be possible. Chronic medical conditions requiring appropriate ongoing treatment are a major reason that early and accessible prenatal care is important.

Another important lifestyle behavior that is important for the health of the mother and child is exercise. Appropriate physical activities during pregnancy can have multiple positive effects including helping manage weight gain, building stamina for delivery, decreasing low back pain and fatigue, and preventing the likelihood of developing gestational diabetes. Exercises to avoid include those that require holding one's breath, contact sports, deep knee bends, and activities that put a strain on the abdomen or where falling is likely.

Environmental/Occupational

Environmental exposures, such as air pollution, have been known to affect fertility and growth of the infant. An often overlooked exposure is **environmental tobacco smoke (ETS)**, also called "secondhand smoke," which is common in areas where the prevalence of smoking is high and there are no regulations in place to protect nonsmokers. The presence of high levels of nicotine in the blood and breast milk of nonsmoking women has been documented. This is a particular problem in developing countries. Exposure to ETS during pregnancy can affect the lung function of the developing child and result in low birth weight, or exposure after delivery is associated with SIDS. Children who live in homes of smokers

sudden infant death syndrome (SIDS): a condition in which an infant stops breathing and dies during sleep

fetal alcohol syndrome (FAS): a group of birth defects composed of physical, social, and learning problems resulting from alcohol use during pregnancy

environmental tobacco smoke (ETS): also known as "secondhand smoke"

or who are exposed to environmental pollution are more likely to develop breathing problems, including bronchitis, coughing and wheezing, and middle ear infections. ETS also acts as a trigger for asthma and may even have a role is causing asthma to develop.

Often workplace exposures to chemicals affect the worker (male or female) and the unborn child. For example, there are several occupational exposures than can affect the fertility of men. These include workplace exposure to chemicals and pollutants that can reduce the number of sperm, enable the sperm to have an abnormal shape, or alter sperm transfer. Some exposures can also alter male hormones that can affect sperm development or sexual performance. The problems caused will depend on the particular chemical, the level and length of exposure, lifestyle (smoking, alcohol use), and medical (co-morbidities).

Personal Characteristics

Maternal age cannot be changed, but it is known that children born to young mothers (younger than age 15 years) or older mothers (age 40 and older) are more likely to have birth defects or to have a lower birth weight than children born to mothers between the ages of 25 and 39 or to succumb to infant mortality. Although age cannot be modified, it is possible to prevent pregnancies at a very young or old age, or at times when it is unsafe for the mother to become pregnant. Other personal characteristics of the mother that may affect the developing child could be chronic disease conditions such as diabetes or hypertension. Managing the health conditions of the mother (e.g., controlling blood sugar levels for women with diabetes or controlling blood pressure for women with hypertension) can help reduce the effect of these problems on the developing fetus.

Prevention

Although the causes of all reproductive health problems are not known, by applying prevention techniques using the known causes, strides can be made in reducing adverse health consequences for the mother, child, and family. Examples of techniques could include education regarding nutrition for men and women before conception; programs to help women avoid drugs and alcohol during pregnancy and breastfeeding; and support for breastfeeding, avoiding excessive weight gain, and avoiding smoking. Many potentially modifiable risk factors may be identified and appropriate interventions taken before problems arise during pregnancy if early prenatal care is available and accessible to all pregnant women.

Of course, even when risk factors are known, it is difficult to change behaviors and, sometimes, policy changes can be more effective. A good example of this is folic acid supplementation. Although it was known that low intake of folic acid just prior and during pregnancy could reduce the risk of neural tube defects in infants, in 1992, only 29% of reproductive-age U.S. women consumed the recommended levels (400 µg) of folic acid daily. Because of this, the

U.S. Food and Drug Administration (FDA) mandated the addition of folic acid to enriched grain products by January 1998. This fortification was expected to add approximately 100 µg of folic acid to the daily diet of the average person and to result in approximately 50% of all reproductive-aged women receiving 400 µg of folate from all sources. The birth prevalence of neural tube defects reported on birth certificates decreased from 37.8 per 100, 000 live births before folic acid fortification to 30.5 per 100, 000 live births conceived after mandatory folic acid fortification, representing a 19% decline, although it is possible that factors other than folic acid could have accounted for some of the decline (Honein et al., 2001).

Almost every risk factor identified for reproductive health outcomes is also associated with low birth weight, suggesting that this is an important marker or perhaps mediator for a number of problems. The potential causes of low birth weight can fall into two general categories: premature delivery or fetal growth restriction. Preventing premature delivery by controlling risk factors associated with preterm birth (smoking, chronic health problems of the mother, alcohol use, infections of the uterus, and placental problems) and preventing fetal growth restriction by controlling risk factors associated with poor fetal growth (birth defects, alcohol use, infections of the fetus, placental problems, and inadequate maternal weight gain) when possible are important in controlling for low birth weight. Intervening on these risk factors would help reduce a number of reproductive health problems.

Issues in Conducting Research

As with most areas of chronic disease research, it is difficult to conduct research to establish causality when there are problems defining outcome (the particular reproductive health issue) and exposure (one or more of the several risk factors). For example, to obtain gestational age, it is necessary to determine the date of conception. This is usually estimated by knowing the date of the last menstrual cycle, but because of various individual differences, this is only an estimate, not the actual date of conception. During the course of the pregnancy, markers based on fetal development can make refinement of gestational age possible. Studies of miscarriage rates are hampered because these data are not routinely collected or because a miscarriage may occur early and before a pregnancy is confirmed. This makes research into early miscarriages/spontaneous abortions difficult to conduct.

Measuring exposures to determine risk factors is very difficult for subjects to remember and to quantify. Many times sensitive topics need to be addressed (e.g., number of sexual partners, abortion, condom use). Other factors, such as nutritional data (alcohol use, folic acid intake) may be hard to obtain, especially in the early months of pregnancy. The dose and the timing of the exposures may also play a role. It may be that prenatal ultrasounds are normally safe, but they may be dangerous to the fetus at certain "windows" of opportunity. In addition, there are numerous confounders (socioeconomic, genetic, and access to healthcare) that must be considered when assessing individual risk factors for reproductive problems.

THE FUTURE

Although with medical advances many of the problems associated with infertility are treatable, the best chance for a healthy family is for the parents to ensure that their bodies are in good health and that they have a nutritious diet prior to pregnancy. During pregnancy, women should take steps to ensure additional iron is in the diet, possibly through a daily vitamin supplement. They should also avoid alcohol consumption and avoid exposure to cigarette smoke. Again, early prenatal care to all pregnant women is of utmost importance. One of the goals of the field of reproductive health is to ensure that children are born healthy and can develop to their full potential. Additional research into the causes of birth defects will lead to more effective prevention techniques.

Summary

This chapter reviewed the scope of the major reproductive health problems facing adults and their children, including the normal and abnormal physiology of the reproductive system. The various types of reproductive health problems encountered were discussed and ranged from minor problems to those with serious lifelong consequences or even death. The known risk factors for the major types of reproductive problems were summarized and preventive measures were discussed. The chapter concluded with a synopsis of some of the issues in conducting research into these problems and what changes may be seen in the future.

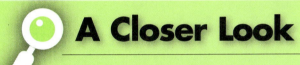

A Closer Look

Teenage Pregnancy

Each year in the United States, there are approximately 750,000 teenage pregnancies. In 2009, 409,840 babies were born in the United States to teenage mothers for a live birth rate of 39.1 per 1,000 teenage girls. **Teenage pregnancy** is classically defined as a pregnancy that occurs in a girl 15–19 years of age. Pregnancy estimates include the sum of the live births, plus the elective abortions, plus the miscarriages. The **teenage birth rate** is the number of pregnancies in women 15–19 years old that go through to delivery divided by the total number of women 15–19 years old. **Teenage abortion rates** include those teenage pregnancies that are electively terminated divided by the total number of teenage pregnancies. In the United States, much of this data is derived from the National Vital Statistics System and the National Survey of Family Growth, as well as from school-based surveys conducted by the Centers for Disease Control and Prevention (CDC) and local agencies included in the Youth Risk Behavior Surveillance System (YRBSS). The Guttmacher Institute and CDC's Abortion Surveillance System provide data on abortions.

teenage pregnancy:
a pregnancy that occurs in a girl 15–19 years of age

teenage birth rate: the number of live births in girls 15–19 years old divided by the number of girls aged 15–19

teenage abortion rate: the number of teenage pregnancies that are electively terminated divided by the total number of teenage pregnancies

Worldwide and U.S. Epidemiology

Worldwide, the highest rates for teenage pregnancies occur in sub-Saharan African where rates in some countries there are as high as 143 pregnancies per 1,000 female teens. Women tend to marry early in that area of the world, and pregnancy early in life is not a cultural stigma but shows fertility. The lowest rates are in South Korea (2.9 per 1,000) and Japan (4 per 1,000). The United States and New Zealand have the highest rates among developed countries. In the United States, the lowest rates (< 25 per 1,000) occur in the northeast (Connecticut, Massachusetts, New Hampshire, Vermont), and the highest rates (> 60 per 1,000) occur across the mid southern states (New Mexico, Texas, Arkansas, Oklahoma). See Figure 14-8.

Continues

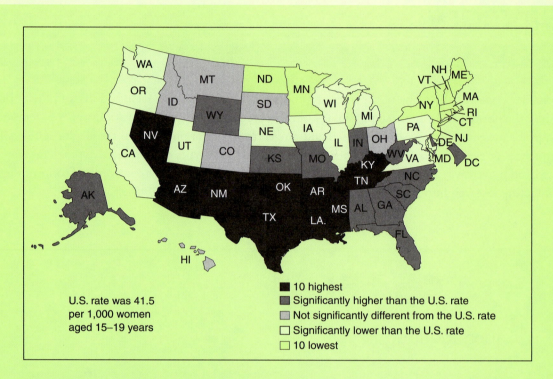

FIGURE 14-8 Teenage Birth Rates by U.S. State, 2008

Note: Data for 2008 are preliminary.

Source: CDC/NCHS, National Vital Statistics System.

Courtesy of Centers for Disease Control and Prevention: http://www.cdc.gov/nchs/data/databriefs/db46.htm

By ethnicity, the teenage birth rates in the United States are higher among Hispanic (127 per 1,000) and black female teens (126 per 1,000) than among whites (44 per 1,000) and Asian Americans (16.3 per 1,000), but there are some variations based on the state populations. See Figure 14-9. Eighty-two percent of teenage pregnancies in the United States are unplanned.

The peak rate for teenage pregnancies in the United States occurred in 1990 when the rate was 116.8 per 1,000 female teens. By 2005, this rate had dropped to 70.6 per 1,000 female teens for an overall drop of 40%. This drop in pregnancy rates was most significant for those girls 15–17 where the rates fell by 48%, whereas the rates for girls aged 18–19 fell by 30%. See Figure 14-10. These drops occurred across all ethnic groups. Teenage birth rates also dropped during this period from 61.8 per 1,000 in 1991 to 40.5 per 1,000 in 2005. There was a brief two-year increase in teenage birth rates between 2005 and 2007, but rates have continued to decline since but at a slower rate. Teenage abortion rates went from the peak of 40.3 per 1,000 in 1990 to 19.1 per 1,000 in 2005. According to data from the National Survey of Family Growth (NSFG), trends in behaviors that may account for 1990–2005 drops include a notable decrease in sexual activity among the younger teenage girls and an increase in the use of contraceptives.

Risk Factors

According to a report published by the American Academy of Pediatrics in 2005, 45% of high school females and 48% of high school males had had sexual intercourse. In this same report, predictors of early sexual activity were early pubertal development, a history

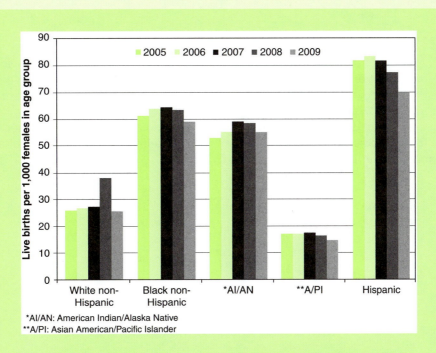

FIGURE 14-9 U.S. Birth Rates for Women Aged 15–19 Years by Race/Ethnicity 2005–2009
Courtesy of Centers for Disease Control and Prevention: http://www.cdc.gov/TeenPregnancy/AboutTeenPreg.htm

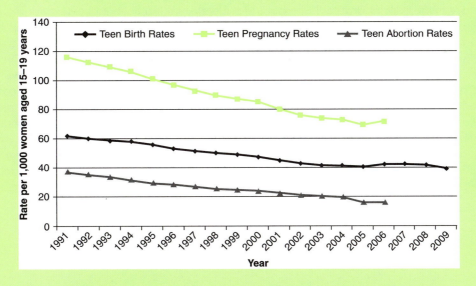

FIGURE 14-10 Pregnancy, Birth and Abortion Rates per 1,000 Women Aged 15–19 Years, All Races and
Origin: United States, 1991–2009*
*Pregnancy and abortion rates only available through 2006

Courtesy of Centers for Disease Control and Prevention: http://www.cdc.gov/TeenPregnancy/AboutTeenPreg.htm

of sexual abuse, poverty, lack of attentive and nurturing parents, cultural and family patterns of early sexual experience, lack of school or career goals, substance abuse, and poor school performance. These predictors of early sexual activity are also predictors of teen pregnancy.

Continues

Outcomes

When looking at pregnancy outcomes in adolescents, 27% of all teenage pregnancies in 2006 ended with elective abortions. Fifty-nine percent of pregnancies ended in birth of a newborn. See Figure 14-11. Adolescents are more likely than women in their 20s or 30s to experience problems during the pregnancy and complications of delivery. The lack of or delay in obtaining prenatal care among this population is the primary factor associated with these poorer outcomes. The more common complications include preterm delivery, delivery of low birth-weight neonates, and a higher risk of infant death.

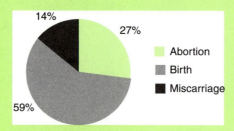

FIGURE 14-11 Outcomes of Teenage Pregnancies
Guttmacher Institute, Community health centers and family planning, *In Brief*, New York: Guttmacher, 2001: http://www.guttmacher.org/pubs/ib_6-01.html

Of those pregnancies that go through to delivery, 90% of the teenage mothers elect to raise their infant themselves rather than to give their child to an adoptive family. These adolescent mothers are more likely to drop out of school and therefore more likely to have lower incomes because of lower education levels. Fifty percent of teen mothers will have a high school diploma by the age of 22. The outcomes in the children of these teen pregnancies are also less than ideal. A child born to a teenage mother is more likely to have lower academic achievement, to quit high school, to have more health problems, to be incarcerated, and to have a pregnancy in her teen years. The financial impact for increased health care and foster care, increased incarceration rates, and lost tax revenue related to teenage pregnancies is more than $9 billion per year. Because of these costs and the personal impact of teenage pregnancies, the Centers for Disease Control and Prevention, in conjunction with the Office of Public Health and Science, is working to implement the President's Teen Pregnancy Prevention Initiative, 2010–2015, aimed at bringing evidence-based prevention and educational programs to the populations at highest risk.

Check It Out

To look at the data for your state or to compare data from your state to other states, go to http://www.thenational-campaign.org or to http://www.guttmacher.org

Review Questions

1. Match the following risk factors and outcomes. (*Hint:* each can be used more than once.)

Risk Factor	**Outcome**
a. Alcohol use	___ Down Syndrome
b. Maternal age	___ Low Birth Weight
c. Lack of folic acid	___ Some other thing
d. Lack of exercise	___ Who knows?

2. Of the following risk factors for low birth weight, which are modifiable? (Circle all that apply.)

    a. Alcohol consumption
    b. Obesity
    c. Drug use
    d. Teenage pregnancy

3. Which of the following are effects of overweight and obesity on the reproductive health of men?

    a. Reduced sperm count
    b. Erectile dysfunction
    c. Altered spermatogenesis
    d. All of the above

4. **True or False** Maternal exposure to environmental tobacco smoke (ETS) can harm a growing fetus, even if the mother does not smoke.

5. A study that follows the lifestyle exposures of pregnant women from conception until the birth of their children is known as a:

    a. Cross-sectional study
    b. Prevalence study
    c. Prospective study
    d. Mother-child study

6. **True or False** The field of reproductive health focuses on men, as well as on women and children.

7. Name one effect of a teenage pregnancy on the mother.

   _____

8. **True or False** Pregnant women have an increased need for iron because the developing fetus draws on the iron stores of its mother to last for the first 4–6 weeks of life.

9. To develop a valid study regarding infertility, which of the following are needed?
   a. Access to a population of women trying to get pregnant
   b. Information on environmental exposures such as lead
   c. Information on the weight and height of the women and their male partners
   d. All of the above

10. Name three reproductive health problems.
    1. _____
    2. _____
    3. _____

11. **For Deeper Thought** Design a campaign that could be used for high school boys or girls with the goal of preventing teenage pregnancy. Who might you target for this campaign? What factors/information might be important to this group?

Website Resources

For general information on reproductive health worldwide: www.guttmacher.org

American Congress of Obstetricians and Gynecologists. (January 2007). You and Your Baby—Prenatal Care, Labor and Delivery, and Postpartum Care: http://www.acog.org/publications/patient_education/ab005.cfm

Birth Defects and Mortality: http://www.cdc.gov/Features/dsInfantDeaths

Centers for Disease Control and Prevention (CDC); Reproductive Health Information Source: http://www.cdc.gov/reproductivehealth/index.htm

Centers for Disease Control and Prevention (CDC). Reproductive Health Atlas: http://www.cdc.gov/reproductivehealth/GISAtlas/index.htm

Centers for Disease Control and Prevention (CDC). Fertility, Family Planning, and Reproductive Health of U.S. Women: Data from the 2002 National Survey of Family Growth, tables 67, 69, 97: http://www.cdc.gov/nchs/fastats/fertile.htm

National Library of Medicine/National Institute of Health. (updated 15 December 2010). Medline Plus— Fetal Development: http://www.nlm.nih.gov/medlineplus/ency/article/002398.htm

National Toxicology Program. Department of Health and Human Services (updated July 14, 2005). Thalidomide: http://cerhr.niehs.nih.gov/common/thalidomide.html

Program for Appropriate Technology in Health (PATH). Reproductive Health Outlook: http://www.rho.org/index.html

<u>Reproductive Health Journals:</u>

American Journal of Obstetrics and Gynecology: http://www.ajog.org

Fertility and Sterility: http://www.fertstert.org

Human Reproduction: http://humrep.oxfordjournals.org

Journal of Reproduction and Fertility: http://www.jri.ir/En

Paediatric and Perinatal Epidemiology: http://www.wiley.com/bw/journal.asp?ref=0269-5022

Pediatrics: http://pediatrics.aappublications.org

Reproductive Health: http://www.reproduction-online.org

United States Agency for International Development (USAID). Maternal and Child Health: http://www.usaid.gov/our_work/global_health/mch/index.html#

World Health Organization (WHO). Reproductive Health and Research: http://www.who.int/reproductive-health/index.htm

World Health Organization (WHO). Trends in Maternal Mortality, 2005–2008: http://www.who.int/reproductivehealth/en

World Health Organization (WHO). Global burden of reproductive ill-health: http://www.who.int/mediacentre/news/releases/2004/wha2/en

References

American Academy of Pediatrics. (July 1, 2005). Adolescent Pregnancy: Current Trends and Issues. Retrieved from http://aappolicy.aappublications.org/cgi/content/full/pediatrics;116/1/281

American College of Obstetricians and Gynecologists. (2009). Adolescent Facts—Pregnancy, Births and STDs; Retrieved from http://www.cdc.gov/nchs/data/factsheets/factsheet_teen_pregnancy.htm

Centers for Disease Control and Protection. (updated November 2, 2009). NCHS Fact Sheet—NCHS Data on Teenage Pregnancy. Retrieved from http://www.cdc.gov/nchs/data/factsheets/factsheet_teen_pregnancy.htm

Centers for Disease Control and Protection. (updated October 20, 2010). NCHS Data Brief, Number 46. Retrieved from http://www.cdc.gov/nchs/data/databriefs/db46.htm

Centers for Disease Control and Protection. (updated January 4, 2011). About Teen Pregnancy. Retrieved from http://www.cdc.gov/TeenPregnancy/AboutTeenPreg.htm

Chandra, A., Martinez, G. M., Mosher, W. D., Abma, J. C. , & Jones, J. (2005). Fertility, family planning, and reproductive health of U.S. women: Data from the 2002 National Survey of Family Growth. *Vital Health Statistics, 23*(25). National Center for Health Statistics.

Guttmacher Institute. (n.d.). Facts on American Teens' Sexual and Reproductive Health. Retrieved from http://www/guttmacher.org/.html

Hamilton, B. E., Martin, J. A., & Ventura, S. J. (2010). Births: Preliminary data for 2009. *National Vital Statistics Reports Web Release, 59*(3). Hyattsville, MD: National Center for Health Statistics.

Health. (2009). United States 2009. Retrieved from http://www.cdc.gov/nchs/hus.htm

Heron, M. P., Hoyert, D. L., Murphy, S. L., Xu, J. Q., Kochanek, K. D., & Tejada-Vera, B. (2009). Deaths: Final data for 2006. *National Vital Statistics Reports, 57*(14). Hyattsville, MD: National Center for Health Statistics.

Honein, M. A., Paulozzi, L. J., Mathews, T. J., Erickson, J. D., Lee-Yang, C., & Wong, M. S. (2001). Impact of folic acid fortification of the U.S. food supply on the occurrence of neural tube defects. *Journal of the American Medical Association, 285*(23), 2981–2986.

Hoyert, D. L. (2007). Maternal mortality and related concepts. *Vital Health Statistics, 3*(33). National Center for Health Statistics. Retrieved from http://www.cdc.gov/nchs/data/series/sr_03/sr03_033.pdf

Martin, J. A., Hamilton, B. E., Sutton, P. D., et al. (2010). Births: Final data for 2007. *National Vital Statistics Reports, 58*(24). Hyattsville, MD: National Center for Health Statistics.

Mathews, T. J., & MacDorman, M. F. (2010). Infant mortality statistics from the 2006 period linked birth/infant death data set. *National Vital Statistics Reports, 58*(17). Available at http://www.cdc.gov/nchs/data/nvsr/nvsr58/nvsr58_17.pdf

Mathews, T. J., Minino, A. M., Osterman, M. J. K., et al. (2008). Special article: Annual summary of vital statistics: 2008. *Pediatrics, 127*(1), 146–157. (Published ahead of print December 20, 2010). Available at http://pediatrics.aappublications.org/citmgr?gca=pediatrics;127/1/146

Merrill, R. M. (2010). *Reproductive epidemiology: Principles and methods.* Sudbury, MA: Jones and Bartlett Publishers.

Mortality and Morbidity Weekly Report. (2009). Abortion Surveillance—United States, 2006. Available from: http://www.cdc.gov/mmwr/preview/mmwrhtml/ss5808a1.htm

Reynolds, M. A., Schieve, L. A., Martin, J. A., Jeng, G., & Macaluso, M. (2003). Trends in multiple births conceived using assisted reproductive technology, United States, 1997–2000. *Pediatrics, 111*, 1159–1162.

Russell, R. B., Green, N. S., Steiner, C. A., Meikle, S., Howse, J. L., Poschman, K., Dias, T., Potetz, L., Davidoff, M. J., Damus, K., & Petrini, J. R. (2007). Cost of hospitalization for preterm and low birth weight infants in the United States. *Pediatrics, 120*(1), e1–e9. doi:10.1542/peds.2006-2386

Staniec, F. O., & Webb, N. J. (2007). Utilization of infertility services: How much does money matter? *Health Services Research, 42*, 971–989.

Teilmann, G., Carsten, B. P., Jensen, T. K., et al. (2005). Prevalence and incidence of precocious pubertal development in Denmark: An epidemiologic study based on national registries. *Pediatrics, 116*(6), 1323–1328. Retrieved from http://pediatrics.aappublications.org/citmgr?gca=pediatrics;116/6/1323

World Health Organization (WHO). (2010). Reproductive Health and Research. Retrieved from http://www.who.int/reproductive-health/index.htm

Chapter 15

THE PRACTICE OF EPIDEMIOLOGY IN DEVELOPING COUNTRIES

Learning Objectives

Upon completion of this chapter, you should be able to:

1. Describe the distribution of diseases in developing countries.
2. Explain differences in the major causes of mortality between developed and developing countries.
3. Name at least two risk factors for the major causes of mortality in developing countries.
4. Describe at least two challenges in collecting health data in developing countries.
5. List at least three problems that involve managing health data in developing countries.

Key Terms

DALY	Health and	population pyramid
developed countries	Demographic	verbal autopsy
developing countries	Surveillance (HDS)	YLD
	life expectancy at birth	YLL

Chapter Outline

INTRODUCTION

This chapter will explore many of the challenges of working with health data in **developing countries**, defined as countries in the process of establishing an economic and medical infrastructure to support health. The social and environmental conditions in these types of countries may make simple tasks, such as recording births and deaths, become huge tasks. The incidence and prevalence of diseases seen in developing countries often differ from those found in **developed countries** (defined as countries with an established economic and medical infrastructure to support health) because of variations in screening, diagnosis, and treatment. Even if the incidence of a disease is the same in developed and developing countries, the mortality rates may be higher in developing countries because of issues related to access to medical care and treatment. Other challenges discussed in this chapter involve collecting and managing health data.

> **developing countries:** refers to countries in the process of establishing an economic and medical infrastructure to support health
>
> **developed countries:** refers to countries with an established economic and medical infrastructure to support health

WHAT ARE DEVELOPING COUNTRIES?

As a starting point to understanding how diseases vary worldwide, some basic information is needed about key differences in developed and developing countries. Keep in mind that there is no universal system to classify a country as developed or developing, but for health data, the classification used considers health infrastructure, data resources, access to medical care, and education. The world map shown in Figure 15-1 provides a general idea of the distribution of countries classified as developed or developing. This figure shows four levels of development from the least developed, to those in transition, to the established economies. Although these

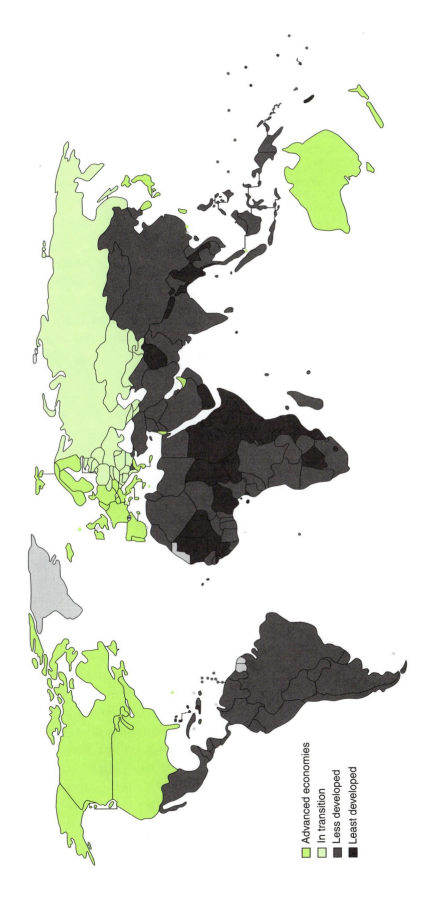

FIGURE 15-1 Geographical Representation of Countries in Various Stages of Development

Wikimedia Commons: http://commons.wikimedia.org/wiki/File:Developed_and_developing_countries.PNG

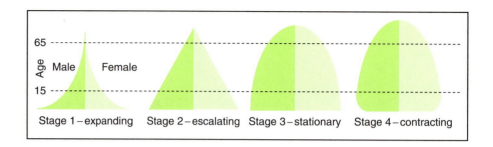

FIGURE 15-2 Population Pyramids for Areas with Various Combinations of High Birth Rate/High Mortality Rate and Low Birth Rate/Low Mortality Rate
Based on: http://en.wikipedia.org/wiki/Population_pyramid

definitions vary depending on whether the focus is on health, economics, industrialization, or productivity, this distribution gives a general idea of where countries lay on this continuum.

Typically, developing countries have a disproportionate number of young people relative to older people. One of the ways to examine this is to look at its **population pyramid**, or the distribution of its population by age and sex. The population pyramids shown in Figure 15-2 depict various stages of population percentages by age groups. The first two pyramids are wide at the base and taper very quickly as the age of the population increases. These pyramids show a very small proportion of elderly people in the population. The next two pyramids show a small proportion of people in the young age groups and a higher proportion in the older age groups. Generally, a pyramid with over 30% of the population between the ages of 1–14 and only 6% at age 75 and above is considered a young population (seen in the first two pyramids). This pattern generally occurs in developing countries, with limited health services, where there is a high birth rate but also a high mortality rate at all ages.

A pyramid with less than 30% of the population between the ages of 1 and 14 and more than 6% aged 75 and above is considered an aging population (seen in the last two pyramids). This pattern is usually found in developed countries with adequate health services, where the birth rate is steady or low and the mortality rate throughout the lifespan is also low. The information on age distribution is very important in understanding the types of diseases that may be present in the population.

Tying into the population pyramid is the concept of **life expectancy**, or a mathematical calculation based on population statistics to estimate the average years a person born in a certain year will live. For example, in the United States, a child born in 2008 would be expected to live an average of 78.4 years. Of course, not all children born in 2008 will live to that exact age; some will die younger and some will live longer, but the average life of all children born that year will be 78.4 years. Considering a country such as Kenya, the life expectancy at birth in 2008 was only 54.2 years. This lower life expectancy is because of the high rate of mortality in childhood or young adulthood as a result of various causes. As shown in Figure 15-3, life expectancy varies throughout the world, but it is typically lower in developing countries.

population pyramid:
a graphical representation of the age and sex distribution in a population, which normally forms the shape of a pyramid

life expectancy at birth:
or a mathematical calculation based on population statistics to estimate the average years a person born in a certain year will live

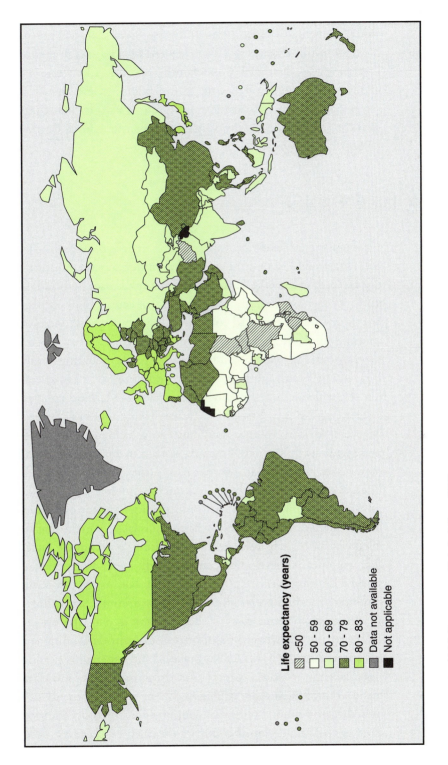

FIGURE 15-3 World: Life Expectancy at Birth, Both Sexes, 2009

Used with permission from World Health Organization: http://gamapserver.who.int/mapLibrary/app/searchResults.aspx. Accessed 1/20/12

Because the number of countries considered developing can be quite large, and without a consistent definition, summarizing data by developing or developed classification might be misleading. Rather than presenting data on hundreds of individual countries or using a classification system that may not be accurate, much of the data in this chapter will be presented by six general regions (Africa, Americas, Eastern Mediterranean, Europe, South-East Asia, and Western Pacific). In addition to these six regions, often data from a high-income area is shown for comparison purposes. This classification by regions is used by many international agencies, including the World Health Organization in its Global Burden of Disease project (World Health Organization, 2008).

DISTRIBUTION OF DISEASES

Although infectious diseases are common in developing countries, the leading causes of death for adults are similar to those in developed countries, with cardiovascular disease leading the way. However, the many diseases that lead to illness or disability are very different. For example, diseases that cause blindness, amputations as a result of injuries or diabetes, and conditions that stunt childhood growth are much more common in developing countries as compared with developed countries. Many of these diseases are widespread because of the shortcomings in the developing countries' public health infrastructure. In addition, there are several infectious diseases that are endemic or habitually present in some developing countries. For example, a disease spread by the tsetse fly, African Trypanosomiasis (sleeping sickness), occurs in several African countries and may cause permanent neurological damage and, if untreated, death. Although malaria, spread by mosquitoes, occurs worldwide, 90% of all cases are found in sub-Saharan Africa, mostly among children. A parasitic disease, onchocerciasis (river blindness) is endemic in Africa, home of most of the 18 million people with this disease. Another parasitic disease that is endemic in many developing countries is schistosomiasis, which causes severe symptoms, including rash, itch, fever, chills, coughing, and muscle aches. Shigellosis infection, common in developing countries with poor sanitation, causes 600,000 deaths worldwide every year. Cholera is another disease spread through contaminated drinking water and poor sanitation with symptoms that include diarrhea, vomiting, and leg cramps. Severe cases of cholera result in dehydration and can be fatal.

One of the challenges of studying diseases in developing countries is that both infectious diseases (HIV/AIDS, malaria, and tuberculosis) and diseases or disabilities as a result of access issues (clean drinking water, immunizations, timely treatment, contraceptives) are problems. These include those diseases that lead to high mortality or disability rates that could be prevented. In addition, common chronic diseases seen in developed countries (heart disease, cancer, diabetes, chronic bronchitis) are also present in developing countries.

A good source of comparative data is found in the Global Burden of Disease project (World Health Organization, 2008). The World Health Organization coordinates efforts to track diseases using standardized methods and summarizes the findings in reports that are updated regularly. One of the ways used to determine the impact of a disease is to use a number that incorporates not only mortality, but morbidity as well. The disability-adjusted life year (**DALY**) is a measure of overall disease burden, expressed as the number of years before age 75 lost because of ill-health, disability, or early death. It is actually the sum of two other measures: **YLL** (years of life lost as a result of premature mortality) and **YLD** (years lived with disability). Using DALYs gives a very different picture of mortality and unhealthy life because they can account for illnesses that result in disability, as well as in death.

> **DALY:** stands for disability-adjusted life year, a measure of overall disease burden, expressed as the number of years before age 75 lost because of ill-health, disability, or early death
>
> **YLL:** years of life lost as a result of premature mortality
>
> **YLD:** years lived with disability

Mortality and Disability

Although the life expectancy for most developing countries is lower than for developed countries, much of the excess mortality is the result of childhood mortality and maternal mortality rather than diseases of old age. Deaths that occur at young ages contribute heavily to overall life expectancy. As shown in Figure 15-4, the deaths per 1,000 children age 0–4 years is very high for the Africa region, yet somewhat lower for the Eastern Mediterranean and South-East Asia Regions. Note that for the high-income comparison group, the mortality rate is very low. The major causes of these deaths include malaria, respiratory diseases, diarrheal conditions, and perinatal conditions, with the "Other" category including such things as injuries, other infectious diseases, and birth defects.

Figure 15-5 displays mortality rates by major cause and by region for adults aged 15–59 years. Again, the death rate per 1,000 adults aged 15–59 years in Africa is much higher than any other region. For high-income countries, the most common causes

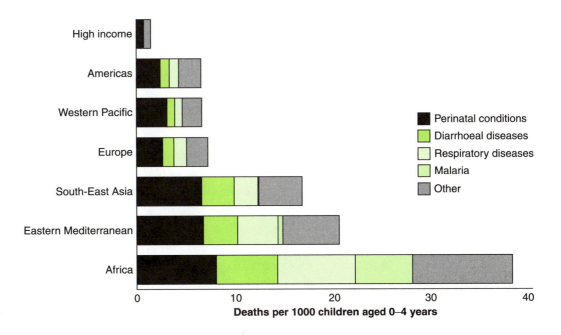

FIGURE 15-4 Child Mortality Rates by Major Cause and Region, 2004

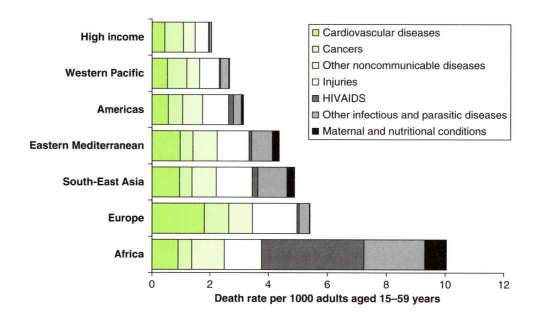

FIGURE 15-5 Adult Mortality Rates by Major Cause and Region, 2004
Used with permission from World Health Organization: http://www.who.int/healthinfo/global_burden_disease/en/index.html

of death are chronic diseases, whereas the most frequent causes of deaths in Africa are HIV/AIDS and other infectious and parasitic diseases. For all countries, chronic diseases, including cardiovascular diseases and cancers, make up a substantial portion of the death rate suggesting that when infectious diseases are more fully controlled, the pattern of mortality will more closely reflect what is seen for high-income countries.

Because we know that mortality is not a complete picture, it is important to look at disability also. When looking at mortality and disability together, as shown in Figure 15-6, the largest burden for the Africa region is premature mortality, whereas in the Americas and the Western Pacific regions, the burden is equally divided between mortality and disability.

Risk Factors

When we think of risk factors for diseases, we usually think of things that are under the control of an individual (such as smoking cessation, healthy eating, and getting enough physical activity). Although numerous risk factors are known for diseases that occur frequently in developing countries, many of these risk factors rely on public health infrastructure rather than on a change in individual behavior. Examples are access to medicines, clean water and air, sanitation, food, and preventive measures (such as nets for malaria prevention). To combat this problem globally and help countries get the most out of limited resources, a collaborative effort from about 200 countries produced a project designed to highlight major preventable problems in developing countries. The result was the Millennium Development Goals (MDG).

Although the MDG are more general in scope than specific diseases, they address topics that account for disproportionate morbidity in developing countries. By focusing attention and resources in eight specific areas, resources could be

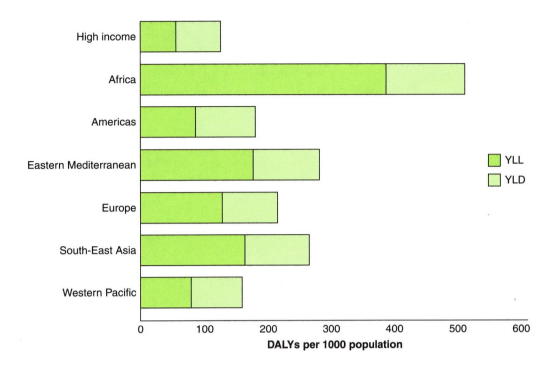

FIGURE 15-6 Years of Life Lost (YLL), Years Living with Disability (YLD), and Disability-Adjusted Life Years (DALY) per 100,000 Population by Region, 2004
Used with permission from World Health Organization: http://www.who.int/healthinfo/global_burden_disease/en/index.html

combined and progress could be tracked. The eight general areas include goals to: eradicate extreme poverty and hunger; achieve universal primary education; promote gender equality and empower women; reduce child mortality; improve maternal health; combat HIV/AIDS, malaria, and other diseases; ensure environmental sustainability; and develop a global partnership for development. Examples of three of MDG that are directly related to health and the progress made in each of them from 1990–2008 are listed in Table 15-1.

Other risk factors, such as cigarette smoking and exposure to environmental tobacco smoke (also called "secondhand smoke"), require a combination of policy and individual behavior changes. A recent report found that tobacco use is a risk

TABLE 15-1 Status of Health-Related Millennium Development Goals

Millennium Development Goal	Progress from 1990–2009
Improve maternal health and reduce child mortality:	
Maternal mortality	Annual global average rate of decline from 1990–2009 was 2.3%, far short of the 5.5% needed to meet targets.
Prenatal visits	From 2000 to 2008, fewer than half of all·pregnant women made the WHO-recommended minimum of four prenatal visits.

Continues

TABLE 15-1 Status of Health-Related Millennium Development Goals (Continued)	
Contraception	The proportion of women in developing countries who report using contraceptives increased from 50% in 1990 to 62% in 2005.
Reduce child mortality.	Annual global deaths of children 0–4 years fell to 8.1 million in 2009—down by 35% since 1990.
Combat infectious diseases:	
HIV/AIDS	New HIV infections have declined by 17% globally from 2001–2009.
TB	TB mortality among HIV-negative people has dropped from 30 deaths per 100,000 people in 1990 to 20 deaths per 100,000 in 2009.
Malaria	The supply of insecticide-treated nets increased, but need outweighed availability almost everywhere. Access to antimalarial medicines increased but it was inadequate in all countries surveyed in 2007 and 2008.

Based on: http://www.who.int/mediacentre/factsheets/fs290/en

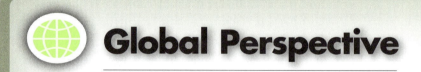

Global Perspective

Worldwide Spread of Infectious Diseases

Although the health problems of developing countries are enormous compared to developed countries, these problems do not exist in isolation. Infectious diseases and environmental pollutants can affect people well beyond the boundaries of the host country. With travel to far corners of the world, infections can be spread to vulnerable populations faster than ever before. Of particular concern is the spread of multidrug resistant infections that do not respond to traditional treatment. Because of this, the problems of developing countries are problems for all countries. A worldwide effort is needed to improve health on a global scale.

factor for six of the eight leading causes of death in the world (Mathers et al., 2006). Because of aggressive policy and social interventions in many developed countries, tobacco use is declining. Unfortunately, the tobacco epidemic is shifting toward developing countries, where it is estimated that 80% of all tobacco-related deaths will occur within a few decades. Because of this, the WHO has identified the six most effective policies that can curb the tobacco epidemic. This program is called MPOWER, and each policy is described in Table 15-2.

These MPOWER policy interventions have significantly reduced tobacco use in the countries that have implemented them. The tobacco use epidemic is man-made

TABLE 15-2 Six Policies to Reduce and Prevent Tobacco Use (MPOWER)

Monitoring tobacco use and prevention	Currently, two out of three countries in the developing world do not have even minimal data about youth and adult tobacco use.
Protecting people from tobacco smoke	More than half of countries worldwide allow smoking in government offices, work spaces, and other indoor settings. Smoke-free policies in the workplaces of several industrialized nations have reduced total tobacco consumption among employees by an average of 29%.
Offering help to quit tobacco use	Among smokers who are aware of the dangers of tobacco, three out of four want to quit, yet comprehensive services to treat tobacco dependence are available to only 5% of the world's population.
Warning about the dangers of tobacco	Graphic warnings on tobacco product packaging deter tobacco use; yet only 15 countries, representing 6% of the world's population, mandate pictorial warnings that cover at least 30% of the principal surface area on the packaging.
Enforcing bans on tobacco advertising, promotion, and sponsorship	About half of the children of the world live in countries that do not ban free distribution of tobacco products. National-level studies before and after advertising bans found a decline in tobacco consumption of up to 16% following prohibitions.
Raising taxes on tobacco products	Increasing tobacco taxes by 10% generally decreases tobacco consumption by 4% in high-income countries and by about 8% in low- and middle-income countries.

Based on: http://www.who.int/features/factfiles/tobacco_epidemic/en/index.html

Check It Out

Go to http://www.who.int to download information on how mobile technology is used to support the Tobacco Free Initiative

and entirely preventable, yet only 5% of the world's population lives in a country that protects its population with any one of these key interventions. If developing countries, even those with meager resources, could focus prevention efforts in these six policy areas, considerable progress can be made in stopping this epidemic. Of particular importance is preventing children and young adults from beginning to smoke because quitting smoking is very difficult once a person is addicted.

DATA ISSUES

Data collection and management are important problems for both developing and developed countries. Accurate information about the population drives the development of health policy and health programs. However, data collection may be more of a challenge in a country with limited resources that are most effectively spent on acute treatment and other infrastructure issues. Even when data are collected, comparing health statistics across countries and over time may be problematic because data may differ in terms of the definitions used, data-collection methods, population coverage, and estimation methods. Organizations, such as the World Health Organization, play a significant role in assisting with data collection and management while providing standardization of methodology.

Availability of accurate data, both in scope and frequency, is the most important obstacle to health data systems in developing countries and particularly in Africa. Although access to up-to-date computer systems is essential, one of the major barriers to setting up and maintaining health data has to do with availability of trained staff. Because this work requires years of experience and training, the number of staff and their level of professional education is important. In addition to the number of staff, turnover may be high and recruitment of new staff with the proper training is difficult. The challenges posed by data collection problems in developing countries often, of necessity, lead to the development of innovative techniques.

Vital Records

To assist developing countries in setting up vital records systems, international standards were developed so that the same data were collected across different countries. However, whether it is because of difficult terrain, political unrest, or lack of an established infrastructure, in much of the developing world, the registration of vital statistics (such as birth or death data) is minimal or nonexistent. This makes it difficult to compare birth or death records with other countries, to evaluate trends, and to calculate stable mortality data. Figure 15-7 displays a world map indicating the proportion of a country that is monitored for vital statistics. You can see from this map that most countries in Africa have vital records coverage for less than 25% of their population.

Data Systems

Even without access to basic birth and death data, there may be access to information collected from health care facilities where people go for treatment. However, information collected in this way provides an incomplete picture of health problems. In Africa, where an estimated 80% of people die outside of such facilities, millions of births and deaths go uncounted. In Chapter 4, Data Sources, we learned the value of surveillance data in tracking disease trends and marking progress over time. We also learned the value of health surveys to obtain detailed information for a particular problem or in a particular geographical area.

Because of the challenge of setting up complete health and surveillance systems in developing countries, innovative strategies such as **Health and Demographic Surveillance (HDS)** is sometimes used (Indepth, 2011). HDS is a way to continuously monitor populations at the household level within a geographically defined area, usually bounded by rivers, roads, or other markers. Every household and its occupants are identified, and all births, deaths, and in-out migrations are recorded. Typically, trained workers visit the same households several times a year and gather information through interviews. If the visits are frequent enough, information on pregnancy is also obtained. Other information of interest to the particular area is also collected, meaning that the data collected may vary from HDS to HDS depending on the needs of the area. For example, there is interest in using an HDS system to monitor the Millennium Development Goals, especially in places where there is no other way to obtain data to track progress.

The **verbal autopsy** is another innovative feature associated with HDS, but it is also used throughout the world when mortality data are not routinely collected. When a death is reported, an interview is done with a close associate of the deceased to ask about the symptoms, signs, and circumstances leading up to the death. The answers usually point to a cause of death. In this way, important information can be collected in areas where no other data exist, which is an advantage of using HDS. There are a few disadvantages also. The defined geographical area may not be representative of the outlying areas so the results cannot be generalized. The personal interviews and repeated visits make this approach expensive. Finally, because a great deal of information is collected from individuals who are then linked to households, the resulting data sets are large and complex, making anything but the simplest analyses difficult.

In the absence of established data systems, there are other ways that health data can be collected in developing countries. Often, as a result of major outbreaks, other countries or agencies will fund a data collection/surveillance effort in the affected area.

Health and Demographic Surveillance (HDS): a system that monitors populations at the household level within a geographically defined area

verbal autopsy: designed to determine cause of death, an interview with a close associate of the deceased

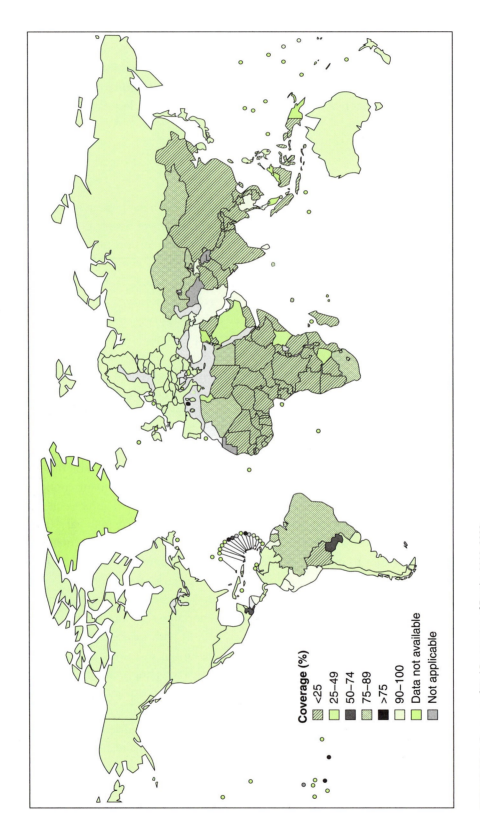

FIGURE 15-7 Coverage of Vital Registration of Deaths, 2000–2008

http://apf.or.id/world-coverage-of-vital-registration-of-deaths-2000-2008.html

For example, some international agencies work with the local ministry of health or a national statistical center of a number of developing countries to conduct several types of studies within a particular region. These studies may be used to determine such things as critical health and nutrition information. These studies are also useful to assess residents' knowledge of particular diseases (such as AIDS and malaria) and their understanding of protective measures, as well as to help the local health officials interpret data and to assess the effectiveness of interventions. The strength of this approach is that data are collected in a standardized manner and can be compared with data from other countries. The disadvantage of this approach is that once the particular problem or event is completed, the country may find itself without the resources to continue the effort.

Data Management

Even when it is possible for local health officials to collect data, other challenges remain before the data can be useful. The costs of setting up a strong data management facility may be prohibitive. First of all, the computer system must be able to

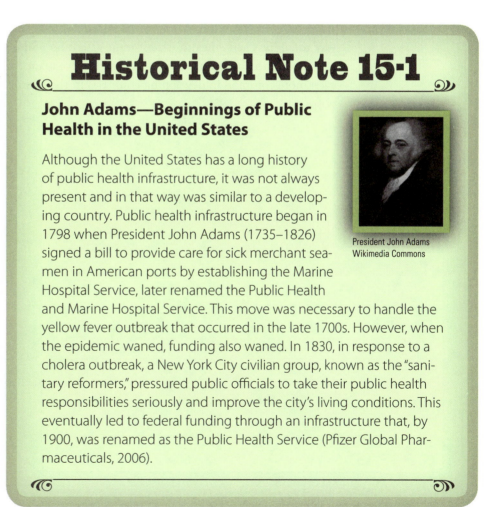

Historical Note 15-1

John Adams—Beginnings of Public Health in the United States

Although the United States has a long history of public health infrastructure, it was not always present and in that way was similar to a developing country. Public health infrastructure began in 1798 when President John Adams (1735–1826) signed a bill to provide care for sick merchant seamen in American ports by establishing the Marine Hospital Service, later renamed the Public Health and Marine Hospital Service. This move was necessary to handle the yellow fever outbreak that occurred in the late 1700s. However, when the epidemic waned, funding also waned. In 1830, in response to a cholera outbreak, a New York City civilian group, known as the "sanitary reformers," pressured public officials to take their public health responsibilities seriously and improve the city's living conditions. This eventually led to federal funding through an infrastructure that, by 1900, was renamed as the Public Health Service (Pfizer Global Pharmaceuticals, 2006).

President John Adams
Wikimedia Commons

handle the latest software and have enough storage for large data files. Next, the appropriate database system software and statistical analysis software must be purchased and updated regularly. Then, the staff must be trained to use the database system to enter and process data files. Because regular reports are a critical part of the process, staff must be trained in analyzing data and providing statistical summaries.

Once a system is in place, all of the potential problems that face developed countries are also present in developing countries. Major among these are quality control issues. These include the completeness of the information, the consistency of collecting data (whether monthly, annually, or other regular schedule), and the accuracy of data entry.

THE FUTURE

Although the burden of disease is disproportionately high for some regions, the global projections from 2004 to 2030 suggest that diseases such as HIV/AIDS, respiratory infections, tuberculosis, and malaria will decrease, whereas diseases that affect older adults, such as heart disease, stroke, and cancer will increase. This scenario suggests that along with the prevention strategies that are currently underway to address acute health issues, some attention will need to be paid to address chronic health conditions, common now in developed countries, that will become even more common in developing countries in the future.

Summary

In this chapter, we learned about the factors that distinguish developing from developed countries. In addition, some of the health infrastructure issues facing developing countries were explored. We also learned some key characteristics of countries, such as the age distribution and life expectancy. Although many of the diseases are the same in both developed and developing countries, there are many more challenges to treating diseases in developing countries because of the lack of medicines, access to health providers, and education. Global strategies to tackle these problems from a policy level were also described. Obtaining regular and accurate data on basic vital statistics is another challenge for developing countries, and innovative ways to collect and manage data and provide basic health data for an area were also described.

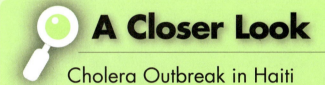

A Closer Look

Cholera Outbreak in Haiti

An unfortunate epidemic of cholera occurred in Haiti in 2010. Discussed in "A Closer Look" are some basic characteristics about this country and its public health system, which will set the stage for understanding how the natural disasters that hit this country and destroyed a fragile public health system led to the cholera epidemic.

Haiti

Haiti, a Caribbean country slightly smaller than the state of Maryland, occupies the western portion of the island of Hispaniola, which it shares with the Dominican Republic. This independent country is known for years of political upheaval. Haiti has a population of nearly 10 million and is the poorest country in the Western Hemisphere with 80% of the population living below the poverty line. More than two-thirds of the working people do not have formal jobs, and most Haitians live on less than $2 a day. The Haiti telecommunications infrastructure is among the least developed in Latin America and the Caribbean. Haiti has 14 airports, but only four have paved runways.

Public Health Infrastructure prior to 2010

Haiti's capital, Port-au-Prince, is a coastal city with about 2 million inhabitants. Before 2010, about 86% of its residents were living in slum conditions—mostly tightly packed, poorly built concrete buildings, of which half had no access to latrines. Using 2008 data from the MDG, 24% of urban and 10% of rural inhabitants had access to adequate sanitation facilities, and 50% of urban and 4% of rural Haitians had access to tap water (WHO/UNICEF, 2010). Because of this, fecal contamination of drinking water was common and diarrheal disease was a leading cause of childhood deaths. For example, the childhood mortality rate was 171

Continues

per 1,000 live births (compared to 14 per 1,000 live births in Europe). By all public health indicators, Haiti lagged behind most other countries in the Americas. Diseases that had been controlled in many other countries (such as malaria and rabies) were common in Haiti. The vaccination rate for measles-rubella was only 58%, and national surveillance systems were unable to provide adequate data for planning purposes.

Earthquake

On January 12, 2010, a massive 7.0 magnitude earthquake hit this small country with the epicenter near the capital city, Port-au-Prince. According to records, this was the strongest earthquake in this area since the 1770s. The Haitian government estimated the death toll to be around 220,000 to 270,000; but since many people were buried in common graves, the true number may never be known. It is estimated that as many as 300,000 were injured, making the Haiti earthquake one of the deadliest natural disasters in modern history.

Earthquake Aftermath

As a result of the earthquake disaster, the already meager public health infrastructure of Haiti was further damaged. Initially, 1,500,000 Haitians were living in tent camps. Prior to the earthquake, approximately 380,000 children were in orphanages; and after the earthquake, an unknown number of children (estimated at many thousands) joined these ranks. About 40–50% of all buildings were destroyed, and many people were homeless. In addition to the problem of tracking its residents, the public health officials had a massive task ahead. The tent cities needed basic public health facilities such as clean drinking water and basic sanitation. The residents needed a way to link families with each other (who may be in another tent city or living on the streets). Public health workers had to find people who had been being treated for tuberculosis and HIV so that the treatment could continue. Schools had to be set up for the children. Although there was an enormous amount of work to do, other countries worldwide contributed technical staff and millions of dollars of aid, some of which was used for immediate needs and some of which was used for public health infrastructure projects, including surveillance. The Haitian Ministry of Public Health and Population began to plan how to use this opportunity to strengthen public health so that it would be better than it had been prior to the earthquake.

Basic Facts about Cholera

Cholera is an acute intestinal infection caused by bacteria transmitted through contaminated water or food. The source of contamination is usually feces of infected people. This disease causes acute diarrhea and vomiting, but about 75% of people infected do not show symptoms even though the bacteria are present in their feces for 1–2 weeks and can spread the disease to others. Among those who do have symptoms, about 20% will have acute watery diarrhea and severe dehydration that can be fatal. Although cholera is treatable by rehydration and antibiotics, it is extremely potent and can kill within hours. Particularly at risk are those with low immunity levels, especially those with other diseases such as HIV, or malnourished children. The best way to control this disease is through prevention. Access to clean water, a major element of public health, is required. However, once an outbreak occurs, the response is to provide prompt treatment and safe sources of drinking water (see Figure 15-8).

Cholera Epidemic

The devastation from the earthquake, poor sanitary facilities, and lack of access to clean drinking water set the stage for the outbreak of cholera that was confirmed on October 21, 2010, by the Haitian National Public Health Laboratory. Initially, more than 3,500 people

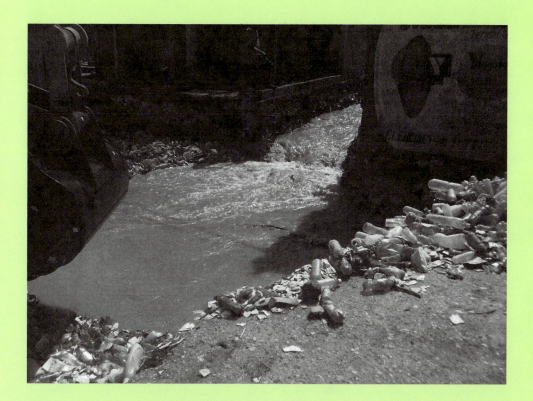

FIGURE 15-8 Unclean Water Sources Following the Devastating Earthquake Set the Stage for a Cholera Outbreak in Haiti
Courtesy of Centers for Disease Control and Prevention: http://blogs.cdc.gov/publichealthmatters/2010/12/haiti-cholera-response-stories-from-the-field/

in a region to the north of Port-au-Prince were treated for diarrhea, acute fever, vomiting, and severe dehydration. Officials believed the cholera outbreak had been caused by people drinking infected water from a local river. This situation was exacerbated in early November 2010 when Hurricane Tomas hit the nation, causing widespread flooding. There were fears the outbreak would reach tent cities housing survivors of January's quake. By December 3, the toll had climbed to 91,770 cases from all 10 health departments in the country and the capital city of Port-au-Prince (see Figure 15-9). During this time, 43,243 (47.1%) of those affected had been hospitalized and 2,071 (2.3%) had died (MMWR, 2010). By February 2011, the outbreak had continued with a reported 230,000 cases and more than 4,500 deaths. Although the officials knew what to do to stem this outbreak, resources were limited and a higher proportion of deaths occurred in rural areas than in urban areas.

This is an example of how important it is to maintain the public health infrastructure. Even in the face of these natural disasters, had more resources been available to provide proper sanitation and clean drinking water, this outbreak might not have happened or could have been reduced in scope. If the ability to monitor those who were ill and provide early treatment, the death toll would have been lower.

Continues

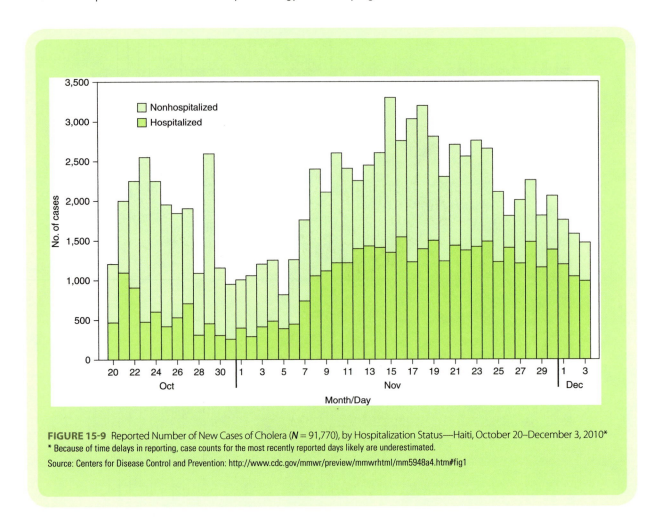

FIGURE 15-9 Reported Number of New Cases of Cholera (*N* = 91,770), by Hospitalization Status—Haiti, October 20–December 3, 2010*

* Because of time delays in reporting, case counts for the most recently reported days likely are underestimated.

Source: Centers for Disease Control and Prevention: http://www.cdc.gov/mmwr/preview/mmwrhtml/mm5948a4.htm#fig1

Review Questions

1. Name three challenges to collecting health data in developing countries.

   1. _____
   2. _____
   3. _____

2. **True or False** Infectious diseases are difficult to treat in developing countries because there is lack of access to medicines and health care workers.

3. Which of the following are characteristics of a developing country?

    a. Low life expectancy
    b. Lack of access to medical treatment
    c. High smoking prevalence
    d. All of the above

4. **True or False** A population pyramid with a large base is indicative of a high birth rate.

5. **True or False** Even though it is difficult to collect data in a developing country, excellent records are maintained for births and deaths.

6. Which of the following diseases are more common in developing countries compared to those in developed countries?

    a. Heart disease
    b. Malaria
    c. Tuberculosis
    d. Arthritis

7. Name three reasons that the childhood mortality rate is so high in developing countries.

    1. _____
    2. _____
    3. _____

8. Name one advantage in using DALYs instead of mortality rates when assessing the health status of a population.

    _____

9. Which of the following are problems that public officials face when collecting data about health?

    a. Lack of a trained work force
    b. Difficulty in traveling to rural areas
    c. Language barriers
    d. All of the above

10. **True or False** Prevention efforts targeting specific risk factors, such as smoking, are more effective if they include behavior change and policy change approaches.

11. **True or False** The Millennium Development Goals were established to set common priorities by highlighting the major problems in developing countries.

12. Which one of the following diseases can be avoided by using recognized public health sanitation techniques?

    a. Cholera
    b. Pneumonia
    c. Diabetes
    d. Cancer

13. Which of the following refer to data management issues in developing countries?

    a. Developing trained staff
    b. Assuring quality control
    c. Entering data in a computer
    d. Dealing with missing data
    e. All of the above

14. Name three innovative features of an HDS (Health Demographic Surveillance).

    1. _____
    2. _____
    3. _____

15. Match the problem in column A with the solution in column B.

Column A (Problem)	Column B (Solution)
___ Cholera	a. Clean drinking water
___ Lack of vital records on cause of death	b. Verbal autopsy
___ Control tobacco use	c. MPOWER program
___ Control of morbidity/mortality	d. Millennium Development Goals

16. **For Deeper Thought** A developing country has received a large grant to support public health efforts. This money must be used over a three-year period, and there will be no additional funds from this source after that time. A preliminary survey indicates that the country has many problems ranging from lack of data to monitor the health of its population to high death rates from potentially preventable diseases. How should the health officials go about developing a plan to prioritize spending this money?

Website Resources

For additional information on world health statistics: http://www.WHO.int

For additional information on developing countries: http://www.worldbank.org

For additional information on infectious diseases of developing countries: http://www.infoplease.com

For additional information on tobacco use globally: CDC: http://www.cdc.gov/tobacco

For additional information on the 2010 earthquake in Haiti: http://hubpages.com/hub/Haiti-Earthquake-Facts

References

Dowell, S. F., Tappero, J. W., & Frieden, T. R. (2011). Public health in Haiti—Challenges and progress. *New England Journal of Medicine, 364,* 300–301.

INDEPTH Network. (2011). Retrieved from http://www.indepth-network.org/index.php?option=com_content&task=view&id=13&Itemid=28

Jordans, F. (February 18, 2011). UN: Cholera eases in Haiti but rural deaths high. *Associated Press.* Retrieved from http://hosted2.ap.org/APDEFAULT/cae69a7523db45408eeb2b3a98c0c9c5/Article_2011-02-18-Haiti%20Cholera/id-db92390be30a4dafb10ee7e613f55465

Mathers, C. D., & Loncar, D. (2006). Projections of global mortality and burden of disease from 2002 to 2030. *PLoS Medicine, 3*(11), e442.

Morbidity and Mortality Weekly Report (MMWR). (December 10, 2010).Update: Outbreak of cholera—Haiti, 2010, 59(48), 1586–1590. Retrieved from http://www.cdc.gov/mmwr/preview/mmwrhtml/mm5948a4.htm

Pfizer Global Pharmaceuticals. (2006). Chapter 11, U.S. public health infrastructure. New York: Pfizer Inc., 213–214.

World Health Organization. (2008). Global Burden of Disease. Retrieved from http://www.who.int/healthinfo/global_burden_disease/2004_report_update/en/index.html

World Health Organization (2010). Millennium Development Goals. Retrieved from http://www.who.int/topics/millennium_development_goals/about/en/index.html

World Health Statistics. (2010). Retrieved from http://www.who.int/whosis/whostat/EN_WHS10_Full.pdf

WHO/UNICEF Joint Monitoring Programme (JMP) for Water Supply and Sanitation. (2010). Progress on sanitation and drinking water: 2010 update. Retrieved fromhttp://www.wssinfo.org/fileadmin/user_upload/resources/1278061137-jmp_report_2010_en.pdf

Glossary

A

abortion   refers to any termination of pregnancy, but most often applies to intentional termination of pregnancy

acanthosis nigricans   a skin disorder found commonly in obesity and diabetes; dark, velvety patches found in body creases

accuracy   the degree to which a measurement or an estimate based on measurements represents the true value of the attribute that is being measured

Acquired Immunodeficiency Syndrome (AIDS)   the most severe stage of HIV infection

active carrier   an infected individual capable of transmitting disease during and after clinical disease

active immunity   when the host's immune system responds to an invading organism or antigen and produces its own immune response

adenocarcinoma   cancer that starts in gland cells (cells that normally secrete a substance)

adjusted rate   a rate that is mathematically transformed to provide a summary rate for an observed population after differences in specified characteristics are removed

adjustment   mathematical transformation of rates or measures of association to account for external variables

adverse event   includes *any* event that occurs following an immunization

adverse reaction   an event that occurs following immunization and that is actually *caused by* the vaccine; also known as a "side effect"

aerobic exercise   includes activities that improve cardiorespiratory capacity and endurance

age-specific mortality rate   death (mortality) rates for specific age groups calculated by the number of deaths in a particular age group divided by the midpoint population in that age group (multiplied by 1,000 or 100,000)

agent   capable of causing an illness

alternative therapy   used as a substitute for mainstream treatment and is meant to achieve a cure

amniocentesis   procedure that collects a sample of the amniotic fluid that surrounds the developing fetus; fluid then used to perform laboratory tests to detect genetic and other diseases

analytic study   a study that tests one or more hypotheses about the relationship between risk factors and disease, generally looking for causation

angina   the most common symptom of coronary artery disease; caused by reduced blood supply to the heart muscle and manifested as chest pain

anovulatory   not accompanied by the release of an egg from the ovary and therefore not capable of resulting in pregnancy

antibodies   protein molecules produced by B lymphocytes in response to an antigen

antigen   substance that is capable of producing an immune response; may be live or inactivated

antigenic drift   minor mutations in the hemagglutinin or neuraminidase protein antigens of influenza A virus that occur continuously; results in new strains of the virus

antigenic shift   an abrupt, major change in the protein antigens that produces a novel influenza A virus subtype in humans that was not currently in circulation

antiretroviral therapy (ART)   combination of medications used to combat HIV infection

arrhythmia   a change in the normal electrical impulses of the heart that cause a change in rate or rhythm of the heart beat

assisted reproductive technology (ART)   all fertility treatments in which both eggs and sperm are manipulated

atherosclerosis   fat, other cells, and debris deposits under the lining of the arteries, causing narrowing of the vessels; also known as "hardening of the arteries"

attack rates   rates of disease during short periods of time or when the entire population is available to observe

attributable risk (AR)   the amount of risk in a comparison group that can be eliminated if the exposure of interest is removed from that group

autoimmune   an immune response against one self's cells or tissues

B

bacille Calmette-Guérin vaccine (BCG)   a live, attenuated vaccine using *Mycobacterium bovis*, or a cow tuberculin bacterium, as the antigen; used globally to prevent TB meningitis and disseminated TB in infants worldwide in high-risk areas

basal cell carcinoma   a type of non-melanomatous skin cancer that arises in the base layer of cells of the epidermis

benign   noncancerous

beta cells   specialized cells, found in the islet of Langerhans regions of the pancreas, that produce insulin

bias   any systematic error in the design, conduct, or analysis of a study that results in a mistaken estimate of an exposure's effect on the risk of disease

birth defects   faults or imperfections present in a baby at birth

blood pressure   a measurement of the force the circulating blood exerts on the arterial walls

bone marrow stem cell transplant   a treatment that restores blood-forming stem cells destroyed during chemotherapy or radiation therapy

BRCA1 and BRCA2   genes that when mutated or damaged put a woman at higher risk for breast or ovarian cancer and possibly men at higher risk for prostate cancer

C

cancer   cells characterized by uncontrolled growth and the ability to spread to other parts of the body

carcinogen   a substance that causes cancer or helps it to grow

carcinoma   cancer that arises in the epithelial cells

cardiac arrest   total stoppage of all heart function

cardiopulmonary resuscitation (CPR)   the method of doing chest compressions and rescue breathing to resuscitate a person who has had a heart attack

cardiovascular disease (CVD)   a generic term that includes several different conditions that affect the heart and blood vessels

carrier   person who has been exposed and infected by the etiologic agent and who is capable of transmitting the disease to others for a prolonged period of time

case   refers to a person in the population or study group identified as having the particular disease, health disorder, or condition under investigation

case control study   a study that allows the comparison of the attributes of a group of cases (subjects with the outcome of interest) to a group of controls (subjects without the outcome of interest)

case definition   characteristics or condition of an individual who will be considered a case for the purposes of surveillance or research

case severity   a measure of adverse events resulting from the disease that can be identified by measuring results such as length of hospital stay, number of follow-up visits, recovery time, disability, or death

causality   refers to determining the cause of a disease

cause   something that brings about an effect or a result

cause-specific mortality rate   the number of deaths as a result of a specific disease divided by the total midpoint population (multiplied by 1,000 or 100,000)

CD4 T cells   T-helper cells; specific immune cells that are infected and destroyed by HIV

cell-mediated immunity   the system that eliminates antigens with specific cells, but not antibodies

cerebrovascular accident (CVA) caused by a sudden impairment of cerebral circulation; also called a "stroke"

cerebrovascular disease disease that involves the blood vessels of the brain; stroke

cesarean section (C-section) refers to a surgical procedure in which one or more incisions are made through a mother's abdomen and uterus to deliver one or more babies

chemotherapy treatment of cancer with drugs

cholesterol a waxy, fat-like substance needed by the body in certain quantities

chorionic villus sampling procedure that collects a small piece of the placenta from the uterus; used for laboratory testing for genetic and other diseases early in pregnancy

chronic disease refers to a disease that is long-lasting

clinical the stage of disease when signs and symptoms appear

cohort study a study that compares subjects according to exposure status

common source outbreak occurs when all cases of the infection are acquired from the same source in a limited period of time and in a limited geographical location

complementary therapy treatment taken along with the standard prescribed treatments; not meant as a cure

conception the joining of an egg and sperm; interchangeable with "fertilization"

confidence interval for a measure of association a range of values that include the calculated estimate of the measure of association and represent the variability likely in the estimate

confidence interval for a rate or proportion a range of values that represents the variability likely in any measurement of disease or exposure occurrence

confounder a variable that is not the hypothesized exposure of interest or the outcome of interest but one that causes confusion or distortion of the measures of association

confounding the confusion or distortion of measures of association between exposure and outcome as a result of third (or more) variable(s)

congenital heart defects malformations of the heart or major blood vessels that are present at birth

construct validity the degree to which a measurement (questionnaire item, for example) correctly identifies the trait that it was designed to measure

contingency table a table in that it arranges data, allowing the comparison of exposure and outcome. A special case of a contingency table is a 2 × 2 table, which has just two rows and two columns.

contraception also called "birth control"; refers to any strategy that reduces or eliminates the chance of fertilization

controlling mathematical transformation of rates or measures of association to account for external variables; also known as minimizing confounding, holding confounders constant, and eliminating the effect of confounding

convalescent carrier a person who can transmit the etiologic agent while recovering from the disease

convenience sampling a method by which volunteers are approached and asked to participate

coronary arteries the arteries that supply the heart muscle

coronary artery disease (CAD) the most common type of cardiovascular disease; occurs when the coronary arteries that supply the heart muscle become stiffened and narrowed by atherosclerotic plaque

coronary heart disease (CHD) *see* coronary artery disease (CAD)

corpus luteum ruptured ovarian follicle after the release of an egg; produces the hormone progesterone

cross-sectional study a study design that investigates the relationship between existing exposure characteristics and existing outcome information in a group of subjects

crude birth rate the total number of live births divided by the total midpoint population (multiplied by 1,000 or 100,000)

crude mortality rate (same as crude death rate) the number of deaths in a period of time divided by the total midpoint population during that same time (multiplied by 1,000 or 100,000)

crude rate also referred to as a raw rate, a rate from the entire population under observation, consisting of a numerator that is all events from the population and a denominator that is the entire population under observation

D

DALY stands for disability-adjusted life year, a measure of overall disease burden, expressed as the number of years before age 75 lost because of ill-health, disability, or early death

dependent variable something that we are studying, usually called an "outcome"

descriptive epidemiology the pattern of disease occurrence from the perspectives of person, place, and time

descriptive study a study intended to determine the distribution of disease in a population

determinants physical, biological, social, cultural, and behavioral factors that influence health

developed countries refers to countries with an established economic and medical infrastructure to support health

developing countries refers to countries in the process of establishing an economic and medical infrastructure to support health

diabetes mellitus group of disorders characterized by high blood sugar resulting in polyuria

diarrhea passage of three or more loose or liquid stools per day

diastolic blood pressure the pressure circulating blood exerts on the arterial walls when the heart is at rest

difference measures rates or proportions that are compared to each other by the mathematical method of subtraction

differential bias systematic errors resulting in bias, which affect the comparison groups of a study differently

direct adjustment a process that eliminates the effect of extraneous variables; involves selecting a standard population and applying the rates from the populations under comparison to establish new rates that would be expected from the standard population

direct cause refers to a factor that causes a problem without any intermediate steps

disease outbreak the occurrence of cases of disease in excess of what would normally be expected in a defined community, geographical area, or season

distribution refers to time, place, and types of persons affected by a particular disease or condition (demographics)

E

ecological study an observational study where the unit of analysis is the population of a community rather than an individual

efficacy the measure of how well a vaccine performs by calculating the reduction of disease of vaccinated persons over unvaccinated persons as a percentage of those at risk (unvaccinated)

electronic cigarettes (e-cigarettes) resemble actual cigarettes but use an atomizer to heat a solution containing nicotine and other substances

encephalitis inflammation and swelling of the brain

endemic the normal occurrence of a disease or condition common to persons within a localized area

endocrine system of glands that produce hormones that regulate functions of the body

enterocolitis/colitis infections affecting the intestines/colon and causing diarrhea

environmental tobacco smoke (ETS) also known as "secondhand smoke"

epidemic refers to a disease or condition that affects a greater than expected (normal) number of individuals within a population, community, or region at the same time

epidemic curve the plot of time trends in the number of cases for a defined population and time period

epidemic threshold upper end of the normal endemic level of infections

epidemiology the study of the distribution (who has the problem) and determinants (things that influence the problem) of health-related conditions in human populations and the application of this method to the control of health problems

epidemiology triangle a graphic demonstration of the relationship between the agent, environment, and individual as a function of time

estrogen a female hormone produced by the ovary

etiology the biological cause of a problem or disease

exercise a subcategory of physical activity that is planned, structured, and repetitive

experimental study study in which the investigator intervenes with the subjects in some way

exposure also known as a "risk factor" or an "independent variable"

exposure odds ratio   an odds ratio that can be calculated by comparing those with the outcome to those without the outcome using the cross-products ratio from a 2 × 2 table

external validity   the extent to which the (internally valid) results of a study can be generalized beyond the study sample or for different people, places, or times

F

fecundity   difficulty conceiving or bringing a pregnancy to term

fertility   the ability to produce children

fertilization   the joining of an egg and sperm; interchangeable with "conception"

fetal alcohol syndrome (FAS)   a group of birth defects composed of physical, social, and learning problems resulting from alcohol use during pregnancy

fetal death   death prior to completed delivery of a fetus of 20 or more weeks of gestation; also called "stillbirth"

fetal death rate   the total number of fetal deaths divided by the total number of live births, plus the total number of fetal deaths (multiplied by 1,000)

folic acid   one of the B vitamins that is a key factor in preventing neural tube defects

follow-up period   the length of time that study subjects are monitored in a prospective cohort design

fomite   an inanimate object that may serve as an intermediary for transmission of an infectious disease between an infected person and a susceptible host

food borne intoxication   toxins in the contaminated foods, rather than the infecting organisms, produce the disease

food-specific attack rate   a rate of disease among those who have eaten a specific food item

Framingham Heart Study   a study designed by Boston University and the National Heart Institute in 1948 to study cardiovascular disease and its risk factors; has involved multiple generational cohorts

G

gastritis   infections targeting the stomach and causing vomiting

gastroenteritis   infections that affect the stomach and intestines and cause both vomiting and diarrhea; also known as the stomach flu

genotyping   detection of abnormalities in the genes of cancer cells

gestation   the period during which an embryo/fetus develops; also called "pregnancy"

gestational diabetes   occurring during pregnancy, gestational diabetes is similar to Type 2 diabetes in that the glucose intolerance is caused by insulin resistance

glucose   sugar used by cells for energy for cellular processes

glycosuria   glucose in the urine

grading   a classification used to differentiate how much a cancer cell varies from a normal cell

Gram stain   stain used in a microbiology lab to help classify bacteria according to the property of whether the bacteria take up the stain (Gram-positive) or not (Gram-negative)

H

Health and Demographic Surveillance (HDS)   a system that monitors populations at the household level within a geographically defined area

health-related states or conditions   diseases or events that cause illness, death, or disability. Examples are heart attacks or car accidents that can cause death, illness, or disability. Conditions that may not cause death but are very important because they cause disability include autism or arthritis.

healthy or passive carrier   an infected person who never gets clinically ill but who can transmit the etiologic agent to others

heart attack   also known as a "myocardial infarction (MI)"; caused when blood supply to the heart is severely reduced or completely blocked; the muscle cells do not receive enough oxygen and begin to die

heart failure   occurs when the heart muscle becomes ineffective at pumping enough blood and oxygen to meet the needs of the body

hemorrhagic stroke   a stroke caused by local bleeding into brain tissue from a weakened blood vessel

herd immunity   when hosts depend on the immunity of those around them in the community for their protection

high blood pressure (HBP) defined as systolic pressure above 140 and diastolic pressure above 90

high-density lipoproteins (HDL) carry cholesterol back to the liver to be removed from the body; high levels are protective from cardiovascular disease and stroke

horizontal transmission transmission of disease from person to person; may be directly from one person to another or indirectly from one person through an intermediate item to another person

hormone therapy use of hormones to treat cancers such as prostate and breast

human immunodeficiency virus (HIV) RNA virus that infects human immune cells and destroys them

human subject any person that is observed for purposes of research

hyperglycemia high blood glucose (sugar)

hypertension high blood pressure

hypoglycemia low blood glucose (sugar)

hypothesis a tentative explanation for a scientific problem that can be tested by further investigation

immunity the ability of the human body to accept the presence of substances that are part of the body ("self") and attempt to eliminate substances that are foreign to the body ("nonself")

immunization the stimulation of the immune system; used interchangeably with the terms "inoculation" and "vaccination"

immunoglobulins protein molecules produced by B lymphocytes in response to an antigen

immunotherapy treatment designed to boost the cancer patient's own immune system to help fight off the cancer

impaired fasting glucose (IFG) fasting glucose level that is above normal (70-100 mg/dL) but not in the range for a diagnosis of diabetes

impaired glucose tolerance (IGT) glucose level taken two hours after a glucose load—either a meal or a liquid glucose solution—(two-hour postprandial level) that is above normal (<140 mg/dL) but not in the range for a diagnosis of diabetes

inactivated vaccines vaccines made from inactivating the organism with heat or chemicals

incidence the number of new cases of a disease in a specified time frame

incident cases cases that are enrolled as the outcome of interest occurs

incidence density ratio a measure of association between exposure and outcome that provides strength and direction using two incidence densities

incidence rate the number of new cases of disease in a specified time (usually one year) divided by the population "at risk" to develop the disease

incubation period the time between infection and clinical disease

independent variables risk factors or exposures that we think might affect the outcome

index case the first case of a disease that is identified in a population

indirect adjustment a process to mathematically transform rates to hold constant some key differences in populations so that the rates can be compared

indirect cause refers to a factor may cause a problem, but through an intermediate step

infant mortality an infant death during the first year after live birth

infant mortality rate the number of deaths among infants less than one year of age divided by the total number of live births (multiplied by 1,000)

infectious disease refers to a contagious or transmissible disease

infertility inability to conceive after 12 consecutive months

information bias a large category of systemic errors in the performance of epidemiology studies that result in reduced validity of the information gathered from study subjects

informed consent the subject understands the scope of the study and can make an informed decision to participate

inoculation the procedure of administering the substance that will stimulate the immune response; used interchangeably with the terms "immunization" and "vaccination"

insulin a hormone produced by the pancreas that is involved in the uptake of glucose by the body's cells to be used for energy

insulin resistance state in which the pancreas produces insulin but the body cells do not respond to it as they should to allow for glucose uptake

internal validity   the degree to which what you did in the study *caused* the effect you observed

International Classification of Disease (ICD)   a standardized format for recording deaths and diseases; revised periodically (last revision, ICD-10, in 1994)

inter-rater reliability   the degree to which independent raters score the same information in the same way

intima   inner layer of the wall of an artery made up of the endothelium

ischemic stroke   a stroke resulting from a blood clot that causes obstruction to cerebral blood flow

islets of Langerhans   area of the pancreas that is related to its endocrine function, including the production of insulin; comprises only 1-2% of the mass of the pancreas

K

Koch's postulates   four rules that establish the causal relationship between an infectious agent and a particular infection

L

latency period   the time from the start of a disease process until signs and symptoms appear

latent TB infection   when infectious organisms are kept in check by the immune system and no symptoms of disease are present

leukemia   cancer of the white blood cells

levels of prevention   refers to three types of prevention: primary, secondary, and tertiary

life expectancy at birth   a mathematical calculation based on population statistics to estimate the average years a person born in a certain year wil live

live, attenuated vaccine   a vaccine made with the wild type organism—or an organism that occurs in nature and causes disease—and modified such that it is still a live organism but is no longer capable of producing significant disease in the host

loss to follow-up   the number (or proportion) of enrolled subjects who cannot be followed for the entire time period of the study

low birth weight   birth weight less than 2,500 grams

low-density lipoproteins (LDL)   make up the majority of the cholesterol circulating in the body; also known as the "bad cholesterol" because high levels are responsible for atherosclerosis

lymphoma   cancer of the lymphatic system

M

malignant   cancerous

maternal mortality   death of a woman while pregnant or within 42 days of termination of pregnancy from any cause related to or aggravated by the pregnancy

measures of association   a tool that enables investigators to describe a relationship between exposure and outcome in one summary number

melanoma   cancer that arises in the pigmented cells (melanocytes) of the skin

menarche   age of onset of menstruation in females

meningitis   inflammation of the meninges, the membranes that line the brain and spinal cord

menses   menstrual periods in females, also known as "menstruation"

metabolic   relating to the breakdown of food and use for energy

metabolic equivalent (MET)   refers to a way to classify physical activities by their intensity of energy expenditure, with sitting at rest equal to 1 MET

metabolic syndrome   also known as Syndrome X or insulin resistance syndrome; a group of risk factors that has been associated with an increased risk of cardiovascular diseases and Type 2 diabetes mellitus

metastasis   distant spread of cancer cells away from the primary tumor

miscarriage   the spontaneous end of a pregnancy at a stage where the embryo or fetus is incapable of surviving, generally defined in humans at prior to 20 weeks of gestation

moderate intensity   includes activities that cause some increase in breathing or heart rate such as walking

modifiable risk factors   those risk factors that can be changed or eradicated with lifestyle changes

morbidity   any departure from a state of physiological or psychological well-being

mortality resulting in death

mother-to-child transmission (MTCT) transmission of HIV infection from an infected mother to her child during pregnancy, labor, delivery, or breastfeeding

mutation change in the normal DNA of a cell

myocardial infarction (MI) caused when blood supply to the heart is severely reduced or completely blocked; the muscle cells do not receive enough oxygen and begin to die; also known as a "heart attack"

N

natural history the course of a disease if left untreated

neonatal mortality refers to the death of an infant within the first 28 days after birth

neonatal mortality rate the number of deaths among infants less than 28 days old divided by the total number of live births (multiplied by 1,000)

neoplasm new growth that may be benign or cancerous

neural tube defects defects that occur early in pregnancy and affect the developing spinal cord or brain; an example is spina bifida

neuroblastoma malignancy arising from the immature cells of the nervous system

nonclinical the stage of disease when clinical signs and symptoms are not present

nondifferential bias systematic errors resulting in bias, which affect all subjects and comparison groups of a study the same

non-melanomatous skin cancers/ carcinomas the more common skin cancers that include basal cell carcinomas and squamous cell carcinomas but not the more invasive melanoma

nonmodifiable risk factors those risk factors that cannot be changed or eradicated

null hypothesis a hypothesis that is stated as if there is no relationship between the study factors and the disease

null value a value that indicates there is no relationship between the study factor (exposure) and the disease

O

observational study study in which the investigator only gathers data from the subjects

odds ratio (OR) a ratio measure of association that provides the strength and direction of the association between exposure and outcome in a population

oncogenesis process of malignant transformation leading to the formation of a cancer

opportunistic infections infections that occur when the immune system is weakened

outcome refers to a particular disease under study

outcome odds ratio an odds ratio that can be calculated by comparing those with the exposure to those without the exposure using the cross-products ratio from a 2 × 2 table (ad/bc)

ovulation release of an egg from its follicle in the ovary

ovulatory cycles menstrual cycles that produce a viable egg capable of being fertilized by a viable sperm and therefore capable of resulting in pregnancy

P

pancreas located behind and below the stomach; a body organ that contains the cells that produce insulin

pandemic an epidemic that has become geographically widespread

Papanicolaou smear (Pap smear) cells from the surface of the cervix are collected and viewed under the microscope for evidence of early malignant changes

passive immunity when immune response products like antibodies, produced by another animal or person, are transferred to another human to provide immune protection

pathogenicity the ability of an agent to cause disease

per-act risk risk of acquiring the infection during an individual episode of exposure to the agent

period prevalence the number of existing cases during a specified time period

peripheral artery disease (PAD) caused by atherosclerotic plaque that occurs in the peripheral arteries (arteries distal to the main arteries such as the aorta), primarily those of the legs and or pelvis

person time   a measure that combines the number of people multiplied by a unit of time

physical activity   refers to any bodily movement produced by the contraction of skeletal muscle that increases energy expenditure

physical fitness   includes health-related aspects such as cardiorespiratory fitness, muscular strength and endurance, body composition, flexibility, and balance

plagiarism   using ideas of others as your own

plaque   formed by cholesterol, fatty acids, immune cells, and debris that collect under the intima of an arterial wall

point prevalence   the count of existing cases of disease at a specific point in time

polycystic ovary syndrome (PCOS)   excess insulin and insulin resistance resulting in overproduction of testosterone in women

polydipsia   increased thirst

polyphagia   increased hunger

polyuria   excessive urine production

population attributable risk (PAR)   a difference measure of association, which identifies the amount of risk that can be eliminated in the entire population (exposed and nonexposed) if the risk factor is removed

population pyramid   a graphical representation of the age and sex distribution in a population, which normally forms the shape of a pyramid

positive predictive value   the proportion of people with positive test results who are correctly diagnosed

power of a study   the probability of finding a positive result, if one is present

precision   how close a measurement is to its true value

preclinical   nonclinical disease because signs and symptoms are not yet present

precocious puberty   defined as puberty occurring before 8 years of age in girls and before 9 years of age in boys

prediabetes   state of impaired glucose tolerance, impaired fasting glucose, or both; blood glucose is higher than normal but not in the range for a diagnosis of diabetes

preterm   delivery occurring before 37 weeks of gestational age

prevalence   the number of existing cases of disease

prevalence proportion   the number of existing cases of disease divided by the population

prevalence ratio   a ratio measure of association that provides the strength and direction of the association between exposure and outcome in a population

prevalence study   another name for a cross-sectional study

primary case   the first case of a specific infectious disease in a population

primary prevention   avoids the initial occurrence of a disease

primary tumor   the tumor growing in the original site of the cancer

progesterone   the female hormone produced by the ovarian corpus luteum and responsible for causing the lining of the uterus to prepare for the fertilized egg to implant

prognosis   the expected outcome of the disease; outlook for chance of survival

propagated outbreak   an outbreak that continues over an extended period of time and includes cases that are transmitted from person to person

proportion   the representation of a numerator as a fraction of a denominator

prospective cohort study   the design considered the "gold standard" of observational study designs; a study design that follows outcome-free subjects into the future to ascertain outcome; measures incidence and can determine risk

prostate-specific antigen (PSA)   normally produced by the prostate at a low level, but this level may raise significantly when cancer is present in the gland; used as a screening test for prostate cancer

public health surveillance   a system for monitoring health events in a defined population

***p*-value**   the probability of obtaining a test statistic at least as extreme as the one that was actually observed, assuming that the null hypothesis is true

R

radiation therapy   treatment with high-energy rays to kill cancer cells and shrink tumors; may be external radiation from a machine or internal from radioactive materials placed directly in the tumor

random sampling   a systematic method of approaching individuals to participate in the study

rate   a proportion measured over a period of time

rate ratio   *see* relative risk

ratio measures   rates or proportions that are compared to each other by the mathematical method of division

recombinant   genetically engineered vaccine that combines DNA sequences from multiple sources

registry   a listing containing information from people with a particular condition or risk factor

relative risk (RR)   also known as rate ratio or risk ratio; a ratio measure of association that uses incidence rates to provide the strength and direction of the association between exposure and outcome in a population

reliability   the consistency of a procedure or a set of measurements to give the same results under different conditions

reportable (or notifiable) disease/condition   a disease/condition that requires reporting to a public health agency

reproductive health   encompasses physical, mental, and social well-being in all matters relating to the reproductive system

research data   studies that focus on finding risk factors for a particular disease

reservoir   the natural host in which an organism grows and multiplies without causing disease to the host; serves as a source of infection for a susceptible individual

retrospective cohort study   a study design that ascertains exposure and independent variable information from the past and outcome up to the present

risk factors   characteristics associated with disease development

risk ratio   *see* relative risk

rubeola   the common measles; also known as the "10-day measles"

S

sample size   number of subjects who participate in a study

sarcoma   a malignant tumor growing from connective tissues, such as cartilage, fat, muscle, or bone

screening test   a test given to people who have no symptoms to check for the presence of a particular disease

secondary attack rate   the rate of disease in an outbreak that results from transmission of the disease from person to person

secondary prevention   limits the effect of a disease by early detection and treatment

sedentary   refers to individuals who do not obtain enough physical activity to achieve health benefits

selection bias   a large category of systemic errors in the performance of epidemiology studies that affect the characteristics of the group of subjects selected for enrollment in a study

sensitivity   the probability that a test defines a person as having a disease when the person does have the disease

seroconversion   occurs when the laboratory test for HIV becomes positive

source population   the population from which the cases are selected

specificity   the probability that a test defines a person as NOT having a disease when the person actually does NOT have the disease

specific rate   a rate comprised of a numerator and denominator that is a subset of the population under observation. The subsets can be variables that may affect the outcome being measured, such as age.

spontaneous abortion   also called "miscarriage"; the loss of a fetus before the 20th week of pregnancy; refers to naturally occurring events, not to medical or surgical abortions

squamous cell carcinoma   a type of non-melanomatous skin cancer that arises from the surface layer of cells of the epidermis

staging   the process of finding out whether cancer has spread and if so, how far

standardized mortality ratio   the ratio between the observed number of deaths as a result of a specific cause and the expected number of deaths as a result of the same cause

statistically significant   the results observed were unlikely to be the result of chance

stillbirth   death of a fetus after 20 or more weeks of gestation, prior to completed delivery

stratification   separating and analyzing data according to categories of a variable or characteristic

stratified random sampling   choosing subjects for the control group from random selections of randomly selected groups such as groups of subjects chosen by age, geographical location, or occupation

stroke caused by a sudden impairment of cerebral circulation; also known as a "cerebrovascular accident"

study population refers to the group of individuals being studied

subclinical nonclinical disease because signs and symptoms will not become apparent

sudden infant death syndrome (SIDS) a condition in which an infant stops breathing and dies during sleep

surveillance data ongoing surveys used to assess population trends

survival rate the percentage of people still alive within a certain period of time after diagnosis or treatment; a 5-year survival rate is usually used in cancers

suspect case a subject who meets all of the characteristics and symptoms of a case but does not have a formal diagnosis

systolic pressure the pressure circulating blood exerts on the arterial walls when the heart is contracting

T

teenage abortion rate the number of teenage pregnancies that are electively terminated divided by the total number of teenage pregnancies

teenage birth rate the number of live births in girls 15-19 years old divided by the number of girls aged 15-19

teenage pregnancy a pregnancy that occurs in a girl 15-19 years of age

teratogenic the ability to produce fetal malformations

tertiary prevention reduces the impact of a disease that has already developed by preventing complications

testosterone a male hormone produced primarily in the testes; a surge in this hormone is responsible for the onset of puberty in males

test-retest reliability can assess the consistency of a measure across time by administering it to the same people at different times

time at risk the time that each individual accumulates between exposure and independent variable

ascertainment and getting the outcome or the end of the study

transient ischemic attack (TIA) a clot that causes temporary obstruction in the brain causing symptoms that last only minutes to a few hours; also called a "mini-stroke"

trimester division of a 9-month pregnancy into three periods of 3 months

tumor mass of cells or growth; may be benign or malignant

2 × 2 table a method to organize and present measures of disease and exposure in an observed population

Type 1 diabetes mellitus disease where no insulin is produced because of an autoimmune response against the beta cells of the pancreas

Type 2 diabetes mellitus disease in which insulin is produced normally, at least initially, but the body's cells do not respond; a state of insulin resistance

V

vaccination the procedure of administering the substance that will stimulate the immune response; used interchangeably with the terms "inoculation" and "immunization"

vaccine-associated paralytic polio (VAPP) polio disease caused by the live, attenuated virus, rather than the wild virus, contained in the oral polio vaccine

validity the degree to which a study accurately reflects or assesses the specific concept that the researcher is attempting to measure

valvular disease disease that affects any of the four major valves of the heart

vector an organism (usually an insect) that transmits or carries an infectious agent from its reservoir to its host

verbal autopsy designed to determine cause of death, an interview with a close associate of the deceased

vertical transmission transmission of disease from mother to child during pregnancy or delivery

very low birth weight defined as weighing less than 1,500 grams or 3 pounds 4 ounces at birth

viable able to survive

vigorous intensity   includes activities that cause large increases in breathing or heart rate such as running

virulence   the degree of pathogenicity possessed by an infectious agent

wild virus   the virus as it occurs in its natural form and causes the disease

World Health Organization (WHO)   the coordinating authority for health within the United Nations system of 193 member countries

YLD   years lived with disability

YLL   years of life lost as a result of premature mortality

zoonoses   infectious diseases that are transmitted from animals to humans

zygote   the cell formed by the union of a sperm and an egg that divides and grows into an embryo

Index